Praise for *Un-Junk Your Diet*

"This is the perfect guide to help one navigate the toxic food environment we live in today. Desiree shows her true leadership by giving readers inspiration, knowledge, understanding, many laughs, and most importantly the (survival) skills to un-junk their own diets, leading them to happier and healthier places."
—Veronica Kacinik, MSc, RD

"As soon as you open this book, you realize Desiree Nielsen is the best friend you wish you had. Written in her voice, *Un-Junk Your Diet* is not out to sell you on some fad diet, but to show you how to change your life in a way you never imagined. The facts will shock you. The self-assessments will open your eyes. The meal plans will inspire you and the more than forty pages of mouthwatering recipes will leave you salivating for a healthier life. We all need a friend to cheer us on and keep us on the right path. When it comes to nutrition, there is no better friend to have than Desiree."
—Jason "The Germ Guy" Tetro, microbiologist and author of *The Germ Code: How to Stop Worrying and Love the Microbes*

"Move over Marion Nestle, Desiree Nielsen is taking the reins in decoding and decluttering nutrition. . . . This book is a journey, one that will wind you down a path where you can feel success—from small, attainable goals to landmark changes. From quizzes and grocery lists to scrumptious recipes, *Un-Junk Your Diet* has it all —it's your one-stop-shop nutrition prescription."
—Wendy Jo Peterson, MS, RD, CSSD, sports dietitian and culinary nutritionist, coauthor of the *Mediterranean Diet Cookbook For Dummies* and *Adrenal Fatigue for Dummies*

T0040161

UN-JUNK YOUR DIET

HOW TO SHOP, COOK, AND EAT TO FIGHT INFLAMMATION AND FEEL BETTER FOREVER

DESIREE NIELSEN, RD

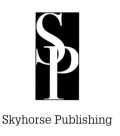

Skyhorse Publishing

This book is dedicated to my husband, Jim, our son, Elliott, and our daughter, Iris.

The information given here is designed to help you make informed decisions about your health. It is not intended to replace the advice of a qualified health professional. If you have a condition that requires care, please seek treatment with your healthcare provider.

Skyhorse Publishing books may be purchased in bulk at special discounts for sales promotion, corporate gifts, fund-raising, or educational purposes. Special editions can also be created to specifications. For details, contact the Special Sales Department, Skyhorse Publishing, 307 West 36th Street, 11th Floor, New York, NY 10018 or info@skyhorsepublishing.com.

Skyhorse® and Skyhorse Publishing® are registered trademarks of Skyhorse Publishing, Inc.®, a Delaware corporation.

www.skyhorsepublishing.com

10 9 8 7 6 5 4 3 2

Library of Congress Cataloging-in-Publication Data is available on file.

Cover design by Jane Sheppard
Cover photo by Joey Armstrong

ISBN: 978-1-5107-1146-4
Ebook ISBN: 978-1-5107-1150-1

Printed in China

TABLE OF CONTENTS

INTRODUCTION: *It's Not One Size Fits All . . .*
(aka How to Use this Book)

PART ONE: *Food for Thought*

1 Overfed and Undernourished 10

2 You Are What You Eat: A Nutrition Primer 26

3 You Are What You Absorb 53

4 Confused Yet? Steering Clear of the Cult of Nutritionism 74

5 Fight Inflammation with Your Fork! 85

6 Stock Your Anti-Inflammatory Arsenal Deliciously 113

7 Start Where You Are 134

PART TWO: *Un-Junk Your Diet Eating Plans*

8 101 Food Swaps and Easy Additions to Make You Healthier Forever! 156

9 Leaving Room for Chocolate: the 80/20 Approach 175

10 Stuck in the Muck?: A Fourteen-Day Kick-Start 184

11 A Twenty-Eight Day Anti-Inflammatory Menu Plan to Make Your Life Simple 194

12 Supermarket Smarts 201

13 Whole Foods for Life 214

PART THREE: *The Recipes*

14 Let's Eat! Whole Food, Plant-Strong Recipes for Life 228

Appendix 277

Photo credits 281

References 282

In gratitude 297

Index 299

INTRODUCTION

It's Not One Size Fits All . . .
(aka How to Use this Book)

Un-Junk Your Diet is all about giving you the tools to transform the way you eat, so each day you get healthier than the day before. It's not about forcing you to eat something you hate or confining you to some strange schedule of mealtimes that won't work for you. As a dietitian, I know that the only way to achieve permanent change is to individualize your eating strategies. While it would take me lifetimes to write a book for each of you, I have tried as hard as possible to create a book that you can use to customize an eating plan for yourself.

Think of this book as a choose-your-own-nutrition adventure!

Sorry, my nutrition geek is showing.

Fad diets work (sometimes). For some people. In the short term. That is why they sell bazillions of copies! And when they fail, there is a new title that promises you the world and sells bazillions more. When a person finds a plan that speaks to their love of number crunching/carnivorous tendencies/ fat phobia, they will make some progress on whatever is trending in the diet world. When the diet doesn't work, it is frustrating. For those who lose weight and regain it after they trail off from the program, it is super frustrating. As your dietitian, I couldn't do that to you. And *Un-Junk Your Diet* is here because I never want you to be frustrated by an eating plan again.

How you engage with this book is up to you, because this is the start of a beautiful and permanent friendship. An anti-inflammatory eating strategy will help you feel stronger and more energetic tomorrow and fight off chronic disease for decades to come.

Interested in nutrition? Start from the beginning of the book, as it is packed full of practical, myth-busting knowledge to help make you a super nutrition whiz.

If years of tweeting have left you with a shorter attention span, and you are eager to get to the "What do I eat?" part, start at Chapter 7. This chapter will help you determine which of the four plans will be right for you.

For those wishing to take the baby steps approach to getting healthy—of which I am a huge fan—start at Chapter 8. It took me fifteen years to transform my own eating habits to their current state. Give yourself some time to adapt.

Are you feeling wretched after a long unhealthy stretch and need to claw your way back to health? Have to get into a bathing suit in two weeks? Head to Chapter 10, and while you are on the kick-start plan, start reading from either the beginning or Chapter 7, because I have big plans for you! Remember, this book is about abandoning diets forever. I'll look the other way if you feel you need a nutritional reset right now.

Ready for a permanent transformation and simply need someone to show you what to eat? Love to cook and hate following rigid meal plans? Meet my 80/20 approach—it is supercharged with anti-inflammatory nutrition that leaves room for the occasional cocktail and burger. I give you the tools; you decide what to eat.

Finally, you might just need someone to take the work out of meal planning for you. You are ready to make a change but don't have the time or energy to figure out the best way to feed yourself. I have given you a twenty-eight-day meal plan in Chapter 11, so you can get healthier ASAP while reading about all the reasons to do so.

Ready to glow? Then turn the page and don't look back. Unless you want to reread something, of course. In that case, look back as often as you need!

PART ONE:

Food for Thought

CHAPTER 1
OVERFED AND UNDERNOURISHED

"We have a health care system that doesn't care about food, and a food system that doesn't care about health." —Wayne Roberts

It's no secret: most of us aren't as healthy as we could be. There have been plenty of times in my life when I haven't been as healthy as I'd like either. Maybe I was working out plenty but drinking a bit too much red wine or eating beautifully but living with so much stress my body was breaking under the weight of it. Our bodies, much like life itself, are a work in progress. This is not about perfection. It is about choosing to stick with a path that leads you to a healthier and happier life. Personally, I went from a kid who liked to eat ice cream for breakfast and bemoaned skim milk to a teenaged, mac-and-cheese obsessed "carb-atarian" to the requisite flings with ridiculous fad diets as a young adult to the plant-based, whole food eater I am now. I still like red wine . . . and potato chips. I have also figured out how to eat so well that I have room for the less-than-stellar choices I make every once in a while. You can get here too. This book can help provide the road map, but it's up to you to take the journey.

The approach you are about to read differs from those found in other books and, frankly, from that all-or-nothing approach that tends to drive so many of us. This is not about overhauling your eating habits until they are no longer recognizable to you. You won't go from eating sixteen-ounce steaks and fries to subsisting on kale and air the next morning, because I am here to tell you an approach like that won't last. And I don't want you to ever go on a diet again.

Instead, I am asking you to hold on, get comfortable, and take the scenic route. We are going to chart a path that meets you where you are and shows you how good the journey can be. Over time, you will leave habits behind that no longer suit the new, healthier you. Life will be filled with great food that energizes, fills you up, and actually tastes amazing. And we're leaving room for a night out with friends or your mother's famous noodle casserole. It's going to take work . . . not sacrifice. Changing your diet for the better requires that you become conscious of your choices, patient with yourself, and accepting of where you are right now. As you read on, you will also have a greater understanding of why a bite of broccoli is really medicine for your cells and why that stuff in the brightly colored box is not actually food.

No, You are NOT too Busy to Eat Well

Life rushes by, and somehow, between work and socializing or making dinner and rushing to soccer practice, food became not something to nourish but something to entertain or fill a void. Fast food and "family" restaurants are now so inexpensive that many of us can afford to eat there all the time. Going out has gone from what was once a rare monthly or perhaps weekly treat to becoming the norm. Canadians spent 28 percent of their food budget on restaurant meals in 2010,[1] and according to the National Restaurant Association,[2] Americans spent 1.7 billion dollars a day at restaurants in 2011. The cobwebs in our kitchens are telling. Your stove misses you! Go warm up the kettle or something and show it some love.

Consumers are coerced by marketers into the cult of convenience to make all that instant junk food seem inevitable and, bizarrely, helpful. Now that we don't have to spend twenty minutes cooking, we can work more, commute longer, and spend more time browsing the Internet and watching TV. We certainly fill our time, but are we truly too busy to cook or are we simply choosing to allocate our time differently? And, are we making these decisions consciously? In fact, we seem to be spending a disproportionate amount of time thinking about food—just not when we are preparing or eating it. Millions of us tune into cooking shows about all the food we aren't eating but would like to and reality programs about losing the weight gained by eating too much food. Hmm . . . just thinking about all those cooking shows is making me hungry . . . you can see how this love affair with a screen turns into snacking.

We are now so "busy" that we have to buy the packaged food and run through the drive-thru or call for takeout. Never mind that in the time it takes for the pizza to arrive, you could have made something. It doesn't have to be anything fancy; a bit of chicken and pasta or some veggie burritos are certainly more satisfying and less expensive to make. Instead, you saved time and spent more money, so you are going to have to work a little longer tomorrow and pick up takeout on the way home. Starting to sound like a mouse spinning a wheel yet?

But It Tastes Soooooo Good!

Once they have their deliciously alluring hooks into you, it is hard to stray from the overprocessed ingredient combinations we currently call food. In a sea of french fries and frozen mac and cheese, broccoli tastes a tad . . . boring. Our collective taste buds crave the salty, sweet, rich tastes of manufactured food and, frankly, don't know what to do with a bunch of parsley or dish of plain yogurt. Those flavors—tart, tangy, bitter, and astringent—are as foreign to us as listening to someone speaking Swahili (assuming you don't, of course).

However, we are not born loving those manufactured flavors; taste buds are made, not born. So we run into the creamy, welcoming arms of a tub of candy-bar flavored ice cream. And that tub of ice cream loves us so much it decides to make a home somewhere around our belly buttons and inside our arteries.

Now more than ever before, we are surrounded by an unprecedented amount of high calorie, high salt, high sugar foods that excite our taste buds and our brains, because that is what they are designed to do. Manufactured foods, which are exactly what all those muffins, chips, sodas, and frozen lasagnas are, are designed with you in mind. Or, to be more accurate, designed for your taste buds and your brain. Flavor scientists (yes, that is a real profession) work hard to perfect just the right combination of flavor molecules along with fat to carry that flavor, sugar to provide a rush of pleasure, and salt to wake up our taste buds so they can take notice. You get a wave of flavor, energy, and comfort that leaves you feeling empty as soon as it passes. You can't really be blamed for not liking cucumbers. They must taste incredibly odd with no sugary dressing on them. That is, until you change your taste buds. There is a lot of food I can no longer eat because it tastes fake to me. Don't get me wrong . . . I still like real ice cream and such. However, that strange big-box store white cake for the office birthday doesn't even hold a second of my attention.

Is There Any Food in Your Food?

Our working definition of what food is has changed now, too. We recognize foods by their familiar packages and shapes, not by the ingredients they contain. Children can recognize the logos for McDonald's, Starbucks, and Dunkin Donuts before many of them know an eggplant or a kidney bean. Flour, salt, sweeteners, stabilizers, and cheap fat come in literally thousands of modern combinations, seemingly different but almost impossible to tell apart by just looking at their ingredients.

Dude, Where's My Cereal?

Below is a selection of common supermarket picks, such as breakfast cereal and crackers. We consider these items to be a reasonable part of our daily diets, but they typify how monotonous and carb-based our diets have become. Sure, from the outside you might recognize these foods as different, but can you tell their ingredients apart? Try and match the food to its ingredients list and see how you score!

This game was inspired by a similar one I found in the excellent monthly Nutrition Action Health Letter.

Food	Ingredients
1. Kellogg's Special K Protein Plus Cereal[3]	A: Whole grain rolled oats, sugar, whole grain puffed cereal (whole grain white corn, whole grain oat flour, whole wheat flour, whole grain brown rice flour, sugar, calcium carbonate, salt, BHT [a preservative]), partially hydrogenated palm kernel oil, high fructose corn syrup, polydextrose, soybean oil, reduced mineral whey, soy lecithin, cinnamon, molasses, natural and artificial flavors, nonfat dry milk solids, dextrose, salt, yellow 5 lake, yellow 6 lake, honey, blue 2 lake, sodium bicarbonate.
2. Keebler Cinnamon Roll Cookies[4]	B: Enriched bleached wheat flour (wheat flour, malted barley flour, niacin, reduced iron, thiamine mononitrate [vitamin B1], enzyme, riboflavin [vitamin B2], folic acid), palm oil, skim milk, sugar, water, soybean oil, egg yolks, contains less than 2 percent of the following: leavening (sodium acid pyrophosphate, baking soda, sodium aluminum phosphate), salt, defatted soy flour, soy flour, soy lecithin, wheat starch, konjac flour, wheat germ, carrageenan, dextrose, natural and artificial flavor, enzyme modified egg yolks, gelatinized wheat starch, colored with turmeric and annatto extracts and beta carotene, defatted wheat germ; dextrose, corn starch, cinnamon, palm oil.
3. Nabisco Ritz Honey Butter Crackers[5]	C: Whole grain wheat, wheat gluten, sugar, rice, soy protein isolate, wheat bran, defatted soy grits, contains 2 percent or less of salt, cinnamon, malt flavor, sucralose, BHT [a preservative].
4. Quaker Cinnamon Granola Bites[6]	D: Enriched flour (wheat flour, niacin, reduced iron, thiamine mononitrate [vitamin B1], riboflavin [vitamin B2], folic acid), invert sugar, soybean and palm oil, sugar, corn syrup, fructose, modified corn starch, contains 2 percent or less of cinnamon, eggs, glycerin, molasses, salt, DATEM, natural and artificial flavors, soy lecithin, baking soda, caramel color, lactic acid, modified soy protein, whey protein concentrate.

5. Dunkin Donuts Cinnamon Cake Donut[7]	E: Enriched flour (wheat flour, niacin, reduced iron, thiamine mononitrate [vitamin B1], riboflavin [vitamin B2], folic acid), soybean oil, sugar, partially hydrogenated cottonseed oil, honey, leavening (calcium phosphate and/or baking soda), salt, natural and artificial flavor (contains soy), soy lecithin (emulsifier), cornstarch. Contains: wheat, soy.

Answers: 1 C, 2 D, 3 E, 4 A, 5 B

Score 5: Nutrition All-Star . . . are you just reading this book for extra credit?

3-4: On Your Way . . . keep reading and you'll be a nutrition whiz in no time

Fewer than 3: Ready for change . . . don't worry, it's designed to be this complicated. Time for some real food rehab.

One of the basic tenets of good nutrition practice is variety—yet most of us are eating just a handful of foods. Wheat, milk, soy, and corn make up the majority of industrialized food ingredients[8] that are assembled into our standard American diet (the acronym SAD says it all!). However, before those four foods become part of dinner, they are hydrolyzed, modified, and esterified within an inch of their lives to create novel tastes, shapes, and textures. As the number of food and beverage products available on North American grocery store shelves skyrockets into the hundreds of thousands, the actual biological diversity of our food is dwindling.

Go and check your cupboards. If our little ingredients game was any indication, your cupboards might feature similar options. In all of the seeming variety we enjoy, we are, in fact, eating just a few common processed foods. From their whole, nutrient-dense state, real food is hyper-processed through milling and extracting, damaged in high heat, and fractioned into basic chemical components. Flour is a great example of this; by the time you take a whole wheat berry and finely mill it into flour, mix it into a paste with cheap fats, and cook it into fun shapes with high heat drying, little of the original bounty of vitamins, minerals, fiber, and healthy fats remains. It's little more than quick sugar for your blood stream. And we call that breakfast. How extensive is the infiltration of wheat, soy, dairy, and corn in our diets? Take a look at some of the common food ingredients that can be made from corn: [9]

alpha-tocopherol (vitamin E), ascorbic acid (vitamin C), baking powder, calcium stearate, caramel, cellulose, citric acid, citrus cloud emulsion, corn flour, corn oil, cornstarch, corn syrup, dextrin, dextrose (glucose), diglycerides, ethylene, ethyl acetate, ethyl lactate, fibersol-2, fructose, fumaric acid, golden syrup, high fructose corn syrup, inositol, invert sugar, malt, maltodextrin, margarine, monoglycerides, monosodium glutamate (MSG), polydextrose, saccharin, semolina, sorbic acid, sorbitol, starch, sucrose, treacle, vanilla extract, white vinegar, xanthan gum, xylitol, zein

Goes beyond corn on the cob as a tasty side dish, doesn't it? Corn, the vegetable, has plenty to offer you nutritionally speaking. However, we have turned corn into a commodity to be bought, sold, genetically manipulated, and value-added. Too bad the values don't include keeping you healthy.

Still wondering why this biological diversity is so important to our health? Each plant and animal on earth has a unique chemical composition; when we consume those organisms as food, we benefit from the complex nutrients, phytochemicals, and cofactors that nature intended us to receive for optimal nutrition. Anthocyanins, phytochemicals that help protect the heart, are found in bright red and purple produce. Vitamin B12, which is essential for forming healthy blood cells, is found only in animal foods. Soluble fiber, which cleanses the digestive tract and helps stabilize blood sugars and lower blood cholesterol, is found in a few grains, legumes, fruits, and vegetables. When we eat only a handful of super-processed foodstuffs, we wind up with a massive nutrient debt to go along with our venti mochaccino-induced financial debt.

Perhaps we should look at our eating choices as an investment strategy in our long-term health. Now, I can't exactly claim to be a money whiz, but I do know that diversification of investments is a pretty standard practice to ensure financial security. So let's diversify! Put down the box, pick up the produce! The next time you go to the grocery store or farmer's market, find the oddest-looking veggie you have ever seen and take it home. With the help of Chef Google, figure out how to cook and eat it. Notice your reaction to the different flavors and textures. Is it love at first bite? Or is the experience the culinary equivalent of having to give a presentation to your boss? As with all things, exploring the unknown can be a little uncomfortable. But soon, the foreign becomes familiar and your body will respond to all of these newfound nutrients and flavors in favorable ways. Eating a variety of real, whole foods will help us load our cells with good nutrition for a rainy day.

Houston, We Have a Problem

Obesity is a staggering concern in North America. Statistics Canada reports that 52.1 percent of Canadians are overweight or obese[10], and according to the Centers for Disease Control and Prevention (CDC), 35.7 percent of American adults are obese.[11] We may be living longer lives, but those lives are sicker than ever before. For many of us, the last half of our lives will be filled with prescriptions, energy deficits, and physical limitations that needn't exist. There is no reason why we can't run marathons at sixty or find the energy to write that bestseller in our spare time.

As we live our lives, so do we teach our children. Never before have health professionals seen children experience the health problems that were once reserved for those in middle age. It's the food, people! Time to lift the veil and realize that what we choose to eat is actually of vital importance to our lives. Night after night of chips and canned soup will take its toll on your health, energy levels, and waistband. Don't have the energy to go for a run? What did you have for lunch? I find it fascinating that foods that pile on the calories (calories represent the energy from food that your body can burn for fuel) can leave you feeling like you have no energy to spare. So we look to stimulants, such as energy drinks, to prop us up, but these short-term strategies only mask the deep imbalance that is causing our energy crisis in the first place: a nutrient-depleted body.

For your children, growing up with nutrient-depleted foods loaded with calories fuels poor quality growth with metabolic and chronic consequences we are only just starting to understand in our society. Along with the love we give them and the rules we create to keep them safe, what we choose to feed our children is one of the most important decisions we make as parents, Helping your kids transition to a healthy diet or starting them out right will keep their lives healthy and happy and provide a better future for us all.

The cost of obesity to our economy is just as enormous—the CDC estimates place the cost of obesity at $147 billion dollars (year 2008 dollars) in the United States.[11] Chronic disease, of which obesity is a primary risk factor, limits our ability to focus and work hard, limiting our productivity. Chronic disease leads to more sick days, higher medical costs for our employers and our health care systems, and when we are no longer able to work due to illness, it becomes a drain on our families. Not to mention that chronic disease destroys our ability to enjoy this precious gift of life that we have been given. In our current food system, food is seen as profit-making for a lucky few. We might remark at the cost of food or how our food-related stocks are performing, but perhaps what we choose to eat should be viewed as its own issue of economics after all. As the saying goes, you can pay your farmer now or pay your doctor (and the pharmaceutical company) later . . . it's your choice.

Now, before I go any further into the obesity discussion, I should clarify. While many of us fret about the ten or twenty pounds that might stand between us and looking celebrity skinny, a few extra pounds aren't really going to hurt us. In fact, they might actually be good for us as long as we are generally healthy. I have less interest in the number we see on the scale than how our cholesterol is doing or how many veggies we are eating. When I set my sights on obesity, I am talking significant, can't-reach-around-your-belly, wheeze-climbing-a-flight-of-stairs obesity. This is the type of weight that dramatically increases your risk of chronic disease later in life and makes you feel crummy right now.

What's Your BMI . . . and What Does It Mean?

The Body Mass Index (BMI) is a tool that tells us what our risk of chronic disease is over time based on the ratio of our height to our weight. It doesn't really tell us how healthy we are right now. Two people with the same BMI might be a salad-munching marathon runner or a super-value meal munching couch potato. BMI also doesn't distinguish muscle from fat. Wait, have I talked you out of caring yet?

Why BMI is interesting, to a health professional at least, is that it acts kind of like an early warning system for your health. If your BMI is on the higher side, you have the heads up that some change might lie ahead. So give it a go. Find your height on the left side of the chart and follow it until you find your weight. At the top of the column is your BMI.

BMI	19	20	21	22	23	24	25	26	27	28	29	30	31	32	33	34	35	36	37	38	39
Ht (in)																					
60	97	102	107	112	118	123	128	133	138	143	148	153	158	163	168	174	179	184	189	194	199
61	100	106	111	116	122	127	132	137	143	148	153	158	164	169	174	180	185	190	195	201	206
62	104	109	115	120	126	131	136	142	147	153	158	164	169	175	180	186	191	196	202	207	213
63	107	113	118	124	130	135	141	146	152	158	164	169	175	180	186	191	197	203	208	214	220
64	110	116	122	128	134	140	145	151	157	163	169	174	180	186	192	197	204	209	215	221	227
65	114	120	126	132	138	144	150	156	162	168	174	180	186	192	198	204	210	216	222	228	234
66	118	124	130	136	142	148	155	161	167	173	179	186	192	198	204	210	216	223	229	235	241
67	121	127	134	140	146	153	159	166	172	178	185	191	198	204	211	217	223	230	236	242	249
68	125	131	138	144	151	158	164	171	177	184	190	197	203	210	216	223	230	236	243	249	256
69	128	135	142	149	155	162	169	176	182	189	196	203	209	216	223	230	236	243	250	257	263
70	132	139	146	153	160	167	174	181	188	195	202	209	216	222	229	236	243	250	257	264	271
71	136	143	150	157	165	172	179	186	193	200	208	215	222	229	236	243	250	257	265	272	279
72	140	147	154	162	169	177	184	191	199	206	213	221	228	235	242	250	258	265	272	279	287
73	144	151	159	166	174	182	189	197	204	212	219	227	235	242	250	257	265	272	280	288	295
74	148	155	163	171	179	186	194	202	210	218	225	233	241	249	256	264	272	280	287	295	303
75	152	160	168	176	184	192	200	208	216	224	232	240	248	256	264	272	279	287	295	303	311
76	156	164	172	180	189	197	205	213	221	230	238	246	254	263	271	279	287	295	304	312	320

Body Weight in Pounds

How Health Professionals Interpret the Results:

BMI lower than 18.5: underweight and increased risk of chronic disease over time
BMI 18.5–24.9: healthy weight and lowest risk of chronic disease over time
BMI 25.0–29.9: overweight and increased risk of chronic disease over time
BMI 30.0 or greater: obese and greatly increased risk of chronic disease over time

If you fall into an increased risk category, that might strengthen your motivation to change. The good news is that you don't have to change overnight or lose forty pounds in a month to be healthy. All you need to do is move toward better choices that will, over time, bring your weight into a healthier zone. If you don't get all the way to an ideal weight, it doesn't matter. Sometimes, simply preventing future weight gain is a powerful indictor of better health choices. Chronic disease takes decades to develop. Don't stress yourself out thinking you have to reach some unattainable notion of perfection overnight. This is about progress, remember?

Digging Deep

How did we get into, to quote Kris Carr, this shit pickle anyway? Because the food we eat is hyper-caloric, utterly devoid of nutrition, and we are being bullied into eating more and more of it. That's right. We are malnourished in a sea of cheap, "tasty" food. In university, malnutrition was a state we learned about in the presence of starvation. Now, for the first time, obesity is a larger global problem than starvation.[12] However underfed or overfed, many North Americans are greatly malnourished.

Here is how it happens: real food, the kind that grows in the ground or lives as an animal, has nutrients! There are hundreds of naturally occurring components in a single blueberry. Nature designed all of these organisms to have the components they need to grow and thrive, which makes them more valuable for us. Nature is also wise enough not to waste precious energy on creating too many energy stores within these plants . . . just enough to survive common pests or a few days without rain. So these foods tend to have a lot of nutrition without a lot of energy, or calories. In fact, we call these nutrient-dense foods because they are full of nutrients, not calories. Our human bodies were designed to eat this type of food. However, when human hands and industrial machines start manipulating, extracting, and concentrating aspects of our food, we disconnect the foods we create from the natural order of things. We create calorie-dense foods that starve our cells of nutrition while piling on massive energy stores we don't even need. The remote control is just not that heavy.

While technology has rapidly evolved, our bodies are greatly lagging behind. We still share the same DNA that hoarded as much energy as it could when food was plentiful so you could survive when it wasn't. However, for those of us lucky enough to put food on the table without too much trouble, food is always there. We don't have to work very hard to grow or process the food—we just drive our SUVs to the store, or better yet, pick up the phone and the food comes to you. Manufacturers have made food so convenient that we don't even need a twenty-minute cooling off period before our desired snack is ready. Food can be ready in just sixty seconds, which is fast enough to indulge a whim and be finished before your belly even registers what just happened.

I like to eat. My Portuguese grandmother's kitchen was a place that greatly formed my food culture and practices. I grew up in a family where people who were "too skinny" were just fed more; as a skinny kid, I was fed a lot. The kitchen was the center of family life. We cooked, sat around the kitchen table, and ate, and when the food was gone, we just talked . . . and eventually my grandmother brought out more food. If you just arrived in my grandmother's home, "you must be hungry." If there were leftovers on the table, you didn't eat enough, but lord help you if there were no leftovers . . . because "someone must have gone hungry!" To make a long story short, I didn't grow up nibbling like a bird, nor do I think you should have to.

So why do I care so much that you are a healthy weight? Because the more you weigh beyond your healthy weight range, the greater your risk of chronic disease. Now, there are plenty of folks who weigh more than their ideal weight yet are fit as a fiddle. If this is you, you probably already know it—and your checkups will show it. But for the rest of us, being significantly overweight often means that our bodies aren't running at their best, we feel terrible, and disease can follow. Cancer. Heart disease. Type 2 diabetes. Alzheimer's disease. These are the biggies: the diseases that affect almost every single one of us at younger and younger ages. We used to call type 2 diabetes adult-onset diabetes because it was a disease associated with getting older and heavier. Now, we see grade school kids with type 2 diabetes. In just eight or nine years, they have assaulted their cells so profoundly that the cells no longer want to listen to the insulin knocking down their doors. This just shouldn't happen. Period. No excuses. Time to pull up our collective big boy pants or big girl panties and fix this mess! Chronic disease is running rampant in industrialized nations, tanking our quality of life, keeping us filled up with prescriptions, and costing us, our bosses, and our healthcare system billions of dollars a year. We are living longer . . . but what is the quality of those lives?

Let me not get ahead of myself—I see you, immediate gratification gene— eating crap food also makes you feel awful. That value meal might taste delightful right now, but, in fact, even if you look healthy on the outside, living a crummy lifestyle makes you feel crummy, too. When was the last time you felt truly energized and vibrant? Do you wake up with a smile on your face, or do you stumble out of bed toward the coffee pot and wait for the caffeine to hit? Do you enjoy running around with your kids or going to the latest fitness class with friends, or do you try and minimize the amount of time you spend upright? We have gotten to the point where it doesn't even seem normal to feel healthy and energetic but it is, indeed, possible. Feeling good is the body's natural state. A body filled with poor–quality food, stuck in a chair all day, and stressed out constantly is a tired, broken, sick body today. . . not just twenty years from now. So changing your ways, gradually so it doesn't sting, will make you feel better in a week. Not bad, I think. Might be worth the trouble of making change, yes?

Resisting the siren call of the cheesecake is one of the challenges of preaching good nutrition. Don't worry; I know what I am up against! When I ask you to eat your broccoli, I know that I am asking you to defer the delights of instant gratification in hopes of a payoff tomorrow, next year, and twenty years from now. Our culture has us hardwired to want everything now. Get your news as it happens, get your food as soon as your craving hits, and lose weight just as fast by starving yourself. Taking care of yourself requires you to put the brakes on a bit. Think about what your goals are and what you truly want for your life and your health. Decide to love your body instead of treating it like a hollow vessel for your overstimulated brain. You're going to have to slow the train down a touch. Putting the smart phone down for a while might help. And yes, you have the time. If you had the time to watch *The Bachelor* last night, you have the time. You just need to shift how you spend it.

Chronic Disease is a Long-Term Annoyance, Not a Life Sentence

In our typical medical model, we live ourselves (remember how we call many chronic diseases "lifestyle diseases"?) into oblivion, get a diagnosis, get the prescription or the surgery, and call it a day. When we get worse or feel worse, we can try to patch it up with more pills. They don't solve the problem; they just blunt the symptoms and, in fact, those pills are putting a massive dent in our wallets. Americans spent 325.8 billion dollars on prescriptions in 2012.[13] Think of all the fancy acai berry smoothies you could buy with that! Heck, you could move to the Amazon basin and buy your own acai berry plantation with all that dough.

We accept our health conditions as permanent, inevitable, and unchangeable. But what if they *were* changeable? Would that change how you live?

Let me rephrase that: they are changeable. But you will have to change, too.

Time to live well.

You can start to deliver clean, anti-inflammatory nutrition to your cells so they can grow and repair properly. You can teach your cells to listen when insulin comes calling. You can tell your blood pressure to calm down. And you can certainly mop up that cholesterol mess. If you can do it before the medications come calling, even better. But you can also make changes that alter your metabolism (and perhaps even reduce or discontinue some of those meds) even after chronic disease decides to hunker down. You can get healthier tomorrow, instead of less healthy . . . which is the path that most of us are tripping along. It all starts with a single choice to have some spinach alongside your steak. Tomorrow, we'll introduce you to quinoa. The cure comes one day at a time, just as the disease did.

It's Not You, It's the Food . . . Well, Part of it is You (and That's the Exciting Part!)

Don't get me wrong—in most circumstances, no one is holding a gun to your head trying to get you to eat that double cheeseburger. We place so much emphasis on individual responsibility, but in reality, our culture builds an environment that only the most disciplined (and educated . . . which is what this book is for) can resist the temptation. That's convenient—for those who make money off of us being sick and overweight. Our food system creates the 500-pound weight, drops it on you, and blames you when you can't lift it off yourself.

Hyper-processed foods are designed in laboratories by the brightest minds in food science to ensure that your brain gets the biggest rush possible from each bite. That rush comes from a magic combination of sugar, fat, and salt, which sends a message to your caveman brain letting you know that you hit the energy jackpot. "You had better eat as much as you can because this will be good fuel for the next famine!" Except that the famine never comes! This gastronomic rush, also known as the bliss point, can be akin to an addiction for some people.[14] In fact, this blissed-out sensation stimulates a chemical reward pathway in the brain that we want to experience again and again.[14] I can speak as an interesting test subject; as someone who lives a real food lifestyle, on the occasion that I find myself confronted with a bag of chips, I always eat more than I expect, because I am compelled to have that flavor experience again and again. We are surrounded by cheap, easily available, and—to our acclimated taste buds—unbelievably delicious food. Modern food is stuffed with more calories than nature could even come close to approximating. So we become driven to these modern foodstuffs subconsciously, and that mindless munching is creating real trouble for our bodies.

Where the exciting part comes in is that, with a little bit of knowledge and enthusiasm for change, you can transform your relationship with food. You can swap the Honey Smacks for oats and get that mocha half sweet. You can choose to nourish your body with foods that create health instead of disease. You can gaze lovingly at a bowl of berries and realize that you will be just fine. There are no pills to take, shakes to buy, or self-loathing necessary. Show yourself a little nutritional TLC and your body will thank you for years to come.

Looking for Answers? Ponder the Broccoli

One of the great riddles of modern food is how foods that require far more ingredients, fancy factories to manufacture, and multi-million dollar marketing

The Commodification of Food, aka "Food"

Slowly and stealthily over the past thirty years, food has been transformed to contain less actual *food*. One by one, from the ice cream and cheese to the bread and juice, food processors have decided that instead of worrying about food quality, they would design food to focus on the bottom line. Industrialized food ingredients, such as hydrogenated oils, high fructose corn syrup, whey solids, and wheat gluten, are chemically consistent, have a long shelf life, and are somehow, bewilderingly, cheap to buy. Food processors can concoct flavors so enticing that you are going to want to eat more and more and therefore buy more and more. Food manufacturing became a volume business. To keep all that volume chugging along, they need to secure market share through brilliant marketing campaigns designed to show you how much better and tastier life is with their product. Just how much does big food spend to entice you to buy more? Take a peek . . .

Coca Cola Company Advertising Expenses for 2012[15]

(Owns Vitamin Water, FUSE, Honest Tea, Zico, Fanta, Minute Maid)

3.3 billion dollars

PepsiCo Advertising Expenses for 2012[16]

(Owns Frito Lay, Tropicana, Quaker, Gatorade)

3.7 billion dollars

General Mills Advertising Expenses for 2012[17]

(Owns Betty Crocker, Häagen-Dazs, Yoplait, Old El Paso)

913.7 million dollars

Kraft Foods Advertising Expenses for 2012[18]

(Owns Wheat Thins, Ritz, Nabisco, Boca, Grey Poupon)

640 million dollars

budgets are cheaper to buy in the store than the apple your neighbor grows down the road. Instead of real foods, such as broccoli, apples, salmon, and butter, we have mono- and di-glycerides, high fructose corn syrup, brilliant blue dye, and carrageenan. Ice cream is rarely made from cream . . . in fact, it is hard to find real ice cream anymore. Technically, most of this stuff has to be called frozen dessert because there isn't any real cream or milk in it. I don't know about you, but when I pay six dollars for a pint of ice cream, I want it to be good.

How do you guard yourself against the chemistry experiment that masquerades as sustenance? The answer is real food! Wait, what? No Amazonian spider nectar . . . no ancient mold from Egyptian tombs . . . no everything-free nutrition plan? Nope. Real food. Junk food got us into this mess, and real food will get us out. But we are going to have to relearn what real food is so we can spot a fake. And we are going to have to be patient with our taste buds and ourselves as we navigate the winding road to eating and enjoying healthier foods. We might have to relearn how to boil water. But I promise, this won't hurt a bit.

Overfed and Undernourished: the Bite-Sized Version

Changing your diet for the better requires that you become conscious of your choices, patient with yourself, and accepting of where you are right now. This is not about perfection; progress will do nicely.

We are surrounded by an unprecedented amount of highcalorie, high-salt, high-sugar foods that excite our taste buds and our brains because that is what they are designed to do. Broccoli just can't compete.

Slowly and stealthily over the past thirty years, food has been transformed to contain less actual food. Industrialized ingredients have replaced those that grew out of the ground.

Our human bodies are designed to eat food that is filled with nutrients without excess energy. Manufacturers create calorie-dense foods that starve our cells of nutrition while piling on massive energy stores we don't even need.

Deferring the delights of instant gratification will, most of the time, pay off tomorrow, next year, and twenty years from now with a more vivacious, energetic, and healthy you.

CHAPTER 2

YOU ARE WHAT YOU EAT: A NUTRITION PRIMER

"Food is an important part of a balanced diet." —Fran Lebowitz

What is your best offense in the fight against poor health and crappy food? A solid foundation of nutritional knowledge. We are pumped full of nutrition information on a daily basis online, in the news, and from others. Not always facts, mind you . . . just a lot of information. This access to information has provided us with the remarkable ability to gain knowledge we would not have otherwise been able to obtain to take control of our health.

The flipside is that there is a lot of informational clutter out there just waiting to take up space in our brains and distract us from the truth. We live in an age where anyone can write a blog post or publish an ebook and we just accept that information as true; as it becomes amplified among believers, it becomes hard to tease out fact from fiction. The ironic state of affairs is that as our society becomes less healthy, we seem to be more and more preoccupied with the notion of what health is and how to achieve it—even if we just want to talk about achieving it instead of actually making the effort. The more we do this, the more overwhelming it can seem to actually step up and make change. With all of this complex information about getting healthy, it must be more difficult than simply adding a bit more spinach to our dinner, right? Wrong!

At its core, the gold-standard rules for healthy eating haven't really changed that much—especially where talk of actual food is concerned. When it comes to nutrients, scientists are working hard to understand how every little molecule affects our overall health, and this evolving knowledge has led to a greater understanding of the complexities of the human body. Because really, when your mother told you that you are what you eat, she was right. Our body was made of first what our mothers ate and then what we choose to eat on a daily basis. Our body uses carbohydrates for energy—in fact, our brain is dependent on sugar, and complex biochemical systems ensure that our brain is never lacking the fuel it is so hungry for. Vitamin C is used to build collagen in the skin and support immune cell function. Fats become the lining of each and every one of our cells, and minerals are incorporated into our bones and teeth and even ensure that our blood can carry oxygen. When you can appreciate the remarkable function of food, you have far more respect for the quality of food you choose. Do you want a body made out of cheese puffs and gummy bears or one made out of black beans and pumpkin seeds? Wait! Don't answer that yet . . . you still might need more convincing.

Most of the time, we end up feeling confused about what we should be eating. Is gluten the issue or is it meat? Will soy destroy our immune systems or is it dairy? Should I eat low carb, low glycemic index, and—please tell me—what is a whole grain and why are they in my Lucky Charms? To level the playing field and make healthy eating feel like less of an uphill battle, we need to get back to basics. I am talking about the fundamentals of good nutrition. Meander through the kind of stuff I spent years learning in school and how it applies to our modern, nutrition-obsessed world—and the next time someone dangles a fad diet in front of you, you will have the tools to give them the brush-off.

Carbohydrates: Basic Fuel

Carbohydrate is a dirty word these days. We spent a good two decades extolling the virtues of a diet rich in complex carbohydrates and our ever-expanding waistlines have made us reconsider that information. However, as with most things in nutrition, the spirit of the advice still holds. It is simply how we choose to interpret the advice that needs to change. So what, pray tell, is a carbohydrate?

Scientists don't mince words—a carbo-hydrate is a molecule that contains carbon and water (it's hydrated, get it?). Thanks to research, our knowledge of what they are and how they affect our body has greatly evolved over time. When I was a kid, we used to think of carbohydrates in terms of simple ones and complex ones. A simple one was a smaller molecule called a sugar. Table sugar counts, as does juice. A complex one is a larger molecule called a starch. Starches can be potatoes, white bread, or brown rice. Our knowledge of carbohydrates at the time was such that we emphasized complex over simple in all their forms.

Carbohydrate foods are broken down into their basic sugar building blocks, and when we eat carbohydrates, those sugars make their way into our bloodstream either slowly or quickly, depending on the type of foods we choose. So you can see how this might be a concern for someone with diabetes, whose main biochemical challenge in life is that their body can't process blood sugars as well as a nondiabetic person can. In the not-too-distant past, health professionals would counsel those with diabetes to avoid dietary sugars and enjoy all the potatoes and white bread they wanted because they were starches, or complex carbohydrates. Yet, we now know that white bread and some types of potatoes can raise blood sugars as quickly as table sugar. See what I mean when I say that nutrition is an evolving science?

Now we understand that there is a little more to the carbohydrate puzzle: not only are we thinking about simple and complex but also whether or not they are hyper-processed or quickly absorbed. Steel-cut oats are a different beast than rice crisp cereal, and an apple is nothing like apple juice. Part of what changed is the realization (common sense alert!) that when you over-process foods, you might strip away substances, such as fiber, protein, vitamins, and healthy fats, that our bodies need for good nutrition and help to fill us up so we don't eat as much. Processing can also predigest the food so all those sugar molecules stored within it are absorbed into the blood stream in seconds. We have another scientific discovery to thank for our greater understanding of how carbohydrates affect our bodies: the glycemic index.

The Glycemic Index: Getting Out of Life in the Fast Blood Sugar Lane

In 1981, Canadian doctor David Jenkins led a team that studied how carbohydrate foods affect our blood sugar in different ways and determined a protocol to measure and document these effects.[1] The team coined the term glycemic index to describe this effect. Foods are compared to pure glucose (our bodies' basic energy sugar) and given a score between zero and one hundred.[2] A low GI food, such as apples, chickpeas, and barley, has a score of fifty-five or less.[2] Middle of the road foods include bananas and sweet corn.[2] Foods with a high GI of seventy or more include white bread, sports drinks, and corn flakes.[2] Generally speaking for a typical carbohydrate-containing food, the more protein, fat, fiber, or acid a food has, the slower it raises your blood sugar. Think of a big spinach salad to which you add tuna, chickpeas, and olive oil and vinegar salad dressing. You have just designed a meal that will fill you up and have a moderate effect on blood sugar because of your healthy additions. The type of starch, the size of the starch particle, and how the food was cooked can also affect its glycemic index, which is why basmati rice has a lower impact than arborio rice and baked russet potatoes have a higher impact than boiled baby potatoes.

Why does this matter? Because the way foods affect your blood sugar affects your metabolism, your appetite, and your weight. When you drink a big bottle of juice, those sugars race through your digestive system and are released rapid fire into your blood stream. Your body senses all the sugar—which is fuel for your cells—and sends a message to your pancreas to release a big parcel of insulin.

Insulin is a hormone that helps your cells take up the sugar in your blood stream so they can run their cellular machinery and live another day. You can think of insulin as a key that unlocks the cell door so it can welcome its sugary friends in for dinner. You want this to happen—without it, your cells starve and can't take care of themselves while that sticky sugar continues to wreak havoc in your blood vessels.

However, it is better if your cells have the opportunity to graze instead of binge. When you eat a handful of berries or a slice of sprouted grain bread with almond butter, digestion and absorption take time. The rate at which sugars enter your blood stream is slower and your pancreas sends out a measured dose of insulin. Your cells are treated to a slow and steady stream of fuel, and your body is comfortable in the knowledge that the fuel will be present for a while. This translates into stable energy levels for you, and if you are the type to get cranky when blood sugar drops, keeping things stable will keep you more, ahem, stable. Slowly digested carbohydrate foods also tend to fill your stomach more so you feel satisfied. Between the full stomach and steady supply of energy, your brain gets the message that you have all the fuel you need so it can hit the pause button on your appetite.

However, if you guzzle that big bottle of juice and get a big rush of blood sugar, a lot of insulin is released right away, and a lot of cell doors open quickly. All of a sudden, your body senses that there is no more sugar in the blood, and you had better replenish the supply, quick! Your body wants to make sure you won't starve to death and ramps up appetite, leading to cravings not for sliced turkey and an apple but for more quick sugars, such as gummy bears and muffins. This is hardwired into us from a time when food wasn't widely available and we needed to be strongly motivated to find more food. The trouble is, most of us have a drawer full of cheap, processed energy waiting to be eaten at whim. Our metabolic survival mechanisms are totally unnecessary and downright troublesome to the modern man or woman. Unstable blood sugars can lead to wanting to eat more food. The foods that typically raise blood sugars quickly don't tend to be satisfying and have a lot of calories. You can see the kind of vicious cycle this turns into.

So what is the take home message? I certainly don't want you to concern yourself with learning the glycemic index of foods. If you have to scrutinize over every single food choice you make, you are going to get bored pretty fast. So let's get back to the food, shall we? In general, whole and unprocessed foods will raise blood sugars more slowly. When it comes to the foods that contain carbohydrates—fruits, vegetables, grains, legumes, and dairy—think unprocessed. You see what I mean about a lot of complex science supporting some simple ideas about what foods to eat? As a dietitian, I am thankful that science is helping us understand the relationship between food and health, but for you, I am always going to distill it back to the food, because you don't eat carbohydrates. You eat bananas and tortillas and cabbage. Thank goodness . . . those foods sound a lot more interesting!

The Not-So-Sweet Life

I can't talk about carbohydrates without talking about sugar. It tends to be the one dietary evil all health advocates can agree on, regardless of dietary creed. Dr. Robert Lustig made waves when he originally publicized the notion that sugar is, in fact, toxic.[3] While catchy, I think the absolute accuracy of that statement, along with the definition of a sugar, is up for debate. Shall I complicate things for you for a moment? Such a simple word as sugar can be used in a myriad of ways. There is sugar—the white or brown stuff you pour into your coffee—and there are sugars—the simple carbohydrates in fruit, juice, sugar, honey, and more. Sugars can be naturally occurring in whole foods or added to processed foods. Which ones do I worry the most about? Added sugars in all their forms.

As you have seen by the discussion of glycemic index above, overloading our system with rapidly digested carbohydrates is going to wreak havoc with appetite and energy levels. Added sugars are also concentrated in calories and almost totally devoid of nutrients, meaning that it is easy to consume far too many calories from added sugars than you need. In addition, they trigger that "YUM" reaction on the taste buds and in the brain that encourages you to overeat whatever food they are added to. We are hardwired to love sugar, as sweet foods were a rare source of concentrated energy back in our hunter-gatherer days. Now we are surrounded by the stuff and our bodies are less in need of concentrated energy, so we end up storing it for a rainy day.

To put not too fine a point on it, the poison is always in the dose. If cakes are reserved for birthdays and you don't drown yourself in cola, a bit of sugar every now and then will have little impact on your health. This will be especially true if you have a diet foundation that is based on whole, unprocessed plant foods—which this book will help you create for yourself. Unfortunately, many of us with the typical Western diet subsist on a daily cycle of foodstuff that is nothing more than a mixture of starches, added sugars, and various flavorings and stabilizers. We eat muffins for breakfast, guzzle juice and coffee drinks, munch granola bars for snacks, eat sandwiches on sweetened bread for lunch, and pour sugary sauces on our dinner. Nutritional zeroes and metabolic foes abound. This is where chronic sugar consumption becomes a chronic poison, to quote Mark Hyman, MD.

When the insult of high calorie, nutrition-poor sugars is added to our overprocessed and underactive bodies, the result can only be disaster. Although some feel that a definitive body of evidence has not yet been reached, early research shows that fructose in table sugars and high fructose corn syrup not only promotes obesity via empty "YUM!" calories, but the fructose sugar they contain may lead to metabolic abnormalities.[4,5] You see, glucose sugar is what starches are made of and our bodies know how to use glucose to fuel our metabolism. Fructose, in contrast to glucose, is nutritionally unnecessary and has to be metabolized by the liver.[5,6] Table sugar contains fructose along with that glucose in equal measure; in high fructose corn syrup, or HFCS, fructose outweighs the glucose. And when you give fructose in high enough doses, the liver can metabolize fructose into glucose, which it pours into the blood stream, even if you don't need it.[5,6] Liver cells can also convert fructose into fatty acids and this liver fat appears to promote insulin resistance and nonalcoholic fatty liver disease.[5,6] It is insulin that promotes the conversion of sugars into fatty acids in the liver. So the very hormone (insulin) we need to metabolize all the excess sugars we are consuming is being stunted by sugar (fructose) consumption. It seems that sugars bite the hand that feeds as they pad your butt for the fall. In addition, high fructose intake appears to put the heart at risk by increasing blood fats called triglycerides in addition to the insult that insulin resistance might pose to your ticker.[5,6]

Reading this, you might galvanize your resolve to switch to alternative sweeteners, such as aspartame, sucralose, and xylitol. Not so fast, caballero! While these sweeteners may win at the calorie game, you might suspect that our body might not be so easily fooled by manufactured sweets. All those sugar-free and no-added-sugar foods? They are typically filled with alternative sweeteners that tantalize our taste buds and may even play their own metabolic role in overeating and obesity. However, to me the biggest problem is not sugar or sweeteners themselves but our sweet tooth. Regardless of their caloric value, artificial sweeteners only feed our love for the sweet stuff. Our world contains such heavily salted and sweetened foods that our taste buds have learned to appreciate only those homogenized, mass-produced flavor sensations. Real food that grew out of the ground can hardly compete. Sweeteners dull the bitter, acidic, and astringent tastes found in many of our healthiest and least processed foods to the point that they taste foreign and unpleasant to us. So, independent of their metabolic effects, sweets (calorie-laden or not) ruin your appreciation for the world of healthy, natural foods that will foster good health.

You might ask, "What if I am diabetic—don't I need artificial sweeteners?" In fact, you don't. It is widely accepted that small amounts of added sugars themselves are not an issue in diabetes;[7] rather, the dosage and the overall effect of carbohydrates on your blood sugar control is most important. This doesn't mean that a diabetic can go and drink Coke with abandon but a teaspoon of real honey on some plain Greek yogurt with berries? Not a

Do Low Carb Diets Really Work for Weight Loss?

In a word, the answer is yes. That was the simple part. Now, let's delve into the grey area of low-carb living.

Carbohydrates do not cause weight gain in and of themselves, and they are not an impediment to weight loss for most. However, when we eat the wrong kind of carbohydrate foods or overdo it, weight gain is often the result. And most of the carbohydrates we eat are the wrong kind—highly refined; doused in sugar, salt, and fat; and essentially pre-digested by machines so we can consume it quickly and send our blood sugars soaring. If insulin resistance or full-blown type 2 diabetes follows, losing weight can be a bit trickier if we are trying to stick to a typical high-carbohydrate plan. Here is why: insulin is what we call an obesogenic hormone. It favors the storage of energy in fat cells and the use of carbohydrates for energy instead of stored fat. We want it to— remember how insulin ensures that sugar in our blood stream can be used by cells for energy? However, if you are consistently flooding your body with rapidly absorbed sugars on a raft of insulin, your metabolism will be favoring fat storage—lucky for you, all those high-calorie foods will provide plenty of excess energy to store!

Typically with type 2 diabetes, you make insulin just fine, but your body isn't responding to it. In order to try and get the job done, your hardworking pancreas will keep pumping out the insulin. The overwhelming flood of insulin is a strong message to your body to stop breaking down energy stores and start storing them instead. If you are trying to lose weight and you are insulin resistant, flooding your system with easily digested carbohydrates in a sea of insulin is a setup for failure.

Low-carbohydrate diets work for a couple of reasons: they 1) force you to stop eating the food that was probably leading to weight gain in the first place, and 2) help keep insulin levels lower to favor the release of energy from fat cells instead of storage. If insulin is low, glucagon—insulin's opponent—comes a-callin'. Glucagon liberates energy from cells for fuel. For those who can't seem to lose weight following a typical healthy eating plan, shifting to a lower-carb (but not no-carb) pattern can help budge the pounds. In order to be healthy, this is not a typical Atkins plan. You cannot eat all the butter, steak, and cheese you want and think you can maintain that way of life healthfully in the long term. In addition, as your body starves for carbohydrates and needs to build fuel for your hungry brain, it chomps up fat in a messy process called ketosis.

Ketosis is touted as the magic of a low carb diet; in the absence of carbohydrates, your body can make usable energy from fat in the form of ketone bodies. However, ketosis is a potentially toxic, acidic state. It was designed for biological emergencies and not with long-term health in mind. Permanent change is what you need to ensure that weight stays off for good. Instead, shift your carbohydrate choices towards fresh produce—vegetables and fruit, legumes, and small amounts of unprocessed grains, such as steel-cut oats and quinoa—and say goodbye to anything processed.

problem. Once again, we see a substance in modern, processed food that is unnecessary to human health and has unknown long-term consequences. Time to eat off the land, not out of the lab.

The Whole Grain Truth

One of the reasons I think it is so important to provide this seeming over-share on nutrition is that without a solid knowledge foundation, your ounce of good intentions can be co-opted by dietary fads and food processors trying to win your grocery buck. Witness the whole grain fiasco: while dietitians, such as myself, have been extolling the virtues of whole grains for a couple of decades, food manufacturers have responded by making all manner of unhealthy processed junk with whole grain. With a little bit of knowledge, you, the consumer, can be duped. We need to drill down to the unalienable truth about whole grains.

When I talk about healthy whole grains, I mean a grain as nature intended: plucked off the plant and cooked or sprouted and eaten. I also think you should be eating a variety of whole grains, so your body can receive all the nutrition nature intended for you to receive. Instead, most North Americans eat highly processed wheat three to six times a day. Even if it is whole grain, it is hardly what I can consider to be good nutritional practice. The reason for this is that when you turn whole wheat into whole grain sugar-sweetened breakfast cereals with little marshmallows or add whole grains to fried and MSG-laden chips, it can't exactly be called a health food. However, if we think whole grains are some sort of magic bullet, we might fool ourselves into believing that those options aren't so bad for us.

Whole grains, when they are unprocessed, possess an incredible nutritional bounty: tons of fiber to help cleanse your digestive tract, plenty of protein to keep you full and maintain stable blood sugars in addition to healthy fats, vitamins, and minerals. Even turning grains into flour can wreak havoc as that once dense and slowly digested grain is now broken into millions of particles that make its digestion and absorption that much faster. As soon as you process these foods, you lose plenty. By only eating one grain, wheat, we lose out on the flavor and nutrition found in the larger world of grains—rye, sorghum, barley, rice, teff, and more. Are you thinking to yourself, "What the heck is teff?" My point exactly! We have to get away from focusing on the nutrients and thinking about the food. So real, unprocessed whole grains are good; processed junk, even "made with whole grain," is not so good.

Desiree's Non-Clinically-Proven, Super (Un)Scientific Carbohydrate Test!

One of my favorite tricks for telling if a grain-based food is good for you is the chew test. Ready to be a food scientist? Get out the lab coat and a few of your favorite grain foods. Now, place the cracker, cereal, bread, muffin, etc. in your mouth (not all at once!). How quickly can you fully chew and swallow it? Will it just dissolve in your mouth without you having to do anything?

The quicker and easier it is to chew and swallow that grain food, the faster your body is going to be able to turn it into a spike of blood sugar. Most processed grain foods are essentially predigested so they go down easy. It's true! Food manufacturers want you to be able to eat more of their tasty product quickly, so you will have to buy more. The grains are finely milled then steamed or cooked to incorporate water and gelatinize the starch. This is like napalm for your blood sugar circuitry. Modern carbs make us super-sized because they don't fill you up, yet they leave you craving their taste; they are easy to overeat and crammed full of calories.

Now try something really grainy—such as some steel-cut oats or a Ryvita cracker. Takes some work, right? Try sitting down and eating a whole container of Ryvita crackers. You can't do it. Not unless you are floating them in nacho cheese.

There—now you are officially a food scientist! Well . . . I suppose not a scientist. But you are definitely a bit more clued in about how to choose a carb when there is no ingredients list hanging around. Fluffy (bread) equals spiky (sugars).

What About Gluten?

Oh gluten. A decade ago, most of us didn't even know what gluten was. Now, gluten is at the center of our carbohydrate aversion. We loathe it, fear it, crave it, and think it might be making us fatter and sicker. What's an eater to do?

We are, for some reason, becoming more reactive to food than any other time in our history. Gluten seems to be one of the key substances in food causing those reactions. Not so long ago, the only people who needed to avoid gluten were those with celiac disease or an autoimmune disease (which is not an allergy) that is triggered by the ingestion of gluten in susceptible individuals. For those with celiac disease, even a crumb of gluten promotes this immune attack and long-term exposure places them at risk for infertility, malnutrition, and digestive cancers.[8] These days, more of us are suffering from celiac disease, and it appears that the difference is not simply one of better diagnosis and detection. One team of researchers, using blood stores from fifty-year-old military samples, found that celiac disease prevalence is indeed higher in modern times.[9]

Alongside celiac disease, nonceliac gluten sensitivity has also risen to prominence. Once the sole domain of alternative medicine, conventional science is now starting to recognize the existence of sensitivity to gluten without an autoimmunity or classical allergy component.[10] And for the rest of us, there are those who believe that gluten is simply bad for you and leads to immune impairment and obesity.

Who's right? We don't quite know yet.

Here are some thoughts on the path to knowing:

—Many of us might actually have celiac disease or gluten sensitivity and not even know it. If we happen onto a gluten-free diet and feel better, there could be a good reason for that! If you think gluten might be causing your issues, get tested for celiac disease before you go gluten free so you can rule it out just in case. Once you go gluten free, it can interfere with celiac disease diagnosis and you might not get the medical care you need.

—If you get a clear bill of health on the celiac front, go gluten free, and feel better, you might have nonceliac gluten sensitivity—which a physician can help you determine for certain.

—However, you also might feel better because the foods that typically contain lots of gluten are terrible for us. Processed snack foods, cheap soft breads, baked goods, and convenience foods cause blood sugar spikes, are too high in salt/fat/sugar/calories, and lead to weight gain. They promote inflammation, impair immune function, and leave you undernourished. Going without these foods and switching to more whole foods in their place will make you feel phenomenal. So it's not always the gluten molecules themselves but the processed foods that also tend to contain gluten that can make us sick.

—We used to only encounter gluten in a few grain foods, such as bread, cakes, or cereal. Now, wheat flour and glutens have been extracted and concentrated and thrown into so many foods[11] that it is possible to eat sources of gluten at every meal and snack without touching a bite of pasta. Gluten is found in trail mixes, barbeque sauces, frozen desserts, and dips. Taken out of the natural context and combined with a body beleaguered by an unhealthy lifestyle, it just might be too much for our bodies.

—It is thought that modern wheat varieties have been bred that contain more immune-stimulating gluten molecules than those we ate one hundred years ago, so the insult might be stronger today than it used to be,[10,12] although not all researchers agree.[13]

—If you have irritable bowel syndrome, gluten-containing grains are also high in fructans, which can exacerbate symptoms.[14] It might not be the gluten . . . it could be the fructans.[14] If this sounds like you, talk to your dietitian about a FODMAPS approach to symptom management.

—A complex interaction of environment and lifestyle might just be changing our bodies to become less tolerant of the gluten we encounter. North Americans generally eat terrible diets and there are implications to our immune health, digestive function, and our gut bacteria that might be determining how our body processes gluten. Time will tell.

Carbohydrates: What's the Bottom Line?

Carbohydrate foods—fruits, vegetables, grains, legumes, and dairy—are not something to be feared. Our challenges with carbohydrates occur primarily due to the abnormal volume of processed carbohydrates we consume. When the carbohydrates in our diet are nothing more than flour, sugar, fat, and food cosmetics in combination, we end up with yo-yoing blood sugars, leading to poor energy levels, weight gain, and lack of good nutrition. Eating real and choosing unprocessed carbohydrate foods (with or without gluten) will set you free.

Protein: Body Building

Carbohydrates are the nutrients du jour, but protein won't stand to be ignored. Should we eat more or less? Animal or vegetable? Is that protein eco-friendly or humanely raised? Most people agree that protein is an important part of a healthy diet, but there are many shades of grey to this story. So let's start with the basics: what is protein and why do we need it?

Protein is built of amino acids in the same way that carbohydrates are built of sugar molecules. There are amino acids that are essential, meaning that we need to get them from food, and those that are nonessential because our bodies can build them. Protein is used for building tissues, such as bone and muscle. The collagen and elastin in our skin are proteins, and protein is also important for maintaining healthy immune function. Protein builds blood cells and enzymes for just about every important chemical reaction in our bodies, and protein is also needed to create hormones.

Food Marketing Farce #234

Just like sugary cereals made with whole grain, I love whenever a food or supplement boasts providing "five essential amino acids." Just five? Really? So, in essence, your product has a bit of protein. So do all the rest of them!

Quality Protein: I Just Want the Good Stuff

In school, I learned about protein quality: whether or not a protein food had the full complement of amino acids needed for life and whether the protein was well utilized by the body. In this regard, an egg is practically perfect and all other proteins are compared to it. Meats, eggs, and dairy were considered complete high-quality proteins and veggie sources were considered incomplete and lacking. Doesn't create a strong argument for a plant-based anti-inflammatory diet, does it?

However, the old-school way of thinking doesn't really take into account the total nutrition picture. Time to think of the whole food once again. While meat offers iron, zinc, and some B vitamins, so do legumes and grains. The only nutrient you aren't going to receive from plant proteins is vitamin B12, which can be added in supplemental form. Plant-based proteins take the protein power a few steps further by coming loaded with fiber, vital anti-inflammatory and antioxidant phytochemicals, and other vitamins, such as folate for a healthy nervous system and plenty of potassium for electrolyte balance and healthy blood pressure. Plant proteins offer this goodness for fewer calories and without all the animal fats that can junk up your pipes. Yes, they might not be concentrated sources of protein, but just how much protein do we think we need? Those sixteen-ounce steaks are totally unnecessary from a biological perspective (and you might want to apologize to your heart when you eat one, too). Believe me, protein requirements are not as much as you might think . . . but they are probably a bit more than some plant-based proponents would recommend.

Uh, what did I just say?

I'm just messin' with you! I will stop talking in nutrition circles and get down to business now.

The longstanding rule for protein that I was taught is that you need 0.8 grams of protein per kilogram of body weight, or 0.36 grams for each pound you weigh. So a 175 pound person would need about 64 grams of protein. That number represents the amount that is estimated to support basic function and prevent protein deficiency in most of the population. However, we have come to expect more from good nutrition; I don't want you to simply exist—I want to help you eat to feel amazing and be healthy for life!

In addition to all of the basic functions of protein, there are a few functions that are particularly helpful in our modern eating environment. Protein is satisfying, and when we eat we need to be satisfied to help curb our appetite and get us to put the fork down. In addition, having a good source of protein at each meal will help slow the rise of blood sugars and keep that meal working overtime for you, helping reduce hunger and cravings for more fast carbs. Finally, lean proteins don't tend to have a lot of calories, so you can get a lot of nutrition without a huge calorie spend. So an easier and more realistic rule of thumb (that doesn't require a calculator) is to divide your body weight in pounds by half. So that same 175-pound person would need 87.5 grams of protein per day. In fact, it looks like that short cut might be a more accurate estimate of our true needs, according to one 2010 study.[15]

Next, we have to deal with the question of animal versus vegetable. I am a proponent of plant-based diets and I suspect, since you are reading this, that you might be interested in them, too. However, if you are already mourning the loss of chicken fajitas, relax! I won't make you go full veggie. In fact, the very soul of this book is about choosing the changes that are realistic for you right now . . . not forcing something that sucks the fun out of eating. I do want you to eat more meatless meals for better health, at least a few each week. That shouldn't be too tough. Still need convincing that meatless is the right way to go? Read on . . .

Five Really Good Reasons for Enjoying Plant-Based Proteins

1. They come packaged with slowly digesting carbohydrates for real energy, vitamins, minerals, antioxidants, and filling, cleansing fiber . . . and we all need more fiber.
2. If you are concerned about animal welfare, food safety, and food quality in modern agriculture, plant-based proteins are for you.

3. Plant-based proteins are gentler on the planet, as they require fewer energy inputs and less water to produce pound for pound. They also pump less carbon into the atmosphere so you can breathe easy.[16]
4. Plant-based proteins are cheap and easy (. . . to prepare—get your mind out of the nutrition gutter!). You can enjoy a super star nutrition plan without a big spend or hours in the kitchen.
5. Beans, traditional soy foods, and whole intact grains are incredibly nutrient dense and will help you thrive.

We used to think (and, in fact, one of my old textbook states) that you had to combine plant proteins at each meal to ensure you get the whole complement of essential amino acids for protein power. Yawn! Time to shake out the nutrition cobwebs because thinking has changed. We realize now that our bodies are a wee bit smarter than that, and as long as we are consuming a variety of grains and legumes throughout the day, we will get all the protein benefits we need. Of course, there is nothing wrong with a nice plate of rice and beans. I nearly lived off them during my unpaid nutrition internship. And it leaves room in the shopping budget for wine, that other student essential.

On to the superfoods . . . what about quinoa, hemp, and soy? They are routinely touted as being complete proteins. Well, truth be told, all proteins are technically complete in their amino acids, it is just that plant proteins usually have one or two amino acids that limit your body's ability to use that protein right away for building purposes. The amino acid lysine is usually limiting in grains, and legumes are typically limited in methionine. Quinoa has plenty of lysine, which is why it is usually called a complete protein, but it doesn't actually have that much protein overall—just three grams per half cup—so it cannot be relied upon as a protein source. You've gotta get those legumes on your plate! Soybeans and hemp seeds are far better. They contain substantial amounts of protein and don't have any limiting amino acids.

Cavemen Did It . . . The Promise of Paleo

As far as nutrition trends go, I don't mind the paleo diet in theory. Our carbaholic nation could use a little cold turkey—pun intended! For those of us suffering from digestive concerns, such as IBS, reducing fermentable (i.e. gassy) carbohydrate foods, such as legumes and grains, can offer some relief.

And if you follow it properly, you will be eating enough produce to nourish your cells well. In essence, it is a protein and produce plan, which is a sure bet for weight loss if you can stick with it. Many do, embracing the plan long term—which is a clear indicator that it works, because fad diets can't be maintained for more than a couple of months before you give up, frustrated and hungry and wrestling with the nearest kid for his candy. However, a bunch of misleading nutrition information, particularly on the Internet, bogs down the theory, and the diet does lack the powerful punch of some heavy-hitting plant foods.

In reality, we eat a diet our bodies were not designed for. Don't think for one second that a triple chocolate pretzel cheesecake was part of our original design. (Ooh, but that sounds good!) We didn't used to have Chili's at the ready anytime we needed a Tex-Mex meal. We had to work for our food. It even took a while in evolutionary terms before we figured out that we could make food stay put in one place so we didn't have to walk so far. And it took a long while before we realized how we could manipulate natural foods into a dizzying assortment of different textures and flavors, the likes of which we enjoy today. So we are, in essence, engaging in a massive experiment on diet composition and our health. It's not going well—we need to make changes! Our paleo-loving brethren aren't so different from us plant power advocates because we both love the same thing: natural, unprocessed food. We just take a slightly different approach.

Paleo plans focus a great deal on protein, and we have already mentioned the benefits of protein for the human body. A paleo diet will help you curb those cravings for processed carbohydrates by stabilizing blood sugars and satisfying your appetite with protein. However, we also know the remarkable benefits of legumes and truly whole and unprocessed grains. Their fiber tones the digestive tract, detoxifies, and helps stabilize blood sugar and reduce cholesterol; they contain anti-inflammatory phytonutrients and vital minerals that are important in the fight against environmental assault. So it's not technically accurate to call grains inflammatory foods. Hyper-processed ones? You bet—I won't argue if you want to banish them from your diet.

And let me remind you that back in the Paleolithic olden days, we didn't exactly live that long. We have become more intelligent, taller, and, dare I say, better looking since adopting a more diverse diet. But that's not exactly a scientific argument. As we live longer, our focus turns to the ability of our body to repair the damage of everyday life, and plant foods help us do just that. Meat might help keep you powered up, but it won't protect you from the effects of environmental and diet-induced cell damage. In fact, too much meat might cause it.

While our ancestors might have thrived on a wild meat diet, modern meat isn't even in the same ballpark. Modern meat is fattier; it contains more of the unhealthful omega-6 and saturated fats and is exposed to more pharmaceuticals and toxic components, such as dioxins, than ever before.[16] Humanely raised and processed grass-fed meat is a big step in the right direction, but it is not affordable for most. And while no one will argue with the fact that animal protein was a vital part of our ancestral diet, most ancestral cultures didn't enjoy access to huge amounts of protein at every meal. What you ate depended on where you lived. Our Inuit relatives ate a lot of whale blubber and not a ton of greens. Others enjoyed much more access to plant foods than animal ones. For many ancestral cultures, wild fruit, veggies, seeds, and wild grains made up the bulk of their diet.[17] Wait! They were sort of plant-based!

Where's the Beef? Finding Protein in Animal and Vegetable Sources

While we want to aim to consume a more concentrated protein source at every meal, remember that all foods have some protein, and it adds up over the course of the day to help you fuel your body. Let's take a look at how the various sources of protein stack up.

½ cup cottage cheese: 14 g	¾ cup black beans: 11.3 g	1 can of tuna: 42 g
3 tablespoons hemp seeds: 10 g	100 g steak: 39.5 g	½ cup peanuts: 19.4 g
1 cup quinoa: 6.5 g	100 g halibut: 26.7 g	1 cup whole wheat pasta: 8 g
1 cup skim milk: 9 g	2 slices sprouted grain toast: 10 g	¾ cup extra firm tofu: 28 g
2 eggs: 14 g	1 cup barley: 3.75 g	100 g chicken breast: 30 g
¼ cup almond butter: 9.8 g	¾ cup Greek yogurt: 18–22 g	1 cup steamed broccoli: 4 g
1 cup oatmeal: 4.1 g	1 medium sweet potato: 2.3 g	1 cup edamame: 23.5 g

Data from Health Canada Nutrient Datafile

There is plenty of protein to be had, even from unexpected sources, such as pasta. As you will see later in the meal plans, a day's worth of veggie protein can easily get you to the 70–90 g of protein you might need each day. Protein content is another great reason to choose your plant foods unprocessed—many of the baked goods we consume regularly have little of the protein found in whole grains or the nuts and seeds we could be choosing instead.

Soy Confusing . . .

I have mentioned the "s" word a few times already, so for those of you who are soy skeptics, you are probably expecting an explanation by now. First of all, let me say that a soybean is a *bean*. Not a magic cure-all, nor an evil poison. And the opinions from health enthusiasts seem to fall somewhere along that range of opinions. In the nineties, researchers began extolling the seemingly super benefits of soy foods in nutrition literature, and all of a sudden, soy protein started popping up in all sorts of foods where it didn't belong. How do we get this so wrong? Let's start at the beginning . . .

Soybeans are a remarkable source of protein; a half-cup of green soybeans, or edamame, rings in at almost 12 grams of protein.[18] They contain a good balance of amino acids and have plenty of folate, calcium, potassium, and plant sterols,[18] which help lower blood cholesterol. However, detractors claim that soy contains antinutrients and estrogens, making it a toxic food that will imbalance your hormones. Soy is also a common allergen, and it is becoming harder to avoid in our complex food world. So let's sort through some of the claims to help you make your own decision about soy.

The Antinutrients: Saponins, Lectins, and Phytates

Those that argue that soy is unsafe usually mention substances, such saponins, lectins, and phytates, in their arguments. They are called antinutrients because they typically bind or block some other biological component in the plant. However, nature has its wisdom and, in fact, these antinutrients may have their own health benefits.

Saponins are found in many plant foods, including quinoa, and are easily removed by rinsing and soaking the bean. Bitter in taste, saponins have the ability to form soaps in contact with fats; in the intestine, they can bind bile salts and carry them out of the body, thereby lowering blood cholesterol.[19] Actually, that sounds pretty good to me, so let's move on to lectins, shall we? Lectins are proteins found in grains, mushrooms, and legumes, and they have the ability to bind biological sugars.[20] They are signaling molecules, and for that reason, a small group think they could cause us harm. However, researchers are also hot on the trail of discovering the potentially antitumor and immune-boosting effects of lectins.[20] So I would say the jury is not quite out on those either.

Phytates are found in many plant foods and they have the ability to bind minerals, such as calcium and iron, thereby reducing their availability for the human body—leading to phytates' reputation as an antinutrient.[19] However, the effect only becomes a concern when there are large amounts of phytates consumed without a large amount of minerals.[19] Luckily, many phytate-rich foods are also mineral-rich, and committing to a nutrient-dense diet will help ensure you are receiving the nutrients you need. Phytates are also remarkable antioxidants and may even have antitumor effects.[19] In fact, a common natural supplement taken for cancer care is IP-6, a phytate.

In summary, many of these antinutrients are, in fact, necessary components of the plant that comprise part of the plant's natural defenses against pests, just as many antioxidants and phytochemicals are. We are just starting to understand that these substances may have valuable effects on the human body, although research is just in its early stages. So there is no need to fear the wisdom of nature and eschew plant foods with the power to deeply nourish our bodies. Finally, for those worried about the impact of these substances on their health, rest assured. Soybeans and other legumes are meant to be soaked and cooked; both practices greatly reduce the impact of said antinutrients, as does fermentation. So give sprouted grains or tempeh a chance!

The Phytoestrogens: Genistein and Daidzein

Another component of soy foods that causes concerns for some are the phytoestrogens, such as genistein and daidzein. I have had clients who avoided soy sauce because they thought it would interfere with their bodybuilding efforts. It is important to note that phytoestrogens do not function in the same way that our bodies' estrogens do, and their interactions with hormone levels in the body are complex.[21] Plant estrogens also have antioxidant and anti-inflammatory activity.[21] Both of these factors have huge implications for their potential health benefits.

What does the research say? It's a mixed bag. One of the greatest challenges in dietary research is approximating the realistic, lifelong effects of a diet that includes soy foods in a scientifically rigorous way. Variables regarding soy's effect on the body would include age, genetics, health profile, and even the type of bacteria someone has in their colon.[21] Population studies that have shown reduced breast cancer risk from consuming soy foods are not considered gold-standard evidence. However, providing supplemental doses of phytoestrogens is not the same as feeding whole soy foods daily, nor is it the same as a diet high in isolated soy proteins in processed foods. Studies consistently contradict one another, making it difficult to clarify the effects of phytoestrogens on human health.[21]

Something else to note: other phytoestrogen compounds have received far less of a lashing in the health world than those found in soy. Lignans in flax and resveratrol in red wine are just two phytoestrogen compounds that are celebrated in the human diet, as opposed to being reviled. Interestingly, these substances are far more commonly consumed in the context of the whole food than in isolated forms. I'm just sayin'.

The Whole Soy Advantage

Remember that whenever we isolate and concentrate a substance from a whole food, we cannot predict its effect on the body. Many potent pharmaceuticals are derived from natural sources, as are many poisons. Soybeans are just that, beans. When food manufacturers started isolating phytoestrogens and proteins from soybeans and littering our food supply with them, we had no idea what the outcome would be. In fact, we can't be fully sure if there is an impact at all, given the diverse range of potentially helpful and harmful factors in our everyday diets that muddy the waters.

I encourage you to be more aware of the forms of soy foods you are consuming; you might be eating soy three to six times a day without consciously choosing tofu for dinner. Relying heavily on soy protein and gluten-based meat substitutes might be placing you under a heavy, unnatural soy load with unknown health consequences. Soy oil, ubiquitous in our cheaply processed food world, is high in omega-6 fats and contributes to a pro-inflammatory state in our bodies that promotes disease.[22] Not to mention that the soy typically used for industrial purposes is genetically engineered, pesticide-laden, and processed heavily. I wholeheartedly agree that we should make food choices without isolated soy components as often as possible. This means looking at breakfast cereals, breads, non-dairy beverages, and even meat products, where animal protein might be supplemented with soy protein because it's cheaper. Look for actual soybeans on an ingredient list and steer clear of soy protein.

For me, soybeans are a healthy choice when we eat them as a whole food—always organic or at least guaranteed to be free of genetic engineering. That means choosing tofu, tempeh, or natto; enjoying soy milk made from whole soybeans; and eating miso, tamari, and traditional soy sauce in addition to edamame and whole soybeans. Soy is not essential in the human diet, but on a plant-based plan, it is a nutritious and concentrated source of protein that adds variety. Eating one or two servings of whole soy foods a day shouldn't be cause for concern.

The one potential exception to the soy for all rule is women and men who have survived a hormone-related cancer, such as breast cancer, or have a strong family history of such. If this is you, talk to your doctor or dietitian about making the best dietary choices for your specific needs. In general, the research points to soy being safe—even for this group—but there is some dissent in the literature. Make a choice that feels right for you—and don't let fear of food diminish your enjoyment of eating.

For prevention purposes, there is some indication that regular consumption of soy foods may help.[21] If you still consume animal products, you can choose to avoid soy foods if you feel strongly about it. If you are totally vegan and avoid soy, pay serious attention to other protein sources to ensure you are hitting your targets (it can be done). Another option is choosing fermented soy, such as tempeh and miso, which you might feel is a better choice for you. The human body is not a test tube; if you feel good eating soy, keep it up! If systematically taking soy out of your diet makes you feel better, it's the right option for you—the choice is always yours!

Powering up with Protein

What about protein for the everyday athlete? If you are consuming your half-gram of protein per pound of body weight and you hit the gym a few times a week, you are getting all you need. However, for those who do serious weight lifting or compete in endurance events, such as marathons or adventure races, you may want to eat a bit more.

Protein requirements are highly personalized, so our best data provides nothing more than ranges to estimate requirements. This is why it's a good idea to work with a sport-focused dietitian to help design a killer performance diet that is personalized for you. For endurance athletes, protein needs are estimated at 1.2–1.4 grams protein per kilogram body weight.[23] For strength athletes, needs are slightly higher at 1.4–1.7 grams protein per kilogram of body weight.[23] Divide your weight in pounds by 2.2 to get your weight in kilograms.

It is important to remember that protein doesn't provide you with performance gains; your training does that. Protein ensures that the building blocks are there for repair, to support optimal performance, and help keep the immune system strong as you train.

Protein: What's the Bottom Line?

Protein is critical for the maintenance of healthy tissues, immunity, and hormone replenishment, but more is not always better. Whether or not you are interested in a vegetarian diet, choosing plant-based proteins more often is a healthy, economical, and environmentally sustainable choice. Get a bit of protein at every meal to help keep you full and energy levels stable. Divide your weight, in pounds, in half to give you the average grams of protein you need every day.

Fat: the Good, the Bad, and the Ugly

Why are we so hung up on carbohydrates? Because a few decades ago we thought fat was the enemy and we started going overboard on them. We have learned a thing or two since then. The first lesson we learned? Healthy fats are critical to your health and wellbeing. They help you absorb vital nutrients, such as bone-building vitamin D and skin-loving lycopene, they moisturize your skin from the inside out, and more.

We're going to have to break this one down . . . so let's talk about what fats are used for in the body and all the different types we find in our food supply. Fats are concentrated sources of energy at nine calories per gram instead of four calories per gram for protein or carbohydrates; this knowledge certainly feeds the idea that fat makes you fat. However, dietary fats are integral to our bodies, as each one of our cells incorporates fats into their cell linings. These cell linings help mediate transport of substances in and out of the cells and are the critical site of cell signaling—how cells talk to each other to get the job of living done. Fats are also components of sex hormones, such as testosterone and estrogen, and help our nervous system relay messages.

My healthy eating focus is never on a low-fat diet—instead, I am most concerned about getting the healthiest sources of fat possible. We need all of the different types of fat in varying amounts and foods contain differing combinations of fats; getting too much of some forms of fat can harm our health. So here's the skinny on the good, bad, and the ugly forms of fat found in our food supply.

Trans Fats

Trans fats come from two sources: they are produced naturally in the stomach of ruminants (cows, sheep, and goats) and industrially in hydrogenated fats. The hydrogenated fats are the ones I am worried about. Trans fats are produced when hydrogen is forced into an oil molecule under high pressure; it creates a kink in the structure that turns liquid oil into one that stays solid at room temperature. Good for shelf stability and enhancing profits in your favorite junk foods . . . not so good for your heart. Trans fats have the unique ability to reduce your healthy (HDL) cholesterol, increase your unhealthy (LDL) cholesterol, and promote artery-damaging inflammation.[24] Avoid these junk fats at all costs by looking for the word hydrogenated on the ingredients list. Even trans fat free products might still contain trans fats due to a loophole that grants the claim if a food has less than 0.5 grams per serving. So if a serving is one cookie and you just ate four cookies, you might just have eaten 1.6 grams of trans fats without knowing it. Sounds like a small price to pay for deliciousness but, in fact, experts believe that getting just 1 percent of calories as trans fats is enough to harm your health.[24] Consider trans fats the new cigarettes and steer clear.

Omega-6 Fats

Next come the omega-6 fats . . . another fat that we have evolved our understanding of and stopped cramming down everyone's throats. Omega-6 fats, a type of polyunsaturated fat, were thought to be outstanding for our health, so we promoted the widespread use of all vegetable oils, such as corn, soy, canola, and safflower, to provide us with these little goodies. While there is still some controversy in the scientific literature, I am convinced that we need to lower our intake of omega-6s stat.

Omega-6 fats are essential—remember the drill? Essential means we need to get them from our food because our bodies can't make them. However, they are essential in small amounts, and in the tidal wave we have been consuming, they overpower their partner in crime, the omega-3s . . . more on that in a moment. Omega-6 fats are widespread in the processed, packaged, and fast foods we eat; they are chosen for cooking because they're cheap, and they even lurk in our meat because animals are fattened up quickly on grain instead of allowed to graze slowly on grass. Why all the hubbub? Essentially, (pun intended) omega-6 fats promote a pro-inflammatory state in the body when overconsumed;[22,25] inflammation is an independent risk factor for most chronic diseases and even promotes annoyances, such as acne and wrinkles.

Omega-3 Fats

Omega-3 fats are the darlings of the fat family, and while we absolutely need more in our diets, we still don't need them in huge amounts. Omega-3 fats are found in cold-water fatty fish, such as salmon, herring, and sardines; we find them also in plant sources such as algae, seeds such as chia, hemp, flax, and pumpkin, and even walnuts. Green leafy veggies also contain omega-3 but in tiny amounts. Getting enough omega-3s in your diet helps calm inflammation and support the health of our brains, skin, and hearts. However, too much—more likely to occur when supplementing as opposed to eating whole foods—can cause trouble, as omega-3 fats also thin the blood.

Controversy exists as to whether the form found in most plant foods, alpha-linoleic acid, or ALA, is adequate to provide the outstanding health benefits attributed to omega-3s. ALA is the only form of omega-3 considered essential, as theoretically it can be converted to two other forms of omega-3, DHA and EPA, that researchers and health professionals get really excited about. However, our ability to convert ALA into these other forms is quite low and many factors, such as too many omega-6s in the diet, can reduce our ability to do so.[22] Based on all the work I have seen, I feel that direct sources of DHA and/or EPA are critical to support our crazy-stressed out lives in this modern world we live in. Luckily, even if we don't consume fish, we can get DHA from algae that will help us to make more EPA from the food we eat.

Saturated Fats

Saturated fats aren't as clear-cut as they used to be. Health professionals have touted their dangers for decades but, in fact, recent reviews of the literature have called some of these dangers into question.[26] Saturated fats are known to increase LDL cholesterol, the kind that isn't so great for your heart. But not everyone with higher LDL cholesterol gets heart disease; it is way more complex than that. And the overall diet must be taken into consideration; a diet high in saturated fats is likely a diet too high in meat and dairy and low in the protective effects of plant foods. Will a bit of butter on your broccoli really cause you harm? Not a chance. A flood of steak and egg breakfasts gulped down with full cream in your coffee will.

We also have to consider the animal versus vegetable question. We abandoned tropical oils—palm and coconut oils—in the eighties because of their saturated fat content . . . and we replaced them with hydrogenated oils. Forgive us, we health professionals are learning as we go along, too. Enter the new, less processed coconut oils, which are rich in saturated fat but also in other unique fats, such as medium chain triglycerides, which the body burns as energy instead of stored energy. The research is not abundant on this topic, but it appears that if you are healthy, modern coconut oil doesn't raise bad blood cholesterol as much as animal fats do, and it might even raise the good cholesterol, HDL.[27,28] If you already have high cholesterol and other cardiovascular risk factors, I would still be cautious. The clinical significance of coconut oil on the diet isn't well understood. Good quality coconut oil can fit into a healthy diet for flavor, heat tolerance, and variety; just don't consider it your numero uno in the kitchen.

We need a small amount of saturated fats in our diet; our challenge is that the standard North American diet is overwhelmed with them. Consider them an accessory, not an entrée, and favor plant-based whenever possible. A diet too high in animal-based saturated fats is pro-inflammatory, and we want to keep inflammation at bay for a healthy body and mind.

Monounsaturated Fats

Next come the fats that should be the foundation of your healthy fat pantry—the monounsaturated fats. These are found in olives, avocados, nuts, seeds, and, of course, extra virgin olive oil. They are the last uncontroversial, healthful type of fat in our food supply. Why is this? Monounsaturated fats help lower LDL cholesterol when used to replace saturated fats and do not raise LDL cholesterol[29] or cause inflammation. In addition, replacing some excess carbs with monounsaturated fats helps improve blood sugar control, HDL cholesterol, and triglyceride (another type of blood fat) levels. Consider monounsaturated fats your healthy fat foundation.

Quality over Quantity

As I mentioned earlier, I am not a low-fat fanatic. If you are trying to improve your weight, it is easy to get too many calories from fat as opposed to protein or carbs, but this doesn't always play out—particularly when you limit added cooking fats and favor whole food sources of fats, such as nuts, seeds, olives, and avocados. Think of eating potato chips as opposed to almonds: those potato chips are almost infused with oil in a way that provides a lot of fat and calories without being filling. However, munching on raw almonds takes a long time, and their fiber fills you up as those nutrients are slowly released into your system to signal to your brain that you are satisfied and nourished. In fact, there is research to show that adding nuts to your daily diet is actually associated with better weight outcomes over time, whereas french fries and potato chips will help you pack on the pounds.[30]

For better health, you have to remember that foods are a balance of nutrients. Remember those low fat snacks that dominated in the nineties? They had to replace the fat with something . . . and it was sugar and flour. Try to over-reduce fat and you might end up with too much protein or carbs; try and lower carbs too much and you might end up consuming boatloads of fat. Instead, if you are concerned with weight control, ease up on the amount of oils you add to food and focus on munching your healthy fats with plenty of produce instead. Limit cooking oils to one or two teaspoons in a recipe; nix the mayo or butter on sandwiches. Enjoy snacking on foods packed with healthy fat, such as almonds, or slice a bit of avocado into your sandwiches.

Fats Won't (Necessarily) Make You Fat . . . Here's the Bottom Line:

Fats are critical for a healthy nervous system, hormone balance, and overall health and wellness. The key to a healthy fat balance in your diet is choosing high-quality plant oils and foods most often and trying to eat your fats instead of pouring them on. Make extra virgin olive oil your new anti-inflammatory best friend! When cooking, try not to add more than ½–1 teaspoon of oil per serving to your meals; measure it out. That is enough to help boost nutrient absorption and carry flavor and texture without adding too much excess energy to your bottom line.

Keep Your Body Running Swimmingly

Water is the medium in which every reaction in our body takes place. Our body starts to run out of steam when water losses hit just 2 percent; a chronically dehydrated body is sluggish, tired, and toxic. We can mistake thirst for hunger and overeat. We resort to coffee and energy drinks to give us a boost when a cup of water would have done the job. Water also allows our body to detoxify; substances are carried out of the body in a fluid river, evaporating in breath, sweat, and trickling out with each flush.

Off-Duty Dietitian: Desiree's Super Sane Advice for the Avoidance of Getting Sloshed

1. Please, for the love of all things holy, eat something before you have a drink. Don't go to cocktail parties hungry. Have some protein, produce, and a bit of healthy fat to fill your belly and slow down the absorption of alcohol.
2. Avoid sugary blender drinks at all costs . . . they can have as many calories as a double cheeseburger and go straight to your head. Nothing like a week of piña coladas to make your jeans burst their buttons.
3. Avoid high-calorie mixers, such as sweetened sodas and juices. Try club soda or naturally sweetened, low-sugar sodas instead.
4. Wine and beer are fine choices, but watch the serving size. You should get six glasses of wine out of a bottle; newfangled wine goblets can drain half the bottle! And a standard serving of beer is 355 milliliters. A full pint is 500 milliliters.

5. Alternate alcoholic beverages with plain water or seltzer to stay hydrated and fend off the snacking spiral.
6. Regardless of what your favorite drink is, don't overdo it. The recommendation for alcohol intake to minimize health risks is no more than one drink per day for women and those lucky fellas get two drinks a day. You can't really save them up for the weekend; the daily assault you place on your liver counts, too.

Just how much water do we need? Again, the prescription is individual. Our best guesses range from a milliliter of water for each calorie you consume to linking water intake to weight or simply telling people to drink two to three liters, or eight to twelve glasses of water a day and hope for the best. When it comes to real life, as long as your urine is clear or pale yellow, you are hydrated. If you eat a highly processed diet, you will need more water, whereas a high plant foods diet comes with plenty of hydration intact.

Alcohol proves to be a more exciting and controversial topic. Alcohol is thought to help improve heart health and lower your risk of stroke and Alzheimer's disease, but at seven empty calories per gram, it can also pack on the pounds—thereby increasing your risk of chronic disease. Mindless munching usually accompanies the tipple, and the resulting loss of inhibitions sends willpower packing, further increasing risk of weight gain. Alcohol consumption is also linked to increased cancer risk. So what to do? If you don't already drink, don't start. If you enjoy your cocktails, keep it light. Red wine is a great bet for potential health benefits.

Of Substance and Supplements

Vitamins, minerals, and phytochemicals, oh my! These are the fancy appliances in your nutritional house. Yes, that dishwasher will make washing dishes easier . . . but if your foundation sinks, that dishwasher isn't going to help you out much when you're wading in the muck.

I get most excited about vitamins, minerals, and phytochemicals in the context of whole food. No surprises there! The reason for this is that nature designed foods to provide us with almost everything that we could possibly need for life on earth with only a few exceptions. And nutritional science still has a lot to learn about the wisdom of whole foods. Just think, there were antioxidants in blueberries long before we even understood what an antioxidant was! My point here is that purchasing hundreds of dollars worth of supplements when your diet is seriously lacking is not the nutritional insurance you might think.

What if antioxidant x really only works when it is paired with cofactor y, as it is in an eggplant . . . but you just spent $46.99 on a bottle of x on its own? This is what I mean when I preach whole foods. The first priority is to start eating right, then choose additional supports wisely . . . and I will help you do that in Chapter 5. Consider the wise, targeted use of supplements as powerful preventative medicine alongside a core anti-inflammatory diet. Purchasing whatever fad pill you hear about without considering if it is truly right for you is a just a waste of money.

You Are What You Eat . . . So Chew on This

At its core, the gold-standard rules for healthy eating haven't really changed that much—especially where talk of actual food is concerned.

Don't hate on carbs. When it comes to the foods that contain carbohydrates—fruits, vegetables, grains, legumes, and dairy—think unprocessed.

Protein is powerful; it helps you stay full and satisfied, supports immunity, and contributes to a healthy hormone balance. Choose plant-based proteins more often.

Healthy fats are your nutritional friend and won't contribute to weight gain when you focus on whole foods, such as avocados, nuts, seeds, and olives. Stay hydrated to keep your body in tip-top shape and to encourage natural cleansing, and think twice before choosing the correct supplements once.

CHAPTER 3
YOU ARE WHAT YOU ABSORB

"Because of the media hype and woefully inadequate information, too many people nowadays are deathly afraid of their food, and what does fear of food do to the digestive system? I am sure that an unhappy or suspicious stomach, constricted and uneasy with worry, cannot digest properly. And if digestion is poor, the whole body politic suffers."
—Julia Child

I come from the world of health food and integrative nutrition, and here we have a saying, "You are not what you eat, but what you absorb." It is nice to fill your body with all sorts of healthful foods, but if your body cannot properly break that food down and absorb its components, a lot of money is literally going down the drain. And while Julia Child may have been suspicious of our seeming "fear of food," she hit the nail on the head when she mentioned that poor digestion wreaks havoc on the body.

Our digestive system had long been considered conquered by science. We figured that we knew how the body takes the food we eat, breaks it down, and turns those components into energy. What more was there? A whole lot, apparently—particularly in the multitude of ways that the system can go off the rails. In the past fifty years, we have faced an unprecedented upheaval in our collective digestive health. Celiac disease, Crohn's disease, and ulcerative colitis are on the rise. Irritable bowel syndrome wasn't even classified fifty years ago, and food allergies were rare. Something is going on; the food we eat has changed, but so has our ability to digest it. But before we talk about what is plaguing our digestion, we should probably brush up on our understanding of what the digestive system is.

A Magical Tour of Your Mysterious Digestive Tract!
You may think of your digestive tract as inside your body because you cannot see it; however, your digestive tract exists outside your body. How could this craziness be true? Well, from mouth to poop shoot, your digestive tract is continuous with the free-living, outside world! Understanding this will give you a better appreciation of how the digestive tract functions and why malfunctions might occur given the right circumstances.

The first critical function of the digestive system as a whole is providing a barrier between your inner world and your outer world. From the minute those first morsels of food cross your lips, potentially laden with little bacteria coming along for the ride, your mysterious digestive tract welcomes it into its lair, and that food will never be the same again. After a churning roller coaster ride of smooth muscle contractions, acids shoot out into your stomach. Once clear of that, alkaline salts are released that only the hardiest of outsiders can withstand. If still standing, victorious food or bacteria reach your intestines only to be met by iron-clad walls that bar all but the most desirable of guests, who are ushered through by digestive doormen, leaving all others on the slippery slope to the sewer system. That is what happens when your digestive defense system works. If those unwanted guests are bacteria or viruses, you can see how the towering digestive tract of terror might indeed play a critical function to your health. To make matters even more interesting, your digestive tract is intertwined with a large proportion of your immune system and your nervous system.

Immune to Your Advances

Barriers are an important part of immunity; your skin is the other barrier that typically comes to mind. So it's in our best interests to keep our guts healthy and happy and that barrier function intact. In fact, the digestive tract is so important to overall immunity that the overwhelming majority of your immune cells are located within spitting distance of your gut lining. Called the gut-associated lymphoid tissue (or GALT, to its close friends), one of its key functions is determining friend from foe and mounting an immune attack should foes be present.[1] GALT is like the gal who checks your ID once the doorman has let you in the club. When this recognition goes well, we are happy, healthy, and dancing in celebration. When it slips out of regulation, our immune system can mount attacks in response to everyday foods that should be good for us, it can overreact to the normal presence of bacteria in our digestive tracts, or it can even turn its attack on the gut itself—essentially biting off the hand that feeds it. [1]

Gut Instincts

In addition to being flush with immune cells, your digestive tract is also heavily enervated. The enteric nervous system, the part of your nervous system that surrounds your digestive tract, contains more neurons (message carrying cells) than your spinal cord! Those neurons are critical for sending messages to and from the digestive tract and ensuring that everything runs smoothly with digestion, but they also send an enormous volume of messages to the brain from the gut.

Did you notice that in talking about the digestive tract and its functions, we haven't even gotten to the digestion part yet? Maybe we shouldn't call it our digestive tract . . . we could rename it your optimum health highway. But that would be a bit cheesy, I suppose. Let's take a peek into the dark, mysterious world of good digestion and learn a little more about how it all works.

Mouth—Your teeth tear and grind food, and your tongue helps you to taste your dinner (working in partnership with your sense of smell) and mixes food with saliva so it can be swallowed easily. Your saliva, in addition to being wet and slippery, contains enzymes that help to break down carbohydrates and fats in food. Digestion has already begun!

Esophagus—This muscular tube contracts rhythmically to help work food toward the stomach. It is protected from stomach acids by a trap door called a sphincter, which is supposed to open only when food is coming its way. When it malfunctions, stomach acid can irritate the esophagus . . . we call this heartburn.

Stomach—This muscular sac churns and mixes the foods with a heady concoction of acids and enzymes that break down proteins (primarily) and fats. The acids will help kill any harmful microbes that might have hitched a ride with your dinner and are essential for unfolding (denaturing) proteins so digestive enzymes can get ahold of them to do their work. Acid-producing cells also release something called intrinsic factor, which helps us absorb vitamin B12. When the digestive dough is ready, it gets released through another trap door into the small intestine.

Liver—Your liver is the Wizard of your digestive Oz. It slices, it dices . . . well, actually it produces bile, necessary for digestion and absorption of fats, and sends it to the gallbladder. But that's not all! The liver also metabolizes any alcohol, drugs, and many of the supplements that you consume. It activates some vitamins so they can do their good work in the body. Fructose metabolism happens in the liver, and the liver can even create sugars from protein or fat when you're running low. Finally, the liver detoxifies the body and processes dietary fats and blood cholesterol. A happy liver makes a healthy body.

Gallbladder—Your gallbladder receives bile from the liver, stores it for a while, and squirts it out when there is food in the small intestine. Not too exciting. Unless you get gallstones; then it becomes exciting for all the wrong reasons, and you might need to have your gallbladder removed.

Pancreas—Your pancreas aids in both digestion of your dinner and using the energy your dinner releases. Your pancreas makes digestive enzymes to complete the breakdown of protein, fats, and carbohydrates so they can be transported in their simple forms into the body. Your pancreas is also the site of all-important insulin production, so when that energy enters your bloodstream, your cells know what to do with it.

Small Intestine—This is where the magic happens, baby! When that acidic ball of digestive dough reaches the small intestine, the pancreas releases digestive juices that contain enzymes to breakdown the food particles; alkali salts neutralize the acid, and the gallbladder releases bile to help emulsify the fat so the enzymes can get ahold of them. Your small intestine looks like plush velvet curtains; finger-like projections called villi are themselves covered in microvilli, which leads to a surface area for digestion that rivals the size of a tennis court! That velvety surface is where the most of the nutrient absorption (hopefully) takes place.

Large Intestine—We used to think of the large intestine as pretty boring. It re-absorbs water from your waste; if it didn't, you would require a constant hook up to a garden hose for hydration. It also salvages a few vitamins in the mix. Little did we know that, in fact, the large intestine is where the party really starts! It gets exciting when we look at all the bacteria that hang out in its dark, reclusive corners. The bacteria in our colon help us digest and absorb nutrients from indigestible plant fibers, they make vitamins, they help teach our immune system when and where to do its business, and even help keep the bad bacteria from getting cozy. Metabolic products from those critters can help nourish the digestive tract and keep it well—kind of like a good tenant paying its rent.

Rectum—At this point, your stool has been formed and it is simply waiting for the most inopportune moment to make its presence known. Like in a big, important sales meeting. Blame that on your enteric nervous system. This underappreciated portion of your digestive tract keeps you from making a mess in your pants. It's worth some respect.

First, Feast with Your Eyes

While the physical mechanics of digestion begins in the mouth, the elegance of digestion is far more complex and subtle. In fact, digestion begins with our other senses. The mere anticipation of food can set the digestive wheels turning: the sights, sounds, and smells of food send a signal to the body that nourishment is on its way. Your emotions and stress level also have a role to play. Digestion is a function of the parasympathetic nervous system—our nervous system at rest. When the sympathetic nervous system gets involved— our flight or fight system—digestion suffers. The rate of transit slows and digestive secretions are halted. This makes sense if you are running away from a tiger; you need the blood to flow away from your stomach to your legs so you can run like hell. However, what if your kids are screaming over who gets to watch TV, and after coming home from work late, you are bickering with your wife as you scarf down the takeout pizza? You know the feeling: food sits like a brick in your stomach, and you end up gassy and feeling terrible all night. Eating and digesting well appear to be a state of mind—after all, we do call the enteric nervous system that lives along the digestive tract the second brain.

The connection between how we eat and how well we digest and absorb is well-documented. Those who eat quickly appear to release fewer of the hunger-controlling hormones than those who eat slowly.[2] In fact, simply chewing more has been shown to increase the satiety hormones that tell you to stop eating.[3] Chewing your food doesn't just help your body digest better—those who chew thoroughly may actually consume less food,[3] a great help in the weight game.

When you mindlessly munch, not only are you robbing yourself of the full pleasure of the food you are eating, you are able to consume more calories before your body registers it's full. In addition, eating too quickly physically hinders the process of digestion. Not chewing food thoroughly makes it more difficult for enzymes to attack food, leading to the potential that large undigested particles of food survive and travel to the lower digestive tract for fermentation by your resident bugs. Do all this under the context of a stressful day, and the future is ripe for tummy trouble.

Nature knows the place of feasting: as I said before, digestion and absorption is under parasympathetic (relaxed state) nervous system control. If you are under a great deal of stress, your body activates the sympathetic, or fight or flight, system, and energy is diverted away from digestion. Does stress put your gut in a knot? Does stress eating leave you feeling like you have a brick in your stomach? Now you know why. No matter what is happening in your day, make the mental and physical space for eating. Take a few deep breaths, take your eyes off your iPhone, and enjoy.

You Can't Trick Your Taste Buds

If sugar is so bad for us, switching to artificial and noncaloric sweeteners should fix things, right? Not so fast. As I have mentioned before, I don't want you going anywhere near artificial sweeteners. Since you might not be convinced, let's go over it again.

One of our greatest challenges to eating well nowadays is learning to appreciate the flavors of real, unadulterated food. There was a time when food was just food. It tasted good, but nothing would convince you to eat it past the point of being full. Now, we have flavors lovingly handcrafted in the finest laboratories that compel your taste buds to crave more and more food. How can you possibly resist the siren call of that giant shrimp scampi platter when your homemade broccoli pasta just tastes so . . . *blah*? Our taste buds have been acclimated to extreme flavor sensations.

We live in a world of uber-tasty food. Our intrinsic love of fat, salt, and sugar has been capitalized into a free-for-all of addictive, over-eatable foods that our taste buds just can't get enough of. If you simply swap sweetened, processed food for artificially sweetened processed food, you are continuing to train your taste buds to respond only to flavors not possible in the natural world. Instead, I would prefer that you gradually wean yourself off the sweet stuff. Get your caramel latte half sweet; note how it is missing something. You will get used to that reduced sugar hit and be able to tease out the caramel flavor after a while. When you are ready, ditch the syrup altogether. When you realize that milk is naturally sweet and goes well with the rich and slightly bitter flavor of coffee, you have graduated real food university!

My next argument is one of passion and not of science. By their very existence, artificial sweeteners are not part of the natural plan for nourishing your body. So your body should not be subjected to them, end of discussion. Research or no, I am convinced that long-term use of any foreign substance can't possibly be benign. I should clarify that I lump in many natural non-caloric sweeteners, such as xylitol and stevioside crystals (refined stevia), into this category. Extracting a sugar alcohol, such as xylitol, from wood pulp is not a natural process, nor is extracting a single chemical out of a natural stevia leaf. Once you take a substance out of the wisdom of the whole food, you cannot predict its effects on the body. My favorite natural sweeteners are honey, maple syrup, and if you truly want something without calories, a bit of traditional stevia tincture or ground whole stevia leaf.

I also want to talk about the interesting research emerging on use of artificial sweeteners and appetite. In the past, we have seen correlational research to show that those who use artificial sweeteners tend to weigh more than those who don't.[4] However, there are lots of confounding variables that could muddy the waters, such as those who feel they need to lose weight may choose more artificial sweeteners. Before we can start declaring them bad for weight control with any certainty, we need to have a deeper understanding of how they might impact appetite. Control of appetite is complex and just as digestion begins with the mouth, so might appetite control.

Researchers are learning more about what compels us to eat and how certain foods might override typical control of appetite. Central to this discovery is the dopamine reward pathway in the brain. Over time, we can have a learned reward response in the brain upon eating certain foods. This happens two ways: both in the actual sensory pleasure of eating the food and in the energy and nutrients that hit the bloodstream following the eating of that food. Where research into artificial sweeteners gets interesting is that artificially sweetened foods provide reward on the tongue but not following the meal, as blood sugars don't rise as the body expects and serotonin release isn't stimulated.[4] So in essence, artificially sweetened foods become fun to eat but are inherently unsatisfying; the only way to keep the reward up is to keep eating.[4] Oops. Real food satisfies in a way that fake foods just can't. In trying to avoid the morsel, you could end up eating the whole cake.

I'm Just a Regular Gal . . . You Can Be, Too

Even if you don't have any major digestive concerns, it is in your best interest to do what you can to keep that gut happy and keep things . . . well . . . moving along. You just can't keep a dietitian away from the poop talk! I care deeply about what goes into and comes out of that miraculous body of yours. Think about it: your digestive tract is designed to remove everything it doesn't need and anything that might potentially be harmful. You don't exactly want waste hanging around for longer than it has to.

When it comes to healthy elimination, there are four foundational habits you need to have to keep things running smoothly.

1. **Move more.** Staying active keeps your digestive system flowing. Work out regularly if you can. If you are sedentary, committing to even a brief daily

walk can help get things moving. Heck, getting up to visit your colleagues instead of emailing them will help. You just need to get that blood flowing and those muscles working.

2. **Eat lots of high-fiber foods.** You must, you must, you must increase your . . . fiber intake! Men need about thirty-eight grams a day, and women need at least twenty-five grams a day. Get yours the whole food way with plenty of whole grains, fruits, vegetables—actually, just follow the food guidelines coming later in this book, and you will be fine. Go slow; switching from a white bread diet to a flax, barley, and All-Bran plan can be a little overwhelming on the old digestive tract.

3. **Stay hydrated.** Adequate water intake ensures smooth passage of stool through the digestive tract; the colon selectively reabsorbs water from the stool. If you are dehydrated, your colon will try and reclaim as much water as it can, leading to hard to pass stool. You need even more water while you are trying to increase your fiber intake; without it, the fiber will more likely lead to constipation than healthy elimination.

4. **Relax already!** You know the drill: stress equals digestive disaster. If you lead a high-intensity life, you have to reach for an antidote daily. Yoga, meditation, deep breathing—whatever you have time for, find a way to manage stress.

Are You Human or are You a Microbe?

It's true—no human is an island; at least, not a deserted one. It is more correct to think of our bodies as ecosystems; ecosystems that are widely populated with bacteria, along with some viruses and yeasts. And we couldn't survive any other way—the proof is in our collective digestive distress. Somewhere along the way, we stopped living in harmony with bacteria and declared war on them with antibiotics and antibacterial home cleaners and personal care. In a foolish bit of fear, we have been eradicating the very critters that keep us healthy, and what we end up with is the hardy bacteria that have survived to make us sick.

Colonization by bacteria starts at birth and our bacterial community evolves as we age and interact with the world around us. Where we live, what we eat, our stress levels, medications . . . all of it impacts our microbiota—what we used to refer to as our intestinal flora. In fact, the bacteria that colonize our bodies overwhelm us in sheer numbers; we have ten times the bacterial cells in us and on us than we do body cells—100 trillion bacteria versus our 10 trillion cells.

We have so much to learn about our relationship with the bacteria that inhabit our bodies that we are only just beginning to explore. We regarded bacteria largely as passive riders in our digestive tract, and any disorder in their community was considered rare. We can't be too hard on ourselves; science is ever evolving! However, now we understand that our first colonization with bacteria is critical to the proper development of our digestive and immune systems; not only do bacteria determine the health of our digestive function, they also educate our immune system to help prevent it from overreacting to harmless stimuli.

So how do we acquire our microbial mix? It all starts with birth; in fact, we are exposed to bacteria before we take our first breath of fresh air. Nature designs our bacterial community before we are even born; as a woman's pregnancy progresses, the bacterial community in the birth canal transforms to include more of a bacterial strain that is commonly found in the small intestine, *Lactobacillus johnsonii,* which helps produce the lactase enzyme.[5] So when we first receive our mother's milk, the bacteria acquired in birth helps us process the vital nourishment we need to survive.

When a baby is born naturally, the bacteria he or she is exposed to begins the process of maturing the digestive tract to receive and process breast milk. When a child is born by caesarean section, its first exposure to bacteria is to species typically found on the skin, such as *Staphylococcus,* or a bacterium found in the hospital, such as *Clostridium difficile,* and the long-term consequence of this difference is not fully understood. [6,7,8] However, children born by caesarean typically have higher incidence of allergies, and it is thought that this initial exposure to bacteria might be the cause.[6] From that first introduction, breast milk continues the exposure to beneficial bacteria and to the fermentable carbohydrates that help foster growth. The air we breathe, the surfaces we touch or that touch us, and the food we consume all contribute to our microbiome.

Bossy Bugs

Those first exposures to beneficial bacteria have a remarkable impact; not only do they help the digestive tract develop normally, but they are also intrinsic to the development of an active immune system.[6] In fact, bacteria are thought to help educate the immune system so it responds to stimuli appropriately and with greater tolerance. It is thought that healthy bacteria primes the immune system so it will function optimally. When it comes to digestion, without the right bacterial mix we may not be able to digest and assimilate food optimally. It is generally accepted that getting first exposure to food through the digestive tract as opposed to skin or airway contact teaches the body to recognize it as safe; what is in the digestive tract that might help teach the body to recognize the food as healthy and safe? Bacteria!

When the bugs aren't right, you aren't right. Colic, that common scourge of sleep-deprived parents everywhere—responds to probiotic treatment.[9] Researchers are noting significant alterations of the microbiome in autism, Celiac disease, and even obesity.[10] We need to do everything we can to foster healthy relationships with bacteria on a daily basis. That means removing antibacterial ingredients from our homes and bodies and eating more food that contains live bacteria. Most of us would probably benefit from a probiotic supplement, too.

Eating for Two

Remember the title of this chapter, you are what you absorb? Well, you are also what your bacteria digest, absorb, and metabolize. Those critters hidden deep in the darkest corners of your digestive tract are hanging out, waiting to feast on the remnants of your dinner. And as it turns out, they are picky eaters. Your bacterial dinner guests are drawn to you based on your genetics, your environment, and your digestive menu. Eat a typically North American high-sugar, high-fat diet and, in fact, you will attract fewer A students and more hooligans that can cause trouble.[11] Eat a more plant-based diet, such as the recommendations in this book, and you will decrease the number of disease-causing bugs and attract more of the bacterial glitterati.[11] Your bugs like plant matter with all of its indigestible (to you) roughage and low concentration of sugars and fats. In the process of eating all that fiber, bacteria produce vitamins such as vitamin K and some B vitamins, in addition to digestive enzymes, such as lactase, so those who lack their own might be less bothered by consuming lactose sugars in dairy. Nice bacteria also make polite dinner guests and always bear gifts for their host. In the process of feasting, healthy bacteria produce short chain fatty acids (SCFA) from dietary fibers, which can be used by the gut cells as fuel to keep them healthy. We didn't think much of SCFA in the past, but now we are researching their impact on obesity, diabetes, blood pressure, and even colon cancer. Friendly bugs also help protect against less friendly invaders; when those bad bugs try and crash the party, they can leave your digestive house in ruins. Instead, healthy bacteria help reinforce the physical barrier of the digestive tract lining, compete for space and food with invaders, and even produce substances that deter their presence, such as hydrogen peroxide. We are just scratching the surface of how bacteria help us thrive—stay tuned.

Put Less Stress on Your Plate

I have already mentioned the impact of stress on our digestive health, but it is worth delving into further. Psychological stress can impact your ability to digest and assimilate the foods you eat in the short term and alter digestive health in the long term. Why? It makes sense from a biological perspective that if a stress is present, your body is best served by mobilizing energy to respond to and remove that stress . . . not digest your lunch. Activation of the fight or flight response diminishes digestion and when the body returns to a relaxed state, digestion can resume as normal. Trouble is, we run through the modern equivalent of a tiger-filled savannah daily—otherwise known as deadlines, bills, chores, and family responsibilities. And we really need to digest that lunch to survive it all with our wits and health intact!

Stress can alter digestive secretions, the motility of the digestive tract, and how the digestive tract responds to its contents.[12] Just think of how nerves can tie knots in your stomach or anxiety can lead to butterflies—intuitively, we understand that stress can affect the digestive tract, but we rarely appreciate the larger picture in terms of how stress affects our nourishment and digestive health.

In the research, eaters who are stressed tend to have altered eating habits, such as eating higher fat foods,[13] altered blood sugar control, and more belly fat.[14] Stress is also suspected in the development of irritable bowel syndrome, inflammatory bowel disease, and peptic ulcer disease, and stress can further exacerbate these conditions once you have them.[12] So no, that bloating and pain you feel is not all in your head . . . but it just might be connected with what's going on in that brain of yours. Because of the connection between the brain and the second brain in your gut, your thoughts and emotions can have real consequences to your digestive health.

Is that burger coming back to bite you? It could be a looming deadline to blame. In this fast-paced world, chronic stress isn't going to go away. If you want to keep your tummy happy, you are going to have to put some mindful eating into practice. Try these tips and relax, already!

Remove screens and excess chatter. If you have an office door, close it. Go sit at the kitchen table. If it is nice out, sit outside away from the din of the workplace. Turn off the TV; silence your phone. Tell the kids to behave and stop shouting (oh, if only it were so easy!). Put on some of your favorite music if you like. Get the environment quiet so your mind can get quiet and your digestive tract can sing!. If you frequently eat in front of your computer and your workload won't allow you the time or space to eat away from it, turn away from the computer, close your eyes, and take a few deep breaths before you choose to eat.

Use the good china . . . or at least a real plate. Don't eat from food packages. Place food thoughtfully on a plate, and while you are at it, use your fancy plates more often. Nourishing your body is a pretty phenomenal gift, so why not make it a special occasion?

Take a minute to actually look at the food you are eating before you eat it. Remember, that we feast with our eyes first . . . even if lunch is just a sandwich. Digestion begins the moment you smell, see, or even think of food. Give your digestive tract some notice that it is going to work by taking a good look at the food you eat before it touches your lips.

Slow down and chew thoroughly. If you are stressed, you are likely to chew less and set yourself up for digestive troubles. Focus on your chewing, and don't swallow until everything feels like a nice smooth paste. Taste your food. Really taste it. Your instinct is to swallow as fast as you can, but resist and persist. It is better to eat one-fourth of your meal in the four minutes you have right now, catch that conference call, and come back to eat more thirty minutes later instead of dumping a heap of underchewed food into your stressed stomach. If you are at home, try to extend eating a meal for at least twenty to thirty minutes.

Fussy Guts

When our digestive tracts are working well, we rarely think of them. When they aren't doing well . . . it is impossible to take our minds off them. Digestive concerns are on the rise: from acid reflux to food allergies to Crohn's disease, our guts are on our minds more than ever before. What's going on? Truth is, scientists and clinicians aren't really sure—the research hasn't reached any confident conclusions. There are plenty of theories: increased pollution, stress, declining food quality and nutrient intake, introduction of genetically engineered foods, vitamin D deficiency, and imbalances in the microbiome are all on the table. So is chronic inflammation in the digestive tract.

Inflammation is a first-response tool of your innate immune system to help arrest disease-causing invaders and stop them from gaining access to your bodily temple. Inflammation is a critical part of your defenses and it keeps you from getting sick; when you cut yourself with a kitchen knife, inflammation goes to work to wall off the infection and speed healing substances to the area. However, when the body is constantly deemed to be under attack, the inflammatory system can work overtime. When this happens in the gut, inflammation can lead to damage in the digestive tract and vice versa. Your digestive tract lining functions as an important barrier between you and the outside world; when that barrier falters, large nutrient particles or microbes that would not usually pass may gain access, inciting a riot when their unrecognizable forms come in contact with your immune system.

What follows is a brief overview of some common digestive concerns; if you feel like your digestion has taken a nosedive that just won't resolve on its own, read on for some helpful tidbits. My hope is that what follows may help you recognize your symptoms so you can talk to your doctor about getting to the root of your troubles and you can focus on living your best (and most delicious!) life. Believe me, in this age of Dr. Google, it can be tempting to want to self-diagnose—but let the diagnostic experts do their job, and then you and I can get down to the business of nourishing your body.

Excuse Me, Your Acid Reflux is Showing

Every once in a while, a little burp will bubble up to the surface. Maybe we ate too quickly, guzzled sparkling water, or some extra spicy food gave our little esophageal sphincter a quiver and our table manners have to take a momentary nosedive. No big deal. In some countries, belching is the sincerest form of flattery to the chef!

What is a big deal is that a staggering number of us seem to be suffering from chronic acid reflux, where the acidic contents of the stomach keep trying to run for daylight. Incidence of chronic severe reflux, or gastroesophageal reflux disease (GERD), appear to be on the rise.[15] Theories for why this might occur include increasing obesity, stress, decreased stomach acid as we age (the esophageal sphincter senses acid), bad bugs in the colon, and use of certain medications.

If your doctor confirms GERD, what lifestyle measures can you take?

1. Make realistic, concrete dietary changes (such as those in this book) to get well-nourished and move toward a healthier weight if you are currently overweight.
2. Chew slowly and avoid overly large meals. This will help prevent you from overfilling the stomach and reduce the likelihood that contents come back to haunt you.
3. Avoid fried, greasy, or fatty foods. In the water-loving environment of the stomach, the cream literally rises to the top and fat takes longer to empty from the stomach than protein or carbohydrates.
4. Watch for trigger foods. Typically, these are caffeine-containing food and

drink, such as chocolate and coffee, spicy foods, or foods such as onion, garlic, and tomato. However, trigger foods can also be as unique as you are; keep a symptom and food diary to spot your potential culprits.

5. Avoid the carminatives—peppermint and cinnamon. These are substances that relax the digestive tract. Good for some, not for reflux.

6. Keep your head elevated for three hours post eating. Give gravity a chance! No lying down for a post-lunch snooze, and no eating within three hours of bedtime.

7. Try everything you possibly can before going on acid-suppressing medication. Your stomach acid is critical to proper digestion. In addition, the parietal cells that release stomach acid also release intrinsic factor, without which you will not absorb vitamin B12 properly. Adequate stomach acid also helps kill bacteria that might linger on food and fosters a healthy stomach environment.

8. Eat in a relaxed environment: our gut is our second brain—if you stress it out, it will come back to bite you in the butt. Turn off any distractions, and focus on enjoying your meal.

Gluten for Nothing: Celiac Disease and Gluten Intolerance

Celiac disease is on the rise, not simply because we are better at catching it, but also because something in the way we live and eat is initiating the disease in more of us than ever before.[16] Sales of gluten-free foods have grown 28 percent each year for the last five-year period.[17] Gluten seems to be the culprit for many of our digestive ills—why now? How could this be?

There are plenty of theories, as we discussed in Chapter 2. We health professionals are just full of theories, aren't we? Let's refresh your memory for a moment. The first is that our wheat has been naturally bred to a point where it contains a super gluten—gluten in larger amounts and with stronger allergenicity than ever before—although that idea is hotly contested.[18,19] Wheat products have become ubiquitous, and some folks might consume them three to six times a day. We are a carbaholic nation—remember when an apple was considered a good snack? Why bother with pitiful fruit when you could enjoy a Scrumptious Apple Caramel Cracker Snack (apple free)? Another theory, you might have guessed, leads back to the bugs. Keep your gut healthy and happy, and your body will be able to process gluten safely—when bacterial-induced inflammation is awry, your gut begins to leak, your immune cells are exposed to this foreign gluten without enough good bugs to calm it down, and now Bob's your celiac uncle.

Let's take a minute though to differentiate between classic celiac disease and nonceliac gluten sensitivity. Celiac disease is not an allergy; it is an autoimmune disease triggered by the presence of gluten. However, it takes more than just the presence of gluten, or we would all have celiac disease. First, you must have the genetic susceptibility; as it turns out, about a third of Caucasian adults carry the genetic risk.[20] But genes are not enough. Genes are kind of an if-this-then-that road map for life. So something needs to turn on the body's utter disdain for gluten. Potentially, this comes in some sort of trauma or change to the body. Celiac disease may occur after a woman gives birth, a car accident, puberty, or if some other disease causes damage to the body. Then, of course, if you didn't eat gluten, your body wouldn't mount an attack. So all three of these things—genes, a trigger, and gluten—need to be in play for celiac disease to develop. When someone with celiac disease strictly avoids every microscopic shred of gluten, their autoimmune attack will cease and healing begins. Celiac disease is quite amazing because it is the only chronic disease that is exclusively managed with diet.

An interesting development in celiac disease is that historically, concrete digestive symptoms were its hallmark: weight loss, malnutrition, and copious diarrhea and digestive distress. Now, silent celiac disease is not uncommon.[20] In fact, a patient who is trying to resolve particularly stubborn, without cause, anemia or joint pain may find his or her doctor cleverly screening him or her for celiac disease just in case and coming out with a new diagnosis.

Next in the gluten parade comes gluten intolerance or sensitivity, which was accepted only in the alternative medical community until recent conventional research started to delve into it. What we see here is that gluten ingestion, again in susceptible individuals, causes adverse effects but does not cause the autoimmune attack on the digestive tract or show the hallmark immune response.[20]

Of course, when these critical shifts in thinking occur, it can launch the most vehement demonization of a foodstuff. Some believe that gluten is the core of all disease and weight gain, and living strictly gluten free will help us to lose weight, become better athletes, and maybe even help us fight cancer. Maybe . . . well, sort of.

I agree that those whom gluten makes sick will likely improve their current and long-term health by eliminating it. However, that is not 100 percent of the world population. The research-based estimates place the numbers closer to 10 percent, or perhaps a third of the population if you link gluten sensitivity to irritable bowel syndrome. Celiac disease is estimated to be present in about 1 percent of the population. At the renowned Center for Celiac Research in Maryland, about 6 percent of patients in a six year period met the criteria for nonceliac gluten sensitivity.[20] People with gluten sensitivity need to be as diligent as those with celiac disease in avoiding gluten to restore optimal health.

The rest of us seem to be able to fight off the gluten scourge. Why? Who knows! Perhaps we have really good bugs that keep our immune system chilled out so it understands that food is our friend, not foe. Maybe our diets are so full of healthy plant foods that they fortify our defenses. Even if gluten doesn't make our bodies sick, I think that for many of us, taking away a lot (but not all) of these gluten-containing foods will makeover our lives. Not because of the gluten per se; but because most of these gluten-containing foods also happen to be the sort of hyper-processed, nutrient-poor swill that is spiking blood sugars, causing us to overeat and become incredibly inflamed, and damage the natural balance in our body. Don't use faulty logic and blame it on the gluten 100 percent of the time. It's like saying that BMWs cause their owners to make more money instead of acknowledging that BMWs are expensive and people who earn more money will be able to afford one.

What to do if you suspect gluten intolerance or celiac disease? First things first: get a simple blood test to screen for celiac disease. Don't stop eating gluten before you do, or you could alter the test results. If celiac disease is confirmed, work with a registered dietitian to help you transition to a totally gluten-free diet and create a gluten-free environment in your kitchen.

If celiac disease is ruled out but you feel certain that gluten is causing your ills, work with your physician and dietitian to do a proper gluten elimination and challenge. It can be hard to tease out whether it is the gluten itself or just the types of gluten-containing foods you eat. Don't do this willy-nilly; save yourself the chronic food phobia and do the elimination and challenge under supervision and know for sure.

Lactose Intolerance

It's no secret—most of us are at least a little lactose intolerant. This is a normal biological state; at least 65 percent of the world's population has a reduced ability to break down lactose in their intestines.[21] Lactose is broken down by the lactase enzyme, which is found at the tips of the finger-like projections of the small intestine. We all tolerate lactose to a differing degree. Some can handle swimming in rivers of triple fudge chunk, while others get the runs just thinking about a cup of yogurt! Where we have an issue is if our own degree of lactose intolerance interferes with the amount of dairy we typically consume.

As with most things in our modern food world, our exposure to lactose and dairy has exploded even though our conscious consumption of the traditional dairy foods, such as milk, might have waned. We are exposed to lactose at many of our meals and snacks, and for those with lactose intolerance, lactose passes through the digestive tract, too big to be transported into the body, and winds up at the colon, where it is feasted upon by the bacteria who live there, resulting in gas, bloating, and for those with serious lactose intolerance, diarrhea.

So what to do? If you feel that lactose is causing your tummy troubles, your physician can do a lactose challenge and a nifty little breathing test to determine how well you digest lactose. Once you know that lactose is your Achilles' heel, you can test your degree of intolerance at home. No really, try this at home!

Just How Intolerant are You? Your (Not Really) Super Scientific Home Experiment

There are varying degrees of lactose in foods, and if you really love dairy, it behooves you to understand where your limits of digestion are. If you don't like dairy to begin with, say goodbye and use quality veggie milk alternatives to get your calcium. No harm done!

For those wanting to continue their love affair with Gouda, start with a no-lactose week to ensure that any symptoms are totally gone before you start, then try the following lactose experiments. If you want to be extra scientific, include a washout no lactose day to be sure that you are really symptom free.

Day One: A small piece (one- to two-centimeter cube) of real Parmigiano Reggiano cheese or a similar hard cheese, such as Grana Padano, with a meal. Hard cheese has very little lactose left in it because the bacteria in the cheese eat it up in the aging process. If you are still feeling good the next day . . .

Day Two: A small piece (one- to two-cenimeter cube) of an unaged cheese, such as mozzarella, with a meal. This has a bit more lactose but not a lot. Ready for more?

Day Three: A half-cup of plain yogurt with a meal. Why all this with-a-meal business? It appears to improve lactose tolerance.

Day Four: Try a half-cup of milk with a meal.

Day Five: You're ready for the big leagues if you made it this far: a cup of milk on an empty stomach.

By now, you should have the sense that one of these stages is definitely your limit. If they all seem fine, it could be that you have a decent ability to digest lactose but need to avoid an all-out orgy of dairy (no cheeseburger and milkshake combos for you!). So save the dairy foods for when they really count, and switch it up with nondairy alternatives once in a while.

Something else you should know is that you can actually buy lactase enzyme to help you digest dairy, like some magical fairy of ice cream land coming to bestow tolerance on your poor digestive tract. And, since I am crazy for beneficial bacteria, know that lactobacillus bacteria actually make lactase, too . . . score one more for probiotics!

Feeling Irritable?

Another scourge of the happy belly is our seeming epidemic of irritable bowel syndrome. A diagnosis that didn't even exist fifty years ago, it is now commonplace: IBS occurs in between 10 to 15 percent of the North American population.[22,23] Doesn't anyone else think this is strange? Shouldn't we be doing more about it?

One of the biggest challenges with all functional digestive disorders is the incredibly subjective nature of the symptoms. Even amongst health professionals, constipation and diarrhea are relatively subjective matters. I think I am constipated if I don't go for a day—but that doesn't exactly match someone else's criteria of constipation. So if you describe cramping, bloating, and urgent needs to go to your doc . . . well, it could be anything. Like stress and a half-digested sandwich. So what are the actual criteria for diagnosing IBS?

Rome III Criteria for IBS:

The Rome Foundation is an expert-based gathering for the study of functional digestive disorders, and they provide diagnostic criteria to help in the care of digestive disease. Here is what they have to say about bestowing the IBS crown on your lowly bowels:

1. First [intestinal] symptoms occurred at least six months ago and in the last three months:
   a. Recurrent abdominal pain or discomfort at least three days per month in the last three months associated with two or more of the following:
      ii. Improvement with defecation (that's pooping, to you)
      iii. Onset associated with a change in frequency of stool (a little or lots of poop)
      iv. Onset associated with a change in form (appearance) of stool (ever-changing poop)

Uh . . . yeah. That's it. For the amazing amount of gastrointestinal distress that someone can be placed under, that's what it takes to be diagnosed with IBS. It is worth noting that as easy as the diagnosis could be to hand off, all other potential digestive concerns should be ruled out before doling out your IBS medal—which is why you can't trust Dr. Google. So, for example, if your doc labels you as having IBS without screening you first for celiac disease or assessing food allergies, it's time to get a more thorough opinion.

So what could be at the heart of IBS? We don't truly know, but research is pointing us in a few interesting directions: stress, food sensitivities, and dysbiosis.

Dysbi-what?

Remember that little chat we had about gut bacteria in this chapter? When those bacteria are out of whack, it is called dysbiosis—essentially, a disorder of life. Not enough of the good guys, too many of the bacterial punks wreaking havoc in your colon. Now, with this emerging theory, it is a bit of a chicken and egg scenario. Did the bad bugs cause the leaky gut that lead to food sensitivities and irritability or the other way around? No matter . . . to help solve the problem, all three need to be attended to.

How do you attend to dysbiosis? A huge influx of healthy bacteria. They will go and clean up the place—you just need to feed them right.

You also need to figure out which, if any, foods are causing you harm at the moment. The only gold-standard way to do that is by elimination of the food and subsequent challenge. Like I said earlier, don't go doing this all willy-nilly. You need to work with a qualified doctor, naturopath, or dietitian who follows your healing philosophy and is comfortable doing elimination diets. Taking allergy blood tests is not enough. A thorough history of symptoms, with or without blood tests, simply helps you design a proper elimination diet to test. It is the elimination diet and challenge that really confirms food troubles. And you can't just decide to eat a piece of bread again if you think it makes you sick—your expectant brain can cause the symptoms.

One of the stronger dietary management strategies for IBS is called the Low FODMAPS diet, which was researched and popularized by two Australian researchers, Sue Shepherd and Peter Gibson. This diet involves altering the amount of fermentable carbohydrates, such as lactose, fructans in wheat and legumes, or excess fructose.[24] In the research, a low FODMAPS approach can lead to effective symptom management in many who suffer from IBS.[24]

Fire in the Hole: Inflammatory Bowel Disease

Not to be confused with IBS (and believe me, it is confusing), the inflammatory bowel diseases, Crohn's disease and ulcerative colitis, are another huge challenge to our digestive wellness. The United States and Canada have the unfortunate honor of having one of the highest rates of IBD in the world according to the Canadian Digestive Health Foundation.

Crohn's disease can occur anywhere along the digestive tract, from mouth to bum, while ulcerative colitis appears in the lower colon and rectum. Inflammation destroys the integrity of the gut lining and can lead to malabsorption of nutrients, malnutrition, and even digestive cancers. The inflammation in

Crohn's disease reaches throughout the wall of the gut, whereas in ulcerative colitis damage is at the surface layer. Other symptoms include pain, blood in stool, abdominal cramping, increased frequency and urgency in bathroom trips, and weight loss.

Could it be something we're eating? People with higher intakes of meat and omega-6 fats have higher rates of IBD.[25] Higher intake of refined sugars might also stoke the fires of IBD.[26] Fiber[26] and fruit and veggie[25] intake appear to be protective. Countries at northern latitudes have higher rates than those in the tropics, and countries with westernized diets appear to have the highest rates.[27] Anti-inflammatory omega-3 fats are being researched as a possible balm for the IBD sufferer. There's a bacterial connection being investigated, too.[27] As you might have guessed, probiotics seem a promising treatment, though the research has yet to convince us of absolute efficacy.

We are a long way from understanding why our digestive tracts are so dysfunctional. In the meantime, doing our best to deliver sound anti-inflammatory nutrition for healing purposes can help support getting well.

Digestion is Complex . . . Here's What You Need to Know!

—Our digestive system health is intimately linked to the health of our entire body, and our digestive tract is connected to our immune and nervous systems.

—To digest well, you need to be relaxed and focus on the pleasurable aspects of eating, taking time to chew thoroughly to avoid digestive distress.

—Bacteria are not our foes; in fact, our digestion-immune-nervous system complex wouldn't function properly without them.

—We need to replenish the good bacteria in our system on a daily basis and stop assaulting our body with antibiotic medications and products.

—When digestion goes sour, getting to the root cause of the problem will allow us to nourish ourselves back to wellness.

CHAPTER 4

CONFUSED YET? STEERING CLEAR OF THE CULT OF NUTRITIONISM

"Indeed, nutritionism supplies the ultimate justification for processing food by implying that with a judicious application of food science, fake foods can be made even more nutritious than the real thing." —Michael Pollan

As a dietitian, my career has been devoted to applying the principles of good nutrition to help people eat well and live healthier lives. This should be a simple task: tell people that broccoli is good, double cheeseburgers . . . well, not so much. However, not all food choices are as clear-cut, and many of them are disguised to fall along the spectrum of healthy eating. Somewhere along the way, the art and science of healthy eating has been coopted by food manufacturers trying to get you to eat more of their unhealthy food by touting some random nutritional property. After spending so much time discussing nutrition and digestion, I think it is time to take a step back to look at the bigger picture for a while before we get too lost in the minutiae of healthy eating.

How does this nutrition confusion happen? First, you need to understand why scientists study single nutrients at all. Why do research on saturated fat when no one eats pure saturated fat? Why research resveratrol when most people get their resveratrol by drinking red wine or eating purple grapes? Because doing so makes for more scientifically valid research—meaning it will help us better understand the role of nutrients in the body.

Let's imagine for one moment that we are budding nutritional researchers wanting to make discoveries about the amazing properties of natural foods so people will eat more of them. First, we have to decide what our research question is going to be.

To do good research, you need to devise a clearly defined question. "Does vitamin C (which, as ascorbic acid, has a distinct and unchanging chemical structure) help prevent the common cold?" is better than "Does citrus fruit or fruit in general help keep you healthy?"

Why? Because there are different varieties of citrus fruit, with differing chemical compositions depending on soils, season, or crop. It would be difficult to tease out what exactly worked in our research, because there are so many variables. Other researchers could easily dismiss our research by correctly assuming that people who eat more fruit are likely healthier and more resistant to viruses in general—leaving our eager scientific rationale for eating more fruit out in the cold. And if there is a reduction in people who get the cold after eating fruit, where do we go with our next research project? How could we know which components of the fruit we should study further?

Is it the fruit as a whole that helps?

Is it one specific citrus fruit or all of them as a group that works?

Is it a specific component of the fruit that provides the benefits?

Since we are clever scientists, we would probably suspect vitamin C as an active ingredient given that other research has pointed to its efficacy . . . but perhaps it is another substance within the fruit, such as naringen (a phytochemical)? Or maybe the vitamin C needs two or three helpers found within the fruit to be active—but what are they?

See how messy this can get? Scientists don't like messy answers—when you are investing precious resources in hopes of making a discovery that can advance human health, messy isn't exactly helpful.

Good research also compares a group that receives the treatment with a group that doesn't . . . but the groups and researchers can't know which is which. This is the gold standard of research: the double-blind, placebo-controlled study. This type of research is important because our minds are so powerful that just thinking we are receiving a therapeutic substance can cause our body to heal. This is an important point to reinforce: when someone swears some supplement or dietary regime worked for him or her, it might have been the change that worked . . . or it might have been his or her brain.

As we plan out our study on vitamin C, we have to design it so the people in the study have no idea whether they are receiving the treatment or a placebo. It is relatively easy to give people a tablet of vitamin C or a placebo that looks just like it. That mimicry will help take the power of the mind out of the equation for the most part. Could you create a fake orange that looks and tastes just like an orange but has no orange in it? Not so much . . . well not yet, anyway. Fake food technology moves pretty fast!

It is also cheaper to provide a chemical substance, and you are more assured that study subjects will take it . . . because what if the subjects don't like oranges? This research business isn't easy . . . so while we need to interpret research headlines with a touch of caution, we ought to applaud those that chose to spend their careers searching for nutritional truth for us. It takes years of confirming research before a health professional such as myself is confident enough to change their practice and use that information to help care for their clients and patients.

Searching for Answers in a Bunch of Broccoli

Given the current miserable state of human health, nutrition is a hot topic. Nutrition is implicated in all of our most troubling chronic diseases, so the more we learn about how nutrition affects our metabolism, genetics, and disease risk, the better. Teams all over the globe are racing to make discoveries about the beneficial properties of food, how they affect and nourish our bodies, and their role in human diseases. From kale for cancer to probiotics for irritable bowel syndrome, the discoveries are ripe for the picking.

Nutrition researchers toil away doing the heavy lifting in the lab so we can live better, healthier lives. This used to go relatively unnoticed. Now, with our hunger for nutrition and food information, we want to be on the cutting edge of research and follow nutrition news as intently as some follow sports statistics. As researchers make new discoveries about nutrition, health professionals and media outlets share the good news about various nutrients and before you know it, the latest nutrient-du-jour shows up in your sugary yogurt. Welcome to nutritionism.

The term nutritionism, coined by Professor Gyorgy Scrinis but popularized by writer Michael Pollan, refers to the reduction of the value of food to the individual nutrients it contains. Sure, food contains nutrients, but the sane among us understand that whole, natural foods are indeed greater than the sum of their parts. Nutrition is a young science, and at the end of the day, we will probably never have all the answers.

In fact, let me share this one, unalienable fact with you:

Mother Nature will always outsmart a scientist.

Doubtful? Let's talk antioxidants, which are certainly a hot topic in the research and the health worlds. There were antioxidants in blueberries before we even knew what an antioxidant was. Scientists are busy isolating and testing potency and delivery methods, but what if they get it wrong for the time being? What if antioxidant A only works in concert with antioxidants B, C, and protein A? But you just spent fifty bucks on a bottle of pure antioxidant A! Or what if the beneficial effect of these compounds is not due to their antioxidant potential but their effect on something else entirely? Fifty dollars buys a whole bushel of locally grown blueberries, doesn't it? Those blueberries will nourish your tissues and provide energy, regardless of the research outcomes.

Our mass confusion over isolated components of whole food has been played out again and again in the scientific literature and media. From soy protein to vitamin A, the research moves from observations that suggest benefit to studies that overwhelmingly support benefits. Then a trickle, a few studies that question the benefits; perhaps, even a potential for harm emerges. Finally, we emerge into a swamp of conflicting information that leaves us all scratching our heads and moving on to the next nutrient-du-jour. No wonder you're confused; I get pretty confused sometimes, too.

Playing into this confusion are all sorts of additional factors. Our DNA interacts with the nutrients we consume, meaning that a bit of vitamin C might supercharge our immune cells but leave our neighbor out with a cold. An older person will react to nutrients differently than a younger person, perhaps not absorbing them as well as they could. Someone with a chronic condition might have need of higher levels of nutrients. Even where we live could affect our nutritional needs! All of this can cause mixed messages in the research world that makes the answers less clear for us as eaters.

The research we are exposed to can even be affected by something called publication bias. When no one was interested in soy, research showing soy did nothing for you wasn't exactly first page news. Talk of soy superpowers was! However, as researchers, health professionals, and the media built up soy's super status . . . NOW dissent becomes interesting; studies that cause discord might be more likely to be published and publicized.

When you are aware of this complex dance, headlines simply become fodder for interesting watercooler chats and you can get on with good old-fashioned healthy eating. When you get too embroiled in the chaos, that's when you can spend a lot of money on useless pills or become so terrified of making the wrong food choice that grocery shopping leaves you anxious.

Some of us are far more trusting of a seemingly sophisticated pill than a humble plant when the opposite should be true. Nature provides . . . and scientists and health professionals just do our best to figure out her plan. Remember, it's just food.

Now with MORE . . . Nutrition!

Here's where we get into the deliciously grey area—yes, nutrients are important. However, the addition of nutrients to an otherwise dead and unhealthy food with the hope that it will make it healthier represents a gross misunderstanding of what our bodies need to be nourished. Let's get super unscientific here for a moment: as creatures of this good green earth, it makes sense that our bodies require the building blocks that can be found also on this earth. When you pick up that box of fruit snacks for your kids that are "Made with Real Fruit" and a "Source of Vitamin C," you assume it must be healthy. It has fruit in it, right? The vitamin C proves it, doesn't it? Not exactly . . . let me tell you why.

When I talk about the health benefits of eating fruit, I mean actual fruit. You know . . . bananas, blueberries, pears, payayas, and such. Actual fruit that grew on a tree or a bush; it was picked, washed, maybe chopped, and eaten. Unfortunately, you can manipulate that original, nutrient-dense fruit quite a lot and still call it fruit in our modern eating environment.

Here's an example: turning fruit into juice is a pretty simple process. You might lose some fiber and be able to drink a larger amount of fruit in one sitting, but you didn't have to mess with the fruit too much to create juice. However, as simple as it is, I would still prefer you eat the whole fruit instead of juice most of the time. The reason for this is that when you free up all those natural sugars from their cell structures, they have a different effect on the body. Those sugars are instantly available to your blood stream and send blood sugars soaring, triggering a metabolic cascade that can leave you feeling pretty hungry and maybe even cranky if you drank a large amount of juice. The calories are concentrated, meaning you are going to have to burn off more energy than if you had just eaten a single piece of fruit. The cleansing fiber was lost, along with who knows what other vital nutrients that might have clung to the pulp or been squashed in heat processing and packaging.

Now, what if you took that fruit juice and removed so much water that what was left looked like a syrup called fruit juice concentrate? Would you still call that product fruit? Food labelers can and do. To me, that is like calling maple syrup a tree. However, when it comes to those fruit snacks in question, creating a gummy candy out of this syrup allows manufacturers to call that candy a fruit snack. Since vitamin C is so delicate and unstable, it is likely that the original vitamin C in the juice concentrate was lost and vitamin C had to be added to the candies.

If you have some of these in your cupboard, check out the ingredients label and see if you can see the C. Those fruit snacks are not necessarily a bad thing—provided that you recognize them as a naturally sourced candy and don't consider them interchangeable with an orange. Therein lies our current problem. We may not consciously do it, but when we see those fruit snacks with vitamin C, they resonate as a healthy option for many of us, and we instinctively think it's okay to eat them every day when it really isn't. Don't even get me started on what passes for a granola bar most of the time.

Crazy Nutrition Claims . . . Blasted!

Ready to go through the silliness of just a few more common health claims? Let's do it! We have already talked about made with real fruit and a source of vitamin C; let's talk about a few more to keep us skeptical and healthy as we shop.

"Cholesterol free"

This pretty standard claim means that a food has no cholesterol, which has the potential to contribute to higher levels of your circulating blood cholesterol, which can lead to clogged arteries. Seems pretty straightforward, right?

What is so ridiculous is that I find this claim most often on potato chips. This is silly for two reasons; the first is that no plant food on earth has cholesterol. Only animal foods contain cholesterol. The second is that it is a health claim on a generally unhealthy food. Its placement is designed to get you to think of that snack food as healthier . . . you see where this is going.

"Trans fat free"

This claim really gets me—because it could be helpful if it meant a food was truly trans fat free. Industrial trans fats are one fat that I will not leave room for in a healthy diet—they are just too caustic to health (see Chapter 2 if you need a refresher). They aren't fit for consumption, even in an occasional treat. So taking the trans fats out of any food should be a good thing.

Trouble is, this claim has a loophole: if a food has less than 0.5 grams of trans fats per serving, it can be called trans fat free. But the food still contains trans fats! For example, if each cookie has 0.3 grams of trans fats and you consume ten cookies—you just ate 3 grams of trans fats— more than I think you should have in a week. How misleading!

"A source of calcium"

The operative word in this claim is source; by definition, a food is a source of a given nutrient as long as it provides at least 5 percent of your daily needs. That's it; just 5 percent. Not super impressive. An excellent source would provide at least 25 percent of your daily needs—now we're talking. Yet, your brain will imprint with the fact that the food you are looking at has calcium . . . leading you to think of it as healthier.

Right about now, you are probably thinking to yourself, "I can't believe there are legal definitions for this kind of stuff!" Welcome to my world.

Decoding Nutrition Information

In the valiant battle to help you understand what is in your food, governments (spurred on by the health professionals who work with them) ensured that all food packages contain ingredients lists in the order of most abundant ingredient to least abundant. This provides you, the consumer, with an opportunity to know that your breakfast cereal has almost as much sugar by weight as it does wheat. This is an important piece of information if you are looking out for it. However, there are ways to manipulate that information and ways that it gets more complex. Of course there are!

What if there were six core ingredients in that cereal (such as crunchy clusters and flakes and blueberry bits) and every one of them contained sugar? But not just plain ol' table sugar. What if there were treacle, honey, glucose-fructose, malt syrup, and invert sugar? Would you know how much sugar was in that product now? Would you even consciously recognize those as forms of sugar as you scan the ingredients? Yikes. That was round one in the battle between health, transparency, and food.

As consumers started worrying more about certain components of our food, such as sugars, saturated fat, and sodium, governments harangued food manufacturers into placing a nutrition facts panel on their packages, too. Now you will know that those six forms of sugar in the ingredients add up to a whopping twenty-one grams of sugars in one cup of cereal. That is more than five teaspoons of sugar in your cereal! "Ha ha!" we health professionals thought, "There is nowhere for food manufacturers to hide now . . . we can see everything clear as day!"

Except that the situation is clear as mud. Many consumers report not really understanding the information presented on nutrition facts panels.[1] In my own practice, I have seen time and time again that people have trouble locating information on the nutrition facts panel, and when they find it, they aren't sure what to do with it. Context is everything. Seeing four grams of saturated fat in a serving of food doesn't really help if you don't understand if that is a lot or a little or a good or a bad thing.

Depending on the nutrition headline of the day, the opinion on saturated fats could change, too. As a health professional, I don't expect you to remember all the stuff I went to school for five years to understand deeply. There is only so much space in our brains! With birthdays to remember, soccer games to attend, grocery shopping, reading for book club, and oh yes, work—let's not waste cognitive energy on how many grams of saturated fat you need to take in! Focusing on the nutrients at the expense of the food is a lot like missing the forest for the trees. And it sucks the joy out of eating.

The other trouble is how food formulas can be altered to provide the numbers you are looking for on the nutrition facts panel. Sugar-phobic? No problem! Take out the sugar and add in some artificial sweeteners and a few other texture-modifying ingredients to make up for it. Want more fiber? Let's put it in your yogurt, in the form of inulin—a prebiotic fiber from Jerusalem artichokes! Never mind that while we know inulin is an effective food for all those healthy bugs in your digestive tract, we don't know if it provides the full spectrum of health benefits to humans as good old dietary fiber from grains or beans.[2] But who needs barley when you have fiber in your yogurt?

Grandma's not sitting in the kitchen creating all of these products from scratch for us. Many foods sitting on store shelves are hyper-processed and would not be possible without a half-century of scientific advances in food manipulation. All of this drama on the nutrition facts panel is meant to distract you from the notion that, sugar or none, those cookies are not a healthy part of a daily diet. They are a treat.

With those caveats behind us, there is definitely merit to the nutrition facts panel, and it can be a useful tool when making decisions about packaged and prepared foods if you are inclined to use it. In Chapter 12, we will discuss what to look for in certain categories of common foods, such as cereals, soups, and breads. My purpose in bringing up the pitfalls of nutrition facts labels is to alert you to the dangers of falling into the nutritionism trap. Remember, our most important question when selecting healthy foods is, "Is this a natural, perishable food?"

Need more convincing? Try my little test.

Can You Spot the Healthier Choice?

Pop Quiz! Here you have two basic nutrition facts panels to help you select the healthier choice. Give them a look and see which one you think is healthiest!

Food One			Food Two		
Calories (kcal)	72.0		Calories (kcal)	80.0	
Fat (g)	0.2		Fat (g)	0.0	
Saturated Fat (g)	0.0		Saturated Fat (g)	0.0	
Trans Fat (g)	0.0		Trans Fat (g)	0.0	
Cholesterol (mg)	0.0		Cholesterol (mg)	0.0	
Carbohydrate (g)	19.1		Carbohydrate (g)	19.0	
Fiber (g)	2.6		Fiber (g)	0.0	
Protein (g)	0.4		Protein (g)	2.0	

If I was just looking at the nutrients, I would be in a debate between fiber and protein. I know that fiber is fabulous for our digestive system, but I also know that the protein in food two will help moderate the carbohydrate impact on my blood sugar; I might lean towards food one. I wouldn't be entirely sure of my choice. I would feel uncertain and a bit confused. This is where focusing solely on nutrients gets you.

Now, if we want to look at the merit of the food itself . . . this will be a much easier choice. Food one is an apple. Food two is Jell-O. There is no way I would ever tell you to eat Jell-O, not even as a lighter snack. You probably don't think of Jell-O as healthy either. But what if that Jell-O came up with a new version that was now a source of vitamin C and made with real fruit? It might make for a healthier dessert, yes? Not a chance. By sleight of food labeling hand, fruit concentrate can qualify as real fruit even though by the time they process real fruit into a concentrate there is nothing left of it but a big hit of liquid sugar.

Nutritionism is confusing. Food is simple.

It's About the Food . . .

Each time you eat, or at least 80 percent of the time, you should make a food choice that is nutrient-dense, meaning that it has a great deal of nutrition for few calories. The only place you will find that magic mix is in whole foods, typically plants. Think of your calorie intake as a food budget: if you have to spend eighty calories of your budget to come up with a paltry added fifty milligrams of vitamin C and another two hundred and fifty calories for a measly three grams of fiber, you are going to eat your way into an overfed, overweight, and undernourished body. Which explains a lot, given our current twin epidemics of obesity and chronic disease! Instead, by choosing a whole plant food like an apple, you get a host of vitamins, minerals, fiber, and phytochemicals that we need to live our best life for that remarkable seventy-two calories. There are probably a whole bunch of other features in the apple that we haven't even discovered yet. That is the power of whole foods.

Should all that other stuff get too confusing, remember this: the healthiest foods don't come in packages or at least not fancy ones. Our healthiest choices are unprocessed foods, such as fruits, vegetables, intact grains, legumes, nuts, seeds, and if you eat them, plain dairy and lean meats. Nutritionism just can't compete in the face of real food. As knowledge grows, theories change. In five years, the theories in this book will probably have evolved. However, when we focus on food—we can't be steered wrong. Eat real food. Be healthy.

My Diet is Better Than Yours . . .

With the current state of our unhealthy nations, it stands to reason that it can take a warrior's heart to resist the crowd and choose a path to a healthier body. The interesting thing about human beings as eaters is that how we choose to eat is held near and dear to our hearts. Food choice is an intimate, personal, cultural, and often spiritual decision.

So if someone cleared her fibromyalgia symptoms with a raw foods diet, it's understandable that she might get a bit preachy. If a paleo plan helped someone lose fifty pounds and normalize his diabetes, he would probably think that paleo is the best thing since sliced bread—well, better than sliced bread by definition! If eliminating gluten-containing foods got someone's blood sugars under control, gluten must be bad for everyone—right?

It seems that nowadays, in order for what we eat to be the right path, others have to be wrong. Really wrong. And we can get a bit uppity about it. I remember back to when I became a vegetarian as a teenager . . . I was preachy and downright annoying! Instead of showing enthusiasm for what vegetarianism meant to me, I simply told others the errors of their ways. Amusingly, I couldn't understand why people didn't understand my choice as I was berating them for theirs.

At the end of the day, if you are at a healthy weight, active, and getting the nutrition that your body needs to thrive, there is plenty of latitude in how you select a diet for yourself. And just because something worked for you doesn't mean it will work for someone else. The amazing thing about the human body is that we are all totally unique—I am talking snowflake-level special! Just as your fingerprint is unlike anyone else's, so too is your body's response to food. That doesn't mean that certain foods are terrible or amazing . . . they just might be terrible or amazing for your unique constitution. There is no one-size-fits-all approach—but there are some basics that everyone needs to follow (such as eating those pesky fruits and veggies).

Did I mention that you really need to eat fruits and veggies? Just checking!

Popular diets tend to work by creating a rigid set of rules to follow that makes it easy for you, the eater, to put willpower aside and just follow along. That cake isn't tasty . . . it's a poison! Meat is toxic—no, grains are! And you are crazy to consume dairy! To make those rules seem more compelling, complex philosophies are doled out and maybe a bit of science is sprinkled in—some of it valid, some of it not.

The flipside is taking the tack of moderation that many health professionals prefer. It's a pretty rational way to go; however, saying, eat as many healthy foods as you can doesn't create a mobilizing cry that compels you to launch headfirst into a bowl of salad for days on end!

Absolutes win in the beginning, but fail in the end.

Every.

Single.

Time.

What matters more than any single food choice you make is the overall pattern of eating you maintain over years. So while a cookie every now and then is no big deal, if you define every now and then to be every day, there might be an issue. That's what this book is here for: to help you create a remarkable everyday diet that gives you the solid nutritional foundation that can withstand a few meatball thunderstorms.

Confusion Is for the Birds . . . Let's Set the Record Straight

—Nutritionism places an individual nutrient above the wisdom of the whole food. Don't buy in.

—Real food—that hasn't been predigested, preseasoned, or pre-formed—is always your best choice.

—Ingredients trump nutrition information. If it doesn't pass the healthy kitchen test, give it a pass. What is the healthy kitchen test? Each ingredient in a food should be found in your healthy kitchen. Last time I checked, there wasn't any diglyceride in your pantry.

—Our bodies are unique, as is the dietary pattern that will nourish them best. Be respectful of others' choices and don't let someone else's philosophy throw your own wisdom into question.

CHAPTER 5

FIGHT INFLAMMATION WITH YOUR FORK!

"Don't dig your grave with your own knife and fork." —English Proverb

Our relationship with food says a lot about our relationship with ourselves. The way most of us live our lives, it seems that our bodies are little more than servants to our brains and mouths. That is, until the body starts rebelling. Placing low priority on the type of food we eat means that we place our health and wellbeing in low priority. Unfortunately, most of these decisions are not being made consciously; we rarely think about the functional and nutritional value of the foods we eat, instead choosing to fetishize fat, sugar, and salt.

When it comes to making more conscious food choices, it is up to you to decide how much are you worth. Healthy eating doesn't have to be expensive or time consuming, but it does demand you shift your priorities to make healthy food possible in your life. Is an extra 50 cents for organic spinach too much? Are you worth the three minutes it takes to make a smoothie (especially considering you will wait four minutes for your breakfast bagel to grill at the coffee shop)? If you swap that $6.99 bag of nasty chicken strips, can you afford a couple pounds of organic tofu? Understand that, in no uncertain terms, the way you eat will impact how the rest of your life will play out.

This is big. Don't freak out!

It is never too late to make a change.

Your body has the remarkable capacity to heal. It was made for this. And should you want to put the book down right now thinking, "I'm not ready for this," know that you are. You know why? Because forever is a long time . . . so there will be room for cake. A margarita every now and then will be just fine. Just like we had to get ourselves past our obsession with nutrients, we also need to get ourselves past our obsession with being perfect. Perfect is rigid; perfect is intimidating. Perfect is the perfect excuse for not changing. And actually, perfect isn't perfect. I won't let you off that easy, but I will make it easy for you to succeed, I promise.

Once you are well-versed in the nutrition basics, we can move beyond the minutiae of nutrients and think about the big picture: food. Food in the context of a lifetime well-eaten! Now that we have had a relaxing break in real food realityland, it's time to build a bit more of your most important healthy eating muscle . . . your brain. This chapter merges both the big picture of a healthy dietary pattern with a lot of scientific detail to explain why I have chosen this as my preferred path to better health. The more knowledge you have, the easier it is to resolve to transform your eating habits for good. So let's train our sights on the ultimate goal of whole food nutrition: eating an anti-inflammatory diet.

"But I don't have arthritis or heart disease," you counter.

"Yet." I reply. We are playing the long game here . . . one of prevention.

Food can enable a remarkable capacity for healing; it is restorative when you are sick, but it is even more exciting to realize how eating well can help prevent you from getting sick in the first place. Eating well provides opportunities for healing from everyday assaults before they accumulate into big trouble. And food has a large role to play in moderating chronic inflammation, the process at the heart of much of what ails us.

So let's start by talking about inflammation: what it is, why we need to care, and how to eat to douse the flames for life. Inflammation is one of our oldest friends, and it is a critical part of our immune system; the one that we are born with, ready to stand guard and attack any invaders that might be storming the gates of our bodily temple. When you cut yourself, the heat, swelling, and redness you see forming around the cut is inflammation at work. More precisely, it is acute inflammation. Acute inflammation helps block invaders from gaining access to the rest of your body, destroys them, and helps heal any wounds that might have formed. Sounds like a good thing, yes? I agree.

So how does inflammation cause us harm? In the case of the cut, when the threat of further injury has passed, inflammation turns off. The job is done, time to pack up the troops and go home. But what if the cut didn't heal? Ever? Or worse yet, what if the body perceived it was under attack, even when it really wasn't? How could you turn inflammation off, and if you don't, what would happen? Welcome to the realm of chronic inflammation.

Inflammation is highly effective in the short term. Without it, cuts would continue to bleed and any bacteria on the surface of our skin would start running marathons in our bloodstream, wreaking havoc wherever they went. Unfortunately, the acute inflammatory process is a bit like sending a bull into a china shop—it can pick up the teacup you asked for, but it will destroy the rest of the shop in the process. In the short term, the end is worth the means. Inflammation quickly resolves and your body can get back to its resting, peaceful state. But if that inflammation continues for weeks or even years, there is going to be a big mess to clean up.

Chronic inflammation is a completely different beast; it's like having termites in a log cabin! Symptoms are rarely seen, but the damage can lead to a massive health problem that would diminish the quality of our precious lives. Interestingly, or alarmingly, chronic inflammation is implicated in almost all of our most common chronic concerns, from heart disease to cancer, irritable bowel syndrome to acne and dementia.[1] We are living lives that stoke the fires of inflammation as we breathe dirty air, eat junk, get frazzled, and crash on the couch. It's worth figuring out where this inflammation is coming from and how we can eat ourselves cool as a cucumber on the inflammation front. Join me now as we wind down the twisted road to chronic inflammation and examine how our waistlines, our guts, our dinner, and even our environment can all lead to inflammation station.

Piling the Pounds on Inflammation

Want to cool off? Start by trimming your waistline. The weight that we carry around our midsections is one of the strongest predictors of our inflammatory state. It's not just getting between you and a clear view of your toes—a beer belly raises a glass to inflammation and invites it over for an extended house stay.

For some time, researchers thought that body fat was a passive storage site for excess energy, or calories, from food.[1,2,3] Kind of like the shopping bag we use to carry food in between the time we purchase it at the store and eat it at home. If we consume more energy than we need, our helpful fat cells simply hang on to it for us, and when we need more energy, they graciously give it back. Unfortunately, it was a naïve view of a potentially hostile state of affairs. How fat cells metabolize and interact with our bodies is incredibly complex. It makes sense, when you think about it: any cell that lives in our body must have a way of communicating with the body it lives in to ensure its survival. A fat cell needs a way of getting what it requires to survive and to design its home to its specifications. We have learned that, in fact, belly fat is incredibly active on the neighborhood block watch. Kind of like the crotchety neighbor with the pink flamingos who blasts his music and leaves his junk all over the lawn.

Fat cells communicate with the rest of your body in all sorts of ways: regulating your appetite and insulin sensitivity, bone formation, and even reproductive functions.[1] Another message that belly fat cells (adipocytes for the smarty-pants out there) send is one that sets off chronic inflammation.[1,2,3,4] Belly fat apparently doesn't like to get cold; it prefers to stoke the fires of inflammation and bask in their glow. How do they make this happen? By enlisting one of the major players in inflammation, a set of immune cells called macrophages. These cells normally attack foreign invaders as part of an immune response and destroy them before they can cause further harm.[1,4] Macrophages are capable of promoting inflammation by sending out their own chemical messengers, appropriately named pro-inflammatory signals, throughout the entire body, making it believe that it is under attack.[1,2] Yet this is nothing more than a subtle trick of the fat cells to ensure they stay happy. This process is known as low-grade inflammation,[1,2] even though over the long term, the effects are anything by minor.

Welcome to the chronic inflammatory state: our ancient defense mechanism confused by a thoroughly modern and foreign environment—fat around our vital organs. Overstuffed fat cells around your waist produce a mob of pro-inflammatory signals with fancy scientific names, such as tumor necrosis factor alpha (TNF-α), interferon-γ, and interleukin-6 (IL-6). [1,2,3,4] You don't need to know how these signals work; what you do need to know is that by stimulating the production of these pro-inflammatory signals, fat cells essentially create a nonexistent enemy of themselves that activates chronic inflammation.

You also need to know the kinds of trouble the chronic inflammatory response creates in its wake. One of the most researched links between chronic inflammation and disease is the relationship between that beer belly and the risk of type 2 diabetes and cardiovascular disease.[1,2] A beer belly leads to the creation of those pro-inflammatory signals. Those signals tell your other cells that there is a problem and normal cellular processes, such as listening to insulin when it comes knocking at the cell's door, should stop. When this happens, it's known as insulin resistance; when the resistance gets out of hand, type 2 diabetes can result.

The bright side? When even a bit of weight loss occurs, insulin resistance improves, as do levels of these pro-inflammatory signals.[1,2,4] Less belly fat, fewer inflammatory problems.

Now that we see the links between belly fat, inflammation, and chronic disease beginning to emerge . . . let's go a little deeper inside the body to another crucial site of inflammation, the gut.

Fire on the Front Lines

Another strategic site of chronic inflammation is your digestive tract; your gut is where you interact with the outside world most intimately. Most of us don't think of it this way; however, the digestive tract is effectively the outside world. Just think of all the food, bacteria, viruses, molds, and fungi that your gut comes into contact with on a daily basis via your mouth. It is the job of the digestive tract to move harmful invaders through a gauntlet of stomach acid and alkaline bile salts and maintain an iron-clad barrier so these harmful substances and organisms cannot gain access to your inner world. Your gut also needs to breakdown your food into absorbable components, somehow selectively accept the nutrients and substances you require to live, and recognize that the healthy bacteria living in your colon are here to help not harm!

It's a tall order for any body system: the digestive tract is ground zero for better health and yet, the barrier between you and the outside world is incredibly fragile. The lining of your digestive tract consists of just a single cell layer standing between you and potential harm; your body has also enlisted an enormous immune police force, ready to engage invaders at the front lines. In fact, roughly 70 percent of immune activity is located just under the surface of your digestive tract lining. When the immune system senses that all is clear on the digestive front, it hangs back and takes a siesta. The healthy bacteria living in your gut even help to pass along the message that everything is on the up and up. However, should the immune system receive warning signals from across the gut or come into contact with invaders it doesn't recognize, it's response is a fiery one.

Much like the police, there are stations for immune cells in the gut. These are collectively known as GALT—gut-associated lymphoid tissue—and are found in multiple sites along and within the digestive tract.[3] Clusters called Peyer's patches are nestled into the lower part of the small intestine; immune tissues are also found in the intestinal epithelium of the colon and within the gut wall structure, called the lamina propria.[3] Think of GALT as digestive law enforcement; when foreign substances or organisms are recognized by the immune patrol within the digestive tract, they are presented to the equivalent of an immune judge for consideration. After weighing the biochemical evidence, one of two things happens—they are tolerated as harmless or the GALT mounts an inflammatory response.[3]

With all the trillions of happy bacteria living in your bowels peacefully, the immune system has the remarkable ability to recognize friend from foe. This is body policing at its finest. GALT has evolved mechanisms for shaping the bacterial community and preventing the bacteria that call you home from breaching the intestinal wall.[5] It does this through production of a progressively impenetrable mucus layer and specialized substances that act like selective antibiotics.[5] But don't think that bacteria are just passive riders; influence is a two-way street.

Without the development of a normal, healthy bacterial community, GALT tissues don't mature or develop properly. [5,6,7] Helpful, healthy bacteria are actually in communication with your immune system to let it know that there is no reason to be alarmed at their presence and promote the strengthening of the gut's barrier function.[7] Healthy bacteria and a strong digestive tract barrier mean a relaxed yet alert immune system. However, your digestive community can fall out of balance, and if that happens, your immune cells use their best, quickest defense to respond—inflammation. The trouble is, when an inflammatory environment is present in your digestive tract, it is tough for it to resolve on its own.[3]

When it's Not All Quiet on the Digestive Front

With all that your digestive tract and immune system have to manage in their interactions with the outside world, there are multiple opportunities for things to go wrong. Here are a few known culprits that stoke the fires of digestive inflammation:

—An abundance of harmful intestinal bacteria that your immune system rightly recognizes as an infection, otherwise known as dysbiosis.

—A diet that is damaging to good digestive health, such as too much red meat, saturated fat, or sugar, and not enough fiber and fresh produce.

—The mortar that holds the gut cells together, called a tight junction, begins to leak, and the immune system is exposed to particles and organisms it doesn't recognize and mounts an attack.[3]

—The immune system mistakenly reacts to the healthy bacteria in your intestine as if they are foes and loses tolerance for them.[3,7]

—Unrecognized food allergies or intolerances damage the digestive tract and launch an inflammatory cascade.[3]

—Chronic stress-induced changes in digestion and the gut itself promote infection, affect intestinal transit, or reduce barrier function.[3,7]

The Bugs That Are Bugging You

Our digestive tracts are a diverse ecosystem; even a healthy person has a few potentially troublemaking microbes hanging around just waiting for their chance to mess with you. When we have an abundance of friendly bugs in residence, they keep the troublemakers at bay. However, when stress, travel, medications, or even diet rough up the neighborhood, the healthy bugs flee, and the nasty ones have the opportunity to take over.[7] This is the attack that you can't see. Stealth mode. But it doesn't escape your immune system—inflammation comes to the rescue and creates a wreckage.

Commensal, or friendly, bacteria usually have little physical interaction with the gut epithelial cell, as they are content to remain nestled within the mucus layer and chat away with their host. This chatting appears to exert a positive pressure on the immune cells, almost like doing training runs in preparation for a marathon.[8] Some superstar probiotic bacteria even appear to be able to turn off or discourage inflammatory activity; the short chain fatty acids they produce are potential anti-inflammatory agents.[5,7,8]

Troublemaking bugs, on the other hand, are maniacally driven to attack the epithelial cells once they get the chance.[6,9] Thankfully, our cells are equipped with their very own alarm system to recognize an intruder. These molecules, known as toll-like receptors (TLRs), sit on the surface of cells and interact with other cells and chemicals. When an enemy of the cell is recognized, the TLRs sound the alarm in the form of pro-inflammatory signals—the same as the belly fat above.[1,6] Once again, the inflammatory response is called to action. The regular cells stop acting normally and allow the immune response to treat the area much like a riot squad, taking down whatever might be in its path. While the gut cells won't be hurt, the same cannot be said for some of the friendly bacteria, which may find themselves killed in the crossfire or sent packing from the body.[6,7,8,9] Most of the time, the area returns to normal; however, some troublemaking bacteria may end up being insurgent, hiding away until the cops are gone or at least on regular patrol. When the coast is clear, they take advantage of the situation and begin to occupy their land.[6,7,9] This is the start of dysbiosis.

Dysbiosis is enough to drive intestinal inflammation; it is the immune system attempting to get the bad bugs under control.[5,6,7,9] Unfortunately, it's pretty difficult to restore a healthy balance when the good guys are beaten down.

Remember that good bacteria help tell the immune system when to back off; if they aren't present in large enough numbers, inflammation can rage on. The inflammatory response depends on a series of checkpoints and patrol cells that the GALT employs to be ready for attacks. For inflammation to resolve, you need a positive balance of pro- to anti-inflammatory messages relayed from immune patrol; the presence of beneficial or disease-causing bacteria will contribute to these messages.[7]

While a civil war on the gut front is bad enough for your digestive health, this inflammatory immune response can go beyond the digestive tissues via systemically active compounds and immune cells triggered at the gut level.[3,5,6] That's the trouble with inflammation; chronic inflammation is like a chronic poison that knows no boundaries within the body. Heard the one about flossing your teeth for better heart health? The link is bacteria and inflammation. Have chronic dry eye? Take omega-3 fats—inflammation is calling the shots there, too, in a condition called blepharitis. We are living in an inflammation nation, and these crazy critters that call us home may call a lot of the shots. What is interesting is that the source of this bacterial riot can be many things—exposure to exotic bacteria is an obvious one, as is antibiotic use. However, stress or a crappy diet (or both) can also promote the growth of the troublemakers and instigate a dysbiosis riot.[6,9]

Picky Eaters . . . Those Bacteria

In the tango involving your gut, the bacteria that live in it, and your immune system, there is another choreographer: your diet. The reason for this is that the bacteria that live in your digestive tract are alive . . . and hungry! They need to eat something to survive, and thankfully, they don't feast on you. So the food has got to come from somewhere; conveniently, all those bacteria live along the same path that food takes through your system. And, brilliantly, friendly bacteria like to munch on the stuff your own body cannot break down: plant fibers.

If you are thinking over your day's menu and all you see is a sea of donuts, hamburgers, and lasagna—not much fiber is going to be available for the hungry bacterial masses. In fact, how you choose to set the table for yourself has a lot to do with which bacterial guests decide to stick around for dinner. You wouldn't take vegetarian friends to a steak house, would you? So you can't expect healthy, helpful bacteria designed to eat indigestible plant fibers to stick around if you feed them a steady diet of fat, over-processed carbohydrates, and salt.

Research validates this picky eaters theory: the way you eat can have a direct impact on the types of bacteria that choose to call your body home.[10,11] In animal models, diets high in fat and sugars have been found to increase potentially harmful bacteria and reduce more helpful strains.[10,11] In addition, a typical high fat diet—particularly in the absence of great prebiotic foods, such as plants—has been shown to contribute directly to inflammation via an increase in lipopolysaccharides (LPS) produced by the more gnarly bacteria in the gut.[10,12] LPS can activate pro-inflammatory pathways, and some research suggests that LPS may contribute to the inflammatory stress of high fat diets as much as, or more than, the nutrient effects of the fats themselves.[12]

Vegetarian diets also appear to promote healthier bacterial diversity (yay plants!) and, in case your crash diet phase is not yet behind you, going on very calorie-restricted diets hurts populations of healthy anti-inflammatory bacteria, including one type that may help protect against inflammatory bowel diseases.[10,11] If you starve, so do your good bugs. Makes sense, doesn't it?

In essence, our modern diet has a multitude of grim effects: it promotes weight gain, sends blood sugars out of whack, causes digestive ills, promotes inflammation, and even angers our bacterial buddies. When we eat the standard American diet, we are not just robbing our bodies of the nourishment they so desperately seek; our hyper-processed diets are also starving the bacteria that seek to protect us. The simple answer? Eat more plants, and introduce more healthy bacteria to your body. That's it, in a nutshell.

Don't worry; the dietary advice and meal plans in section two will give you the long form how-to.

Trust Your Gut

Here is why a preventative approach is so important: without any overt symptoms, you have no idea that all of this inflammatory craziness is occurring until the damage tips you into a chronic condition. Perhaps just a little gas or fatigue will come your way; it could also be more serious, such as chronic acid reflux or irritable bowel syndrome. We rarely think about our digestive tracts until they start causing us trouble—and then we can't get our minds off them. Unfortunately, modern conventional medicine hasn't been able to solve many distressing digestive concerns, and chronic inflammation continues to damage the digestive tract lining, becoming a vicious circle of dis-ease.

No matter what the root cause, inflammation along the digestive tract keeps the immune system intertwined with our guts on constant alert. It's an army with itchy trigger fingers. Our body diverts energy and nutrient resources to fight this attack, and the gut is the battleground. Our gut lining, a complex and fragile barrier between the outside world and our inner sanctum, can become compromised and start to leak. And once the gut starts to leak, the immune system really freaks out as it tries to fight off invaders that have no business making it past the gut wall. Inflammation also damages the absorptive capacity of the digestive tract, meaning all that (hopefully) good food you are sending down the hatch might not be providing you with as much benefit as you might expect. Shifting your dietary habits to a more anti-inflammatory approach could help prevent a multitude of troubles from coming your way in the future.

When the Gut Leaks . . .

The outer, absorptive surface of your digestive tract, which looks like a vast velvety carpet, is just a single cell layer called the intestinal epithelium. But what an impressive bunch of cells! The reason the surface resembles velvet is that these epithelial cells are covered in finger-like projections called villi, which are again covered with tinier finger-like projections called microvilli. The epithelial cells cover the outer layer of the digestive tract; beyond the tract wall lives all of that rich immune tissue. Along the gut edge, thick mucus is excreted that serves to reinforce the defensive barrier and provide a home for the trillions of happy bacteria to cling to.

What we haven't discussed yet is how this seemingly impenetrable layer could actually leak and cause the immune system to freak out. Each epithelial cell is joined together by a locking mechanism called a tight junction.[13] The purpose of the tight junction is to keep out any organism or substance that isn't meant to cross into the mucosal layer. These surface epithelial cells are home to transporters that can accept small molecules, such as amino acids, vitamins, and minerals. Anything larger needs to be broken down first by the enzymes in your intestinal space, or it'll pass on through the poop shoot! In this way, the intestinal lining is like the ultimate velvet rope. Only nutritional VIPs are supposed to pass through.

As we have discussed, infection and dysbiosis can directly alter the barrier function as disease-causing bugs attack the cells and the barrier falters. This is akin to when a bee or a kitchen knife disrupts the barrier of your skin. Inflammation soon follows. Inflammation can also alter barrier function in the absence of overt injury, and when it does, large molecules can make their way past the velvet ropes.[3,13] It is the inflammatory cytokines that are thought to directly increase the permeability of the gut barrier through some biochemical meddling, such as TNF-α, IFN-γ, and those pesky interleukin molecules.[3,13] The exact hows and whys are not quite understood, but the take home message here is that inflammation in the gut is bad for the integrity of the gut barrier.[3].

When the gut leaks, all of that rich immune tissue just below the surface of the epithelium can go into overdrive upon contact with a far greater diversity of substances than it's used to seeing.[3] It becomes this disastrous feedback loop where inflammation reduces barrier function, leading to increased inflammation from foreign substances, thereby further reducing barrier function, and so on.[3] Pro-inflammatory cytokines may also trigger enzymes that can damage tissues, leading to malabsorption.[3] So by now you might be thinking . . . does this have anything to do with food allergy? Perhaps.

Food allergy and intolerance is on the rise, and it is a potential suspect in the leaky gut case, although it is a chicken-and-egg scenario: did the intolerance come because the immune tissue was exposed to undigested food particles, or did existing intolerance cause the gut to leak? In celiac disease, new evidence shows that exposure to gluten causes the excessive release of a molecule called zonulin, which acts like a crowbar in opening up the tight junctions and causing an inflammatory response.[14] Could something similar be happening with other foods? Time will tell. When the gut leaks, immune activation can lead to the immune system tagging otherwise helpful substances or organisms as harmful. In inflammatory bowel disease, one theory of chronic inflammation activation is that the body tags normal digestive bacteria as harmful, creating a permanent state of war.[3] How this occurs is unknown, but a leaky gut, leading to immune activation, is one plausible theory.[14]

Allergy, Sensitivity, Intolerance . . . What Gives?

Sensitivity

Sensitivity is a blanket term that refers to any adverse reaction to a food or chemical in food;[15] however, it is also now commonly used to refer to a reaction that is not a classic allergy (see below). In this modern use of the term, this is where a leaky gut and food reaction makes the most theoretical sense. The gut leaks, the immune system incorrectly tags a nice food as a naughty one, and symptoms build. Heal the gut, take care of the reaction? Hopefully time will tell.

Allergy

Allergy is an adaptive immune response to a protein in a certain food, mediated by the immunoglobulin IgE.[15] The most common food allergens are wheat, soy, tree nuts, peanuts, eggs, milk, mustard, seafood, sesame, and sulphites.[15] Symptoms can range from mild to severe anaphylaxis (fatal shock), and even the tiniest amount of the food sets off a reaction.[15]

Intolerance

Food intolerance refers to an adverse response that is not immune mediated.[15] Lactose intolerance is a classic example; if we lack the lactase enzyme, lactose in dairy products causes us trouble. That lactose travels through the gut, drawing water that might lead to diarrhea or being fermented by our resident bugs, leading to uncomfortable gas and bloating. Typically, trace amounts of the food won't cause harm; there is usually a dose-response reaction.[15] Some people can tolerate a small to moderate amounts of lactose, others can't.

One Man's Food . . . Another Man's Poison?

The tidal wave of people who feel that food sensitivities (not classic food allergies) are undermining their health is a modern conundrum; leaky gut is an interesting theory in how these sensitivities may have come to be. It is thought that a leaky gut allows the immune system to be presented to larger molecules of undigested foodstuff that it is not used to seeing.[14] When this occurs, the immune system can tag a food particle as foreign, creating an inflammatory response to future exposures as long as the gut is still inflamed and leaky. However, at this point we don't really know why so many of us seem to be reacting to otherwise healthy food. Taking care of your gut certainly won't hurt . . . but it might not fully correct the situation either. While we search for more conclusive answers, if food sensitivity is suspected as an inflammation trigger, removing the offending food could provide some relief. Take care with eliminating too much from your diet; doing so could put you at risk for malnutrition, which will also interfere with your healing process. Talk to a dietitian for help if you suspect food sensitivity or intolerance is an issue for you.

How Food Fans the Flames

We have seen that food can influence inflammation via your bacterial world and potentially through miscommunication with a leaky gut. However, even better understood is how the nutrients in food themselves fan the flames of inflammation. From a nutrition perspective, there are two main aggressors in the firefight: unruly blood sugars and poor-quality fats.[1] This isn't new information . . . it's just not widely adopted. Dietary effects on inflammatory pathways have been known for some time, and a couple of pioneering physicians, Dr. Nicholas Perricone and Dr. Andrew Weil, were first to bring these messages to the health-seeking public. For some reason, not enough of us are on the anti-inflammatory train yet. Come on folks, it's time to leave inflammation station en route to greener pastures!

It must have seemed radical that food could alter inflammation and, heck, that inflammation could even exist in the body at a subclinical level. However, our approach to food and nutrition has evolved a great deal. Instead of seeing food as a relatively inert source of nutrients, forward-thinking nutrition researchers and practitioners are instead looking at food as a source of information. The components of food are essentially messages from the environment that our own body interprets and responds to. So from this perspective, the role of food in inflammatory pathways makes a bit more sense. Nutrients and compounds contained in food become building blocks on inflammatory pathways; the types of fats we eat can either discourage or promote pro-inflammatory pathways, and soaring blood sugars can set off an internal alarm that drives inflammation to the rescue. Knowing this, we can figure out how to send the right information to keep our body calm, cool, and collected.

Go On . . . Be a Control Freak

It's time to unleash your inner control freak . . . on your blood sugar. Maintaining stable blood sugars, as we mentioned, is important for stabilizing energy levels and hunger control. To make matters worse, a constant blood sugar roller coaster fueled by hyper-processed carbs, such as granola bars, sugary drinks, muffins, and too much fluffy bread, also stokes the fires of inflammation, and here's how.

Hyper-processed carbohydrates tend to have rapidly digested sugars; between the added sugars and the processed flour that quickly becomes sugar, these types of foods send blood sugar soaring quickly. As I described in Chapter 2, this is called a high-glycemic response, and these foods would have a high glycemic index.

Research has found that a higher glycemic carbohydrate load can actually alter the production of pro-inflammatory signals from within the cell itself! The target is known as nuclear factor kappa b (NF-κB), which is responsible for turning on pro-inflammatory pathways.[16] When there is an inflammatory signal, NF-κB is prompted to start the process. When inflammation is calmed, the process is halted. Now look at what happened in one particular study that focused on diet and NF-κB. The researchers gave subjects either white bread, pasta, or glucose, and after a few hours, they looked at the levels of NF-κB in immune cells. Eating white bread incited an inflammatory riot to equal pure glucose sugar, whereas those who received pasta (a lower glycemic choice) had a much lower response.[16] The amount of carbohydrate received was the same, and these were nondiabetic people![16]

It may seem unbelievable that simply eating what we could consider to be everyday foods could have such an impact on our cells. Yet as you can see, carbohydrates are not created equally and in and of themselves are not inflammatory foods. It's the quality, people! This same pattern is being played out again and again—hyper-processed foods wreak havoc on the body; foods closer to nature keep it cool, calm, and collected.

In our carbaholic nation, even if we don't gain weight or develop diabetes, these foods are contributing to disease development over years through inflammatory modulation. This inflammatory state is probably a lot worse for us than carrying fifteen extra pounds. To compound things, most of the foods that promote inflammation also lack the nutrition found in plant foods that would help us to clean up the mess.

It's Quality, Not Quantity (Mostly) That Counts!

In addition to keeping your blood sugars stable, you also want to take a look at the types of fats you are eating. Here, it is not quantity but the quality of fats you consume that can alter the inflammatory process.

Remember how we talked about toll-like receptors (TLRs), the alarm system on gut cells that can trigger an inflammatory response? Well, it turns out that these gatekeepers are also activated to cause inflammation indirectly by saturated fatty acids.[1,12,17,18] Your body doesn't want bacon double cheeseburgers, and it has defense mechanisms designed to root out those dietary aggressors.

Saturated fatty acids affect inflammatory pathways by helping bacteria produce a part of their anatomy called lipopolysaccharides (LPS). Most nasty bacteria produce quite a bit of this LPS, and when they come into contact with the TLRs,[18,19] well, you know what happens. But here is where it gets worse. Over time, the continual presence of this fat can alter the bacterial community, and not for the better.[12] Now just imagine what it must be like when you have an entire community made up of rabble rousers who are constantly setting off home alarms and bringing out the riot police. After a while, the entire area starts to decline into a war zone. The continual battles begin to affect your entire body, leading to other problems, most specifically, obesity.[12]

You see? What you're feeding your bacteria matters! Mind-boggling, isn't it? Hopefully though, the message is pretty clear. Laying off a diet high in unhealthy fats is probably a good idea!

When it comes to quality, generally speaking, it is the omega-6, saturated, and trans fatty acids we want to see less of in an anti-inflammatory eating plan. Omega-6 fatty acids are essential to our health—essential meaning that we need to obtain them from our diet. The trouble is that they are metabolically connected to omega-3 in almost a seesaw-like fashion. When the two are in balance, the tension between pro-inflammatory and anti-inflammatory pathways is at ease. However, if one or the other gets out of whack, the balance is lost. How does this tie into inflammation? Omega fatty acids are the precursors to a group of molecules called eicosanoids, which can either promote or regulate the inflammatory pathways.[3] In addition, the omega-3 fatty acids appear to increase certain molecules called resolvins, which help to decrease and regulate the inflammatory response.[3]

Currently, it is the omega-6 fatty acids that are dominating our dietary landscape.[3] Most of these fats come from seed oils that are hyper-processed and cheap, making their way into all manner of hyper-processed foods, from artificial creamers to crackers to your value meal. So our body is receiving an overwhelming amount of omega-6 fatty acids and almost no omega-3 fatty acids. Why? Because we find omega-3 fats in natural foods that are not as abundant in our modern diets.

Sources of Omega-3 and Omega-6 Fatty Acids

All foods contain an assortment of different dietary fats; however, these are the foods that feature predominantly omega-6 or omega-3 fatty acids. Generally speaking, we want to eat fewer omega-6 fatty acids and more omega-3 fatty acids. For the purpose of completeness, I have also singled out a particular omega-6 called GLA, which is anti-inflammatory and healing. It is one that you want more of in your diet, too.

Omega-6 Sources

Corn, soy, canola, safflower, sunflower, grape seed, cottonseed oil, processed foods, and spreads containing these oils.

Omega-6 GLA Sources

Hemp, borage seed, and black currant oil.

Omega-3 Sources

Flax, hemp, chia, pumpkin seed, walnuts, cold water fish, such as salmon, herring, and sardines, and some green leafy veggies, such as purslane and kale in tiny amounts.

The saturated fat story is interesting here: as a dietitian, I was taught that saturated fat caused blood cholesterol to rise and lead to heart disease. Now that we have spent a couple of decades researching the link, it is not as clearcut as we used to think.[20,21] So perhaps there is a link between saturated fat and inflammation? It certainly looks like it at this point. Saturated fats are thought to activate inflammation via those toll-like receptors by feeding the bacterial production of lipopolysaccharides (LPS).[12,17,18,22,23]

In the literature, it has been proposed that palmitic acid (a saturated fatty acid found in meat and dairy) also triggers pro-inflammatory pathways directly, but it remains to be proven unequivocably.[12,19] So a diet too high in saturated animal fats might not have a direct link to heart disease, but if you look at chronic disease as being the sum of a number of risk factors (as you should), then saturated animal fats contribute to the risk profile via inflammation and increased cholesterol levels in the blood.

A simple way to look at your chronic disease risk is this: think of your healing capacity as a glass. Genetically, some of us get bigger or smaller glasses than others. Into the glass, you pour all the risks and disease promoters in your life, such as stress, saturated fats, nutrient-poor foods, or a beer belly. For each beneficial habit you engage in, such as stress relief, exercise, or eating your veggies, you can pour a little out. It would be better not to have to engage in this seesaw, but as long as your healing capacity is not overwhelmed, you will be okay. Now, as your glass gets older, crud might build up at the bottom or the top might start chipping away, representing a decreased ability to deal with the insults as time goes on. Over the course of your (hopefully long) life, should you fill your cup faster than you empty it, the cup runneth over and chronic disease results.

By now it should be quite clear that targeting inflammation with an anti-inflammatory diet is not about an overnight cure for disease. It is simply about removing those habits that will fill your cup too quickly and applying plenty of nourishment to help keep your cup from filling again. Nothing about this dietary approach is magic, although healthy eating can feel magical as you let go of poor habits and start to feel amazing. Targeting low-grade inflammation is working at a basic level to remove insults to your body's defense mechanisms, so it can rest and repair and operate as nature intended: strong, healing, and resilient.

Beyond the Belly: Living La Vida Inflammation

Between the fat on our belly, the bacteria underneath our belly, and the food that gets into our belly, there are plenty of inflammatory land mines to navigate. But wait! That's not all! There are plenty of lifestyle and environmental triggers for inflammation that, while not the focus of the book, are worth mentioning as they play a role. If you suspect other lifestyle and environmental factors are contributing to dis-ease for you, take the time to learn more about them and take steps to correct what you can with the professionals and guides that know those realms best.

Stressed to Your Core

Chronic stress is the price of admission to our fast-paced lives. The story here echoes that of inflammation: it is a good thing to have a stress response when you have to run away from a tiger or a purse-snatcher. Unfortunately, our bodies think that we live with virtual tigers every day, in the form of an alarm clock, traffic, catty coworkers, deadlines, and family shouting matches. So the stress response doesn't dissipate and our bodies get broken down in the process.

As I mentioned in Chapter 3, this is of vital importance in digestive health, as stress can physically alter digestive tract function and influence the balance of healthy bacteria in the digestive tract. These alterations can lead to, or exacerbate, chronic inflammation at the gut's edge. In the research, stress has been linked to chronic reflux, ulcers, irritable bowel syndrome and flare-ups, and even incidence of inflammatory bowel disease. While eliminating stress seems possible only for those no longer living, how you interpret and respond to stress is critical in maintaining a healthy digestive tract and reducing inflammation in the body.

Chill Out! Realistic and Practical Approaches to Stress Management

The only person without stress in his or her life is resting in a pine box! While certain stressors can be minimized with conscious life choices, effective stress management is truly the path forward to better physical and mental health. I am not an expert in stress management, so what I share is through my own experiences. I lead a fairly high-paced life with career, travel, and family; however, the amount of stress and my ability to manage it has ranged anywhere from cakewalk to five-alarm fire. The following is a list of stress management techniques that have worked for me at different times in my life and in response to varying stressors.

1. **Spend time outside.** If you live close to something beautiful—a beach, park, mountains, gardens—go there. Leave the phone and the kids at home. Take something to sip, and just sit and be in nature. Fifteen minutes is great, but the more time you can spend, the better.

2. **Have a dance break**. Put on whatever song is making you smile right now; crank it up (watch your hearing if you are using ear buds!) and dance like crazy. This obviously doesn't work well if you don't have a private office. However, you could institute office-wide dance breaks so everyone is shaking a tail feather. Then coworkers will be laughing with you . . . instead of at you.

3. **Honor your inner intro/extrovert:** If you are an introvert like me, time alone recharges your batteries. Lock yourself in the bathroom and have a bath, go for a walk or run, or take a scenic drive. If you are an extrovert, call up a friend or go out with someone who brings you joy.

4. **Breathe deeply.** There are various meditative breathing techniques out there, but one that everyone can do, anywhere, without feeling silly is called square breathing.

   Here is how you do it: Sit comfortably, close your eyes, and breathe in for four counts, hold the breath in for four counts, exhale for four counts, and hold for four counts. Try and do a few rounds of this whenever stress takes hold; it is easy to do several times a day if need be.

5. **Try yoga.** For me, yoga has always been a go-to for managing stress in my life because it combines physical activity, me time, meditative movement, and breath all at once. I cannot recommend it enough and if you have been wary of trying yoga because it is too new age, expensive, or intimidating, I highly recommend seeking out yoga DVDs and online videos by Tara Stiles,

who has a very inclusive, modern approach that is easy to connect with. You can do yoga in the comfort of your own home, so no intimidation!

6. **Sweat.** There is nothing better than a heart-pumping workout to blast the cobwebs out of your brain. Everyone can find time to work out three times a week; it is just a matter of shifting priorities.

7. **Indulge in a favorite hobby.** You know that hobby you had when you were younger that you gave up? If you allowed yourself the time to indulge in a hobby, you would probably feel a lot less stressed than you do now. I love to cook and I love to read; doing either calms me down and makes me feel in control and happy.

8. **Try meditation.** Meditation doesn't have to involve chanting or complicated techniques; meditation is simply bringing one's attention to the present moment. Try Googling "simple mindfulness meditation practice" and see what pops up. The more you practice, the more it will bring you a sense of calm.

> **Want to get started right away?** Set a timer for five minutes and sit comfortably for this basic meditation: close your eyes and simply focus on the sound and sensation of breathing. Focus all your attention on your breath, and when thoughts come, let them go. You don't have to worry about not thinking—just don't get attached to the thoughts that come.

> Pay attention to your inhales and exhales; where does the breath go? Use your awareness to watch it. You are not trying to clear your mind; simply remove attachment to thoughts, allow them to wash over you, and focus on the breath. There! You just meditated for the first time. It might not have felt like much, but as you practice, you will be able to go deeper into the process.

9. **Sleep.** Sleep is reparative; the more stressed out you are, the more you need to sleep. And a cozy bed will provide the comfort that you might have normally sought out in a bag of potato chips. Sleep is healthier.

10. **Start saying no.** I have the disease of yes, and many times, my current stress level and workload are a direct result of taking on too much. Then I start making mistakes, and that stresses me out even more. Start saying no; it's good stress prevention.

11. **Spend time with family and friends.** No matter how busy you are, you need to carve out time in each day to have real quality time with your family or friends. The stronger those bonds are, the happier you will feel, and the more you will feel you can reach out when you need help. Use your commute to connect (hands free) with friends; institute a no-device rule during dinner for some family quality time.

Environmental Attack

The air we breathe can also lead to chronic inflammation. Both carbon dioxide and air pollution have been linked to chronic inflammation; lighting a cigarette is akin to lighting the fire of inflammation.[24] Smoking is toxic to the body, and the inflammatory fallout confirms it: smokers also have higher levels of the pro-inflammatory signals, such as TNF-α.[2,24] This is one inflammatory insult that is just too large and too chronic to ignore. If you smoke, make plans to quit, and perhaps focus your energy on smoking cessation instead of dieting for now. If you live in a polluted area or on a busy thoroughfare, consider investing in air purifiers for your bedroom to clear pollution particulates out of the air as you sleep. And don't add to internal air pollution by filling the house with chemicals! Choose more natural cleaning products to keep your house safer.

Inactivity

Sometimes, it's what you're not doing that makes the difference. Exercise exerts a positive stress on the body that improves its functioning and helps you to manage psychological stressors to boot. Inactivity is also an independent promoter of inflammation.[24] Our incredibly sedentary lifestyles further promote inflammation by encouraging weight gain and poor food choices.

Exercise doesn't have to be expensive, complicated, or even take a long time. Getting your sweat on for just twenty minutes a day is better than nothing, particularly if you can be consistent with it. Walking, running, swimming, and doing exercises with videos you find online are all low or no cost ways to get active on your schedule.

Rest and Repair

Sleep is when the body repairs itself: stress hormones are metabolized and the body heals. However, we tend to place sleep below Facebook and HBO on our priority list. And for all those parents out there, there is usually not much you can do about sleepless nights when a child is the source—I have a preschooler, and I still get woken up at dawn on a regular basis. For those of you without pint-sized alarm clocks, sleep needs to move back to a priority. Lack of quality sleep is an independent promoter of inflammation;[14] try to get at least seven hours of sleep per night. The dishes can wait.

Can't Sleep? Maybe it's Your (Sleep) Hygiene!

Modern life is almost designed to toy with your sleep patterns . . . here are a few ways to ensure a better night's sleep.

1. Turn off all screens for one hour before bedtime.
2. Have a very dark, quiet room. Buy heavy black out curtains if you live on a busy and bright street. Close the windows if there is too much noise from outside.
3. Go to bed at the same time and wake up at the same time. Easy to say, hard to do, but your body loves routine and will thank you for it.
4. Cut out caffeine after noon. The half-life of caffeine is six hours, so that venti Americano you drank at 10 a.m. is still one-fourth in your system at 10 p.m. Ironically, the more caffeine messes with your sleep habits, the more you need caffeine to get you through the next day. Vicious cycle.
5. Watch the alcohol. While a bit can make you feel drowsy, alcohol actually messes with your sleep patterns.

An Ounce of Prevention . . .

So now that we know how inflammation is formed in the body, we need to revisit what the end result of chronic inflammation might be. When inflammation comes home to roost, chronic disease doesn't fall too far behind. Most chronic conditions are what we call multi-factorial, meaning that a wide array of genetic, environmental, and lifestyle factors all combine to fill up your cup toward an overflow of disease.

Chronic inflammation is your new target, to be squashed by flooding your body with nutrient-dense whole foods. The goal is to prevent, improve, or potentially heal chronic conditions that are associated with inflammation, including:

—Skin disorders: psoriasis, eczema, acne, rosacea

—Autoimmune conditions: rheumatoid arthritis, lupus, celiac disease

—Digestive disorders: inflammatory bowel disease, irritable bowel syndrome

—Chronic lifestyle diseases: cancer, cardiovascular disease, type 2 diabetes, stroke, Alzheimer's

It makes good sense that if we want to live a prevention-focused lifestyle, we need to set our sights on eliminating chronic inflammation before the damage is irreversible. We have talked about all the inflammatory pressures on our miraculous bodies, and now we are going to focus on all of the edible anti-inflammatory balms that are available to us to help cool down, soothe, and heal.

Dousing the Flames

The trouble with inflammation is that it takes a great deal of energy in the body; it creates major fallout in our cells and tissues to the point where it promotes chronic disease, and unfortunately, modern life seems designed to build a big old bonfire of inflammation. What is amazing, though, is that we can actually eat in a way that discourages inflammation. Regardless of the initial cause of chronic inflammation, many of the damaging pathways of inflammation are similar—providing an opportunity to target those pathways with the food we eat.[3]

Here is where eating to live and eating to live your best life diverge. Sure, we'll survive for fifty years eating fast food—a testament to our bodies' remarkable ability to clean up the garbage we throw at it. Eventually though, our bodies' repair mechanisms get spent; as our healing processes burn out, so do we. However, we can live longer and healthier lives by opting out of the hyper-processed food world and getting back to what nature intended for us to eat. All the research leads back to a simple place: a largely plant-based diet.

Would you rather spend the last half of your life in declining health or just the last few years? What is most surprising to me is that we have accepted how bad we feel because it is so common. There are twenty-one-year-olds that huff and puff walking up a single flight of stairs. Fifty-year-olds on six different medications after two surgeries. Thirty-five-year-olds who should own stock in antacid companies because they use so many of them. We see evidence of dis-ease everywhere, so much so that we think this is the normal state of affairs. It's not normal—but it is common. Common and normal aren't the same thing.

If your idea of a good life is forty or so decent years followed by a forty year decline in energy, constantly sick, propped up by pills, and hardened by disuse . . . maybe this book isn't for you. Do you want seventy-five or eighty good years? Years when the only pill you might pop is an occasional aspirin because you are out there on the slopes shredding it at sixty? Where you wake up happy and raring to go? If this sounds good to you, it's time to embrace an anti-inflammatory eating plan.

So let's talk about which foods ease inflammation and which supplements might be of help to you in your journey to vibrant health. Remember that too much meat and dairy, overprocessed carbohydrate foods, and poor-quality vegetable oils are your primary aggressors in the inflammation tug of war.

What follows is a brief overview of an anti-inflammatory diet, then in the upcoming chapters, we will visit my top anti-inflammatory foods and describe four practical and detailed approaches to creating an anti-inflammatory eating plan that works for you.

Feast on Anti-Inflammatory Foods

What to eat on an anti-inflammatory eating plan? Plenty of plants! Read on for the anti-inflammatory basics, and if you feel it is light-years away from how you are eating now, don't worry. One whole chapter of the book is devoted to transforming your diet into a more anti-inflammatory one, slowly and painlessly, without deprivation. It's a good route to take as you explore new foods and have fun in the kitchen.

Focus on Fruits and Vegetables

The most important foods you can eat to become healthier right away are fruits and vegetables. Now that you have seen the remarkable ways that food can affect our bodies, you are more likely to appreciate the truly medicinal qualities of fresh produce. Fruits and vegetables come charged with anti-inflammatory nutrients with none of the pro-inflammatory substances common in processed foods. The more you base your meals on produce, the healthier you will be.

Fruits and vegetables contain antioxidant vitamins A, C, and E; the connection to inflammation is thought to be the prevention of oxidative tissue damage that would otherwise require an inflammatory response.[3,25,26] Carotenoids, such as lycopene in red fruits and veggies, beta-carotene in orange and yellow fruits and veggies, and lutein in yellow and green veggies, are all thought to be anti-inflammatory molecules in their own right.[3]

Flavonoids are another group of anti-inflammatory phytochemicals that make eating your fruits and veggies so powerful. This group includes the quercetin in onions, apigenin in celery, and catechins in tea.[3] In essence, eat lots of fresh plant foods, and your cells will be bathed in delicious anti-inflammatory medicine!

Don't get caught up in a nutritionism mindset and go looking for supplemental forms of these anti-inflammatory marvels. Real food is still the best bet for accessing these important phytochemicals, as the research on supplemental forms can produce some surprising results, such as the potential for pro-inflammatory responses to supplemental vitamin E.[3,26] We are not at the point where we understand how best to maximize the efficacy of most antioxidants in a supplemental form. Food provides these potent compounds in naturally designed dosages and in the right biological context . . . which as the research progresses, we may fully understand the wisdom of nature's medicine delivery systems!

Anti-Inflammatory Proteins

Legumes are an important part of the anti-inflammatory diet. A great source of plant protein, fiber for a healthy digestive tract, and slowly released carbohydrates, they also contain a host of anti-inflammatory nutrients. If you are on a gluten-free diet or are choosing to eat fewer grains, legumes can be an excellent and nutritious stand in. Organic tofu and tempeh fit into this category, too, as great plant-based protein options to help keep blood sugars stable and energy levels up. Fish and seafood are the only nonplant proteins recommended on an anti-inflammatory diet, as they don't contain the saturated and omega-6 fats that farmed animals do. Fish are either low in fat or rich in anti-inflammatory omega-3 fatty acids. Sustainability issues do exist with seafood, so look to programs, such as Seafood Watch or Ocean Wise, to help you make better choices for your health and the environment. You can find information on both in the resources section of this book, and both have smart phone apps that help you make shopping choices on the go.

Intact Grains

As we discussed in the section on carbohydrates, grains themselves are not considered to be pro-inflammatory; on the contrary, a diet that includes unprocessed grains is anti-inflammatory! I have to distinguish intact grains from whole grain foods. The healthiest form of a grain is the one that looks similar to what gets picked right off the plant: quinoa, wheat or rye berries, whole buckwheat, steel-cut oats, and the like. Sprouted grain breads and tortillas are also a good choice, as they are made with the intact grain instead of fluffy, blood sugar spiking flour. Pasta is also an acceptable choice on the anti-inflammatory diet, which may surprise you; however, when cooked al dente, it has a moderate effect on blood sugar—keeping inflammation at bay. Choosing 100 percent whole wheat, einkorn, spelt, brown rice, or quinoa pastas makes it even better.

Healthy Fats, Whole Food Preferred

You don't need to fear fat; it is the type of fat that you choose that matters most for good health. Choosing whole food sources of fats—avocados, olives, nuts, and seeds—have the added benefit of being filling in addition to being good for you. Cooking oils and fats, such as extra virgin olive oil, are part of a healthy diet, but they are easy to overdo. Stick to about a teaspoon of fat for each serving of food you prepare, and instead focus on whole foods rich in healthy fats. Avocados are a delicious substitute for butter and mayo on sandwiches and provide fiber, vitamin E, folate, lutein, and zeaxanthin. Olives make a great snack . . . just watch the salt! Nuts and seeds are super nourishing foods in such a tiny package! Fiber, minerals, and omega-3 fats are the stars here. Nuts and seeds also stand in for less healthy snack foods and add texture, flavor, and nutrition to your daily diet.

Fermented Foods

Since such a big part of an anti-inflammatory plan is promoting digestive health and a healthy community of bacteria, I highly recommend eating fermented foods daily. Most cultures have a fermented food that is a daily staple, and most supermarkets have at least one of these options. Health food stores are fermented food gold mines! You can choose from kefir, kombucha, kimchi, traditionally fermented sauerkraut, miso, and apple cider vinegar. If these foods are new to you, I have made recommendations and listed brands and online resources to help you find them. Your grandmother might have a recipe for something fermented, too . . . just ask! Most yogurts on the store shelves are little more than health-washed desserts; however, if you make plain yogurt at home or know of a good local brand of traditionally made organic yogurt, give that a go, too.

Supplements

As a dietitian, I am a food first kind of gal. For the most part, whatever your body requires has been provided by nature, and if you eat a good diet you will be getting what you need. I know that others may refute that statement, but I think that the case can be made that our nutrient deficiencies are largely a result of our deficient diets, not a reduction in the nutrient value of normal healthy foods, such as broccoli (although there is some interesting research on that question).[27,28]

However, there are some supplements that are helpful when targeting specific concerns, such as inflammation, and others that are excellent when bridging the gap between a not so great diet and the amazing diet you will have once you have given yourself time to adapt and progress. I recommend you talk with your health provider before adopting a supplement regime; even quality, healthy supplements can cause issues if they interact with a medication or a chronic condition.

Nutrition Insurance

The first step if you are starting out with a hyper-processed and inflammatory diet is a multivitamin. Dead, hyper-processed food has little nutrition to speak of, so it is worth covering some bases with a multivitamin. I prefer a multivitamin to single nutrients, as it is easy to go overboard on single nutrients, such as B vitamins or zinc, when supplementing without a dietitian or physician guiding you.

Men need a multi without iron, and once you feel your diet is getting up to snuff, a multi is optional. For women of childbearing age (not just those planning a pregnancy because there are plenty of oops! moments), a basic multivitamin is an easy way of getting the iron and folate you need daily for a healthy infant should the time come. Ensure that there is 400 micrograms of folic acid in your multi, and you are good to go. In my resources section, I list my picks for good quality supplements that should be available in your local health food store.

Next on the anti-inflammatory shelf are my three basic daily supplements for pretty much every man, woman, and child: omega-3 fats, vitamin D, and probiotics.

Powerful Oils

Omega-3 fats are helpful if you are not eating fish on a regular basis or don't eat fish at all. I think it is important to load your diet with daily plant sources of omega-3 ALA, such as hemp seeds, chia seeds, ground flax, pumpkin seeds, and walnuts, but I feel strongly that the benefits of long chain omega-3s, such as DHA and EPA, are important enough to supplement.[29-33] EPA and DHA are precursors to substances that oppose inflammation in the body, such as select eicosanoids, resolvins, and protectins; EPA and DHA also have the ability to block the formation of pro-inflammatory cytokines. [31,32]

I recommend, fish eater or not, a plant-based DHA supplement, as they are a more environmentally sound choice. Contrary to popular belief, there really aren't that many fish in the sea; to me, it makes more sense to honor that gift by moderate food consumption of fish—not industrial use of fish stocks. If you do choose to use a fish source, ensure that you are using one made with small fish, such as sardines and herring, instead of larger fish—don't use cod or salmon oils unless the company is committed to sustainable practices that you can verify by third-party certification. Some fish oils are made from flesh that would otherwise be wasted, thereby reducing food waste instead of consuming more valuable fish stocks.

My recommendation is one to three grams of omega-3 oil daily, providing at least two hundred milligrams of DHA (and four hundred milligrams of EPA if taking a fish oil supplement). Check the label to make sure you are getting the right dosage of the active ingredient. Less expensive oils will often provide less EPA and DHA; you will have to take more to get the same active dose. If you eat an omega-3-rich fish three times a week, feel free to skip the supplement. Note that if you are on medications to thin the blood, EPA and DHA can have an additive effect. Discuss your dose with your doctor.

The Sunshine Vitamin

Vitamin D is one of my nonnegotiable supplements. The reason for this is because you can't actually get the vitamin D you need from food; we have evolved to create vitamin D in our skin upon UV exposure, and the natural food supply contains little vitamin D. Milk is fortified at 100 IU per cup; drinking enough milk to get your daily dosage would not be in line with an anti-inflammatory eating plan. Wild salmon is one exception, but we can't rely on daily salmon for our vitamin D. It's just not sustainable.

While we know vitamin D is a bone-builder, the last twenty years of research has shown it to be a whole lot more.[34] Vitamin D is has the ability to modulate the immune system and oppose inflammation in the body.[34] My recommendation is 1000 IU of vitamin D3 in the summer, and 2000 IU of vitamin D3 in the winter. This is a modest but still active dose that is safe for lifelong use and within the upper limits set by the Institute of Medicine.[35] There are conditions where higher dosages of vitamin D3 are advised, but I recommend using them under the supervision of your physician or dietitian, ideally beginning with having your vitamin D levels checked with a simple blood test so you can track how effective your dose is.

Better Bugs

Probiotics are my other nonnegotiable. From all we have learned about the role that healthy bacteria play in better digestion, immune defense, and inflammation, it makes perfect sense to add a probiotic to the mix.

Probiotics are the most perplexing supplement to purchase, because unlike omega-3s or vitamin D, they are not chemically identified, inert substances. Each probiotic bacterial strain is unique and has unique therapeutic properties; making choosing a product complex. You want to ensure that you are buying a good-quality product; otherwise, you could be literally wasting your money on dead bacteria.

Probiotics have the potential to influence inflammation in a multitude of ways: from improving the bacterial community and enhancing gut barrier function to direct modulation of the immune response.[3] Fermented foods provide the innocent bystanders that your digestive tract needs; supplemental probiotics are the Special Forces with the power to keep the peace.

I have provided a probiotics recommendation in the resources section, but I encourage you to do your own research and find the one that is right for you. Take a high-quality probiotic daily in addition to the fermented foods I recommend. Here is what to look for when you are reviewing probiotics online or at the store.

1. A potency of at least ten billion CFU guaranteed until the expiry date. You don't want to spend money on a dosage too low to have a strong impact—kind of like sending a fancy sail boat to defend a coastline against a fleet of war ships! Also, you want a clearly marked expiry date so you aren't buying a product that was effective three months ago.

2. If there are multiple strains in the product, you need to know that they work well together—fermenting them together is a good way to judge this. This also follows the wisdom of traditional fermented foods. Why? We take probiotics because they are bacterial gladiators, able to fight off other bacteria, and help protect your digestive community. If you sprinkle eight bacteria together in a product without fermenting them together and testing it, those bacteria might be killing each other off or simply be useless!

3. A product that has been clinically tested to be effective, as opposed to research-proven strains. What is the difference? It is pretty huge . . . let me explain. There are certain strains of bacteria that have hundreds of research studies to support their efficacy; that makes them pretty popular for manufacturers. The trouble with that is that there are multiple suppliers and products available that may not have been produced as carefully, in the right type of formulation, or at the proper dosages that the research studies have proven effective. So in theory the strain is effective, but the product produced from it actually isn't.

Instead, a retail product that has been clinically tested in humans means that the same product you buy has been put to the test—ensuring you are getting what the research says you are paying for. Every product says it's clinically proven or research-based. . . if it truly is, you can actually find the research on their website. There are a handful of retail products that have actually been tested on humans; choose one of those.

Natural Medicines for Inflammation

Now that we have our basics—multi, omega-3, vitamin D, and probiotics—we can turn to natural therapies to help battle inflammation when and if you need them. A good diet is your first defense against inflammation; natural medicines provide fine-tuning when it is called for. Popular natural remedies for inflammation and gut healing include L-glutamine, Zyflamend, Pycnogenol, boswellia, Recovery, and bromelain. Some of these remedies are more effective than others and are worth researching on quality resources, such as www.medline.gov or www.pubmed.gov.

You don't necessarily need the extra boost that natural medicines provide; I recommend going ahead with dietary strategies first and turning to natural medicines when your condition dictates a stronger approach, preferably in communication with your integrative practitioner—be it a dietitian, physician, or naturopath—who is well-versed in, and supportive of, natural remedies.

Can't Take the Heat? Time to Transform the Kitchen!

—Chronic, low-grade inflammation is a chronic threat to feeling good now and staying disease-free later.

—The food we eat, stress we're under, air we breathe, and couch surfing we do can all stoke the fires of inflammation.

—Keeping our digestive tract in tip-top shape with plenty of plant foods and healthy bacteria can moderate much of the inflammatory pressures in our system.

—Choosing unprocessed plant foods most of the time will provide the body with the building blocks of an anti-inflammatory defense system.

—Create a basic anti-inflammatory supplement kit that meets your unique needs, but don't overdo it; spending two hundred dollars on supplements won't help much if you are on a steady diet of drive-through meals.

CHAPTER 6

STOCK YOUR ANTI-INFLAMMATORY ARSENAL DELICIOUSLY

"Leave your drugs in the chemist's pot if you can heal the patient with food."
—Hippocrates

I feel like we just climbed a nutritional mountain over the past five chapters, and you might be feeling a little weary of talk of nutrition. My hope is that you now understand why it is so important to eat an anti-inflammatory diet, because it can be hard to muster the strength to swim upstream against the strong current of our junk food culture. If you don't know what wonderful rewards lay ahead, it would be easy to just give up every time a bag of Doritos calls your name.

So let's get on with how to eat and what to eat—the fun stuff. To get you inspired on your healthy eating journey, I have chosen twenty-five of my top anti-inflammatory foods for you to experiment with and enjoy on a regular basis. No fuss, no muss, no strict regimes if you don't want them—just a bit of inspiration to get you choosing healthier foods. For each food, I will tell you a bit about why it is special and give you some simple ideas for incorporating it into your daily eating plan. That way, you can enjoy playing with healthy eating while you read on about how to make anti-inflammatory living a life-long reality.

The anti-inflammatory picks in this chapter are truly nourishing foods; have fun and try to incorporate at least a few into your daily regime. No one of these foods is intended to cure—food is incremental daily medicine. Crafting a diet built of these foods with research-proven medicinal benefits will create healing over time; next week, you might feel a little more energetic. Next month, a little lighter and more at ease. Over months or perhaps a year, true healing is possible.

One of the easiest ways to un-junk your diet is to focus on simply adding in more nutrient-dense foods; as they become a part of how you eat, less healthful habits will float away. So start eating some great food now without assigning any particular structure or rule to it—just enjoy it! Part two of this book will provide further guidance on eating strategies and meal plans that make the most of these foods and help you build a truly anti-inflammatory eating plan.

Berries and Cherries

Berries and cherries are standouts for many reasons: they won't spike blood sugars like tropical fruits can, they are fiber-rich, and they are filled with anti-inflammatory plant compounds. They are also crazy delicious! Berries contain anthocyanins, which are plant pigments known to help fight off oxidative damage that can incite an inflammatory response.[1] While anthocyanins aren't readily absorbed across the gut, we now know that gut bacteria metabolize anthocyanins and could potentially be the missing link to their positive effects on the human body.[2] Eating berries regularly is thought to help reduce inflammation, improve vision[3] and brain function,[4] protect the heart,[5] and prevent cancer formation.[6] Raspberries are one of the richest fruit sources of fiber at eight-and-a-half grams per cup. Strawberries contain small amounts of salicylic acid, a natural anti-inflammatory. Berries also contain ellagic acid, an anti-inflammatory compound that supports the natural cleansing pathways in liver. Tart cherries, loaded with anthocyanins, have been a popular folk remedy for inflammation. Eat berries raw, frozen, or even cooked; try to buy organic when they are available and affordable.

Easy ways to enjoy: Make a smoothie, eat as a snack, toss on cereal or salads, coat in dark chocolate as a dessert, cook down for a yogurt or pancake topping.

Turmeric

This golden-hued cousin of ginger is a remarkable anti-inflammatory food worth consuming daily. Turmeric gives curry powder and mustard their signature color thanks to its main medicinal component, curcumin. Curcumin is thought to help prevent oxidative damage and calm inflammation directly through inhibition of pro-inflammatory cytokines, such as NFKB.[7,8] Curcumin has been linked to cancer prevention, Alzheimer's disease prevention, and provides relief in inflammatory bowel disease and rheumatoid arthritis.[7,8,9] Turmeric also supports heart health and liver function.[8] Turmeric can be found as a dried spice or fresh rhizome, and it has a peppery, somewhat bitter flavor, so a little goes a long way. Again, bioavailability of curcumin is somewhat limited; to improve effectiveness, pair with black pepper whenever possible—pepper contains a molecule called piperine that helps with bioavailability.[8,9]

Easy ways to enjoy: Stir one teaspoon ground turmeric into soups and sauces or a half-teaspoon into smoothies, finely chop fresh turmeric and add at the end of cooking to stir-fries and stews, grate fresh turmeric into a smoothie or a salad dressing, or use as a golden-hued marinade for chicken.

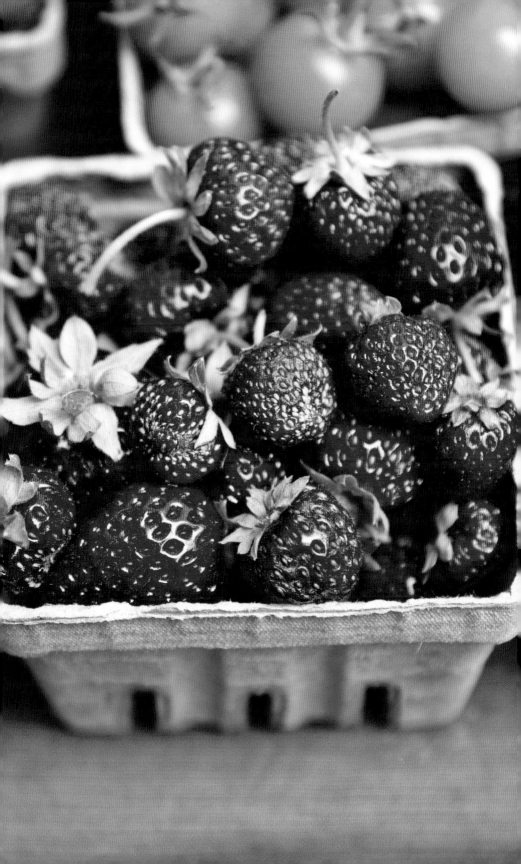

Tomatoes

What's not to love about luscious, ruby red tomatoes? Tomatoes are a low-glycemic fruit choice that are incredibly rich in beneficial plant compounds. Lycopene is really the star here; lycopene is a potent antioxidant and anti-inflammatory compound that is thought to protect prostate health, prevent UV damage in the skin, and support heart health.[10] Tomatoes also contain naringenin, lutein, and zeaxanthin, which also oppose inflammation. Tomatoes are one of those rare foods that get even more nutritious when cooked. Be sure to enjoy tomatoes with a little extra virgin olive oil; lycopene bioavailability goes up with the addition of fat.

Easy ways to enjoy: Chop fresh, in season tomatoes into salads or slice on sandwiches, add tomato paste to marinades, soups, and casseroles, slow roast tomatoes and garlic and toss with pasta, or whip up a gazpacho in your blender.

Ginger

Eating ginger is like fighting fire with fire—this spicy rhizome is a potent anti-inflammatory, just like its cousin, turmeric. Great for digestive distress, ginger has been traditionally used to expel gas from the bowel and soothe nausea and intestinal contractions. The gingerols found in ginger are potent anti-inflammatory agents, which inhibit pro-inflammatory cytokines; ginger has been studied for pain relief in arthritis[11] and cancer prevention.[12,13] Choose the fresh rhizome over the dried spice, and more often than pickled or candied varieties.

Easy ways to enjoy: Grate fresh ginger into stir fries, fruit pies, and smoothies, eat candied ginger after a meal or bake into muffins, enjoy pickled ginger with sushi or in sandwiches, and to boil fresh ginger with lemon and enjoy as a tea with honey.

Oily Cold Water Fish

This is the mother lode of anti-inflammatory, long chain omega-3 fatty acids DHA and EPA. Wild salmon, mackerel, herring, sardines, barramundi, and sablefish, or black cod, all have impressive amounts of omega-3 fats, and if you eat fish, it is worth adding these fish to your diet one to three times a week if you can. DHA and EPA are considered potent anti-inflammatory fatty acids thought to be protective in cancer[14,15] and heart disease.[16] EPA and DHA also

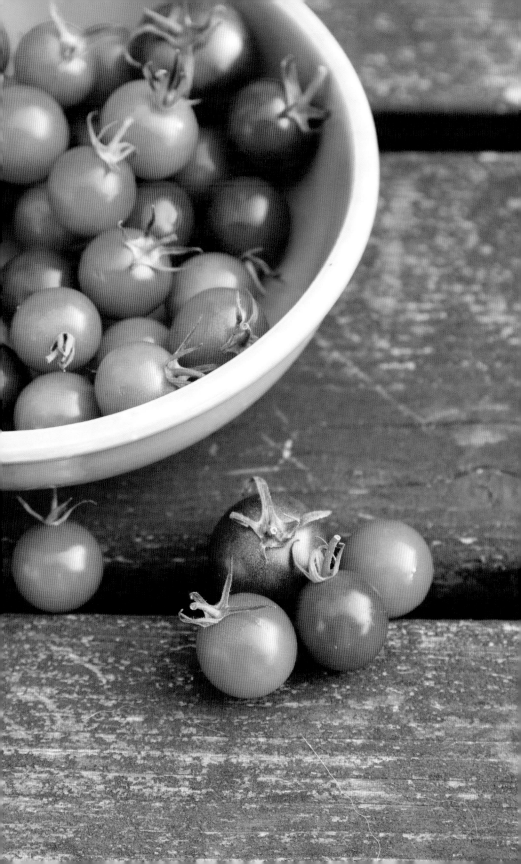

play a role in a healthy brain[17] and mood support,[18] in addition to easing inflammatory disorders, such as arthritis.[19,20] Fish are also a great source of anti-inflammatory protein, and salmon contains a superstar antioxidant called astaxanthin. Because of the sustainability issues surrounding fish stocks, choose only sustainably caught wild or eco-farmed fish.

Easy ways to enjoy: Add canned wild salmon to salads and sandwiches, grill fresh herring on the BBQ with a lemony marinade, broil salmon for fish tacos, or poach sablefish with wild mushrooms and edamame.

Living Fermented Foods

Belly, meet your makers! Living fermented foods need to be a daily part of your diet to help boost your level of commensal and potentially probiotic bacteria. These foods have been a part of traditional diets for millennia and their lack in the North American diet is contributing to our intestinal dis-ease. What are commensal bacteria? They are the friendly bacteria that do no harm but aren't necessarily therapeutic, either. Whether your fermented food contains probiotic bacteria (the therapeutic critters) depends on what you buy or whether you live in a lucky bacterial environment (if you are fermenting at home). Buy your fermented foods raw and unpasteurized to keep the bacteria intact.

Fermented foods are common to food cultures all over the world. Kefir is a Russian fermented milk drink, although water kefir and coconut kefir are now available. Ensure you are getting true kefir grain, as some commonly available kefirs are little more than drinkable yogurts and don't contain the unique yeast strains that true kefir does. Kefir should be slightly fizzy and have just a hint of a yeasty smell.

Kombucha is a wonderful fermented fizzy tea that is an energizing, low-sugar alternative to sodas and coffee drinks—I make it myself at home! Look for kombucha in stores or use a high-quality SCOBY, purchased from a reputable supplier, to start making some at home. Kimchi is a spicy, pungent pickle native to Korea that can be found in Asian food markets, miso is a fermented soy paste that hails from Japan, and sauerkraut is fermented cabbage native to Europe. Note that most commercial sauerkraut is pickled, not fermented, so read labels.

To save money, you can make most of these foods at home, but ensure that you practice good canning hygiene if you are going to be canning them for storage instead of eating them right away. Fermentation classes are becoming more popular and are a great place to start to ensure you are fermenting safely. The recipe section of this book includes a recipe for making your own kimchi, so you can get started on your fermented foods road trip!

Easy ways to enjoy: Sip kombucha instead of soda, add sauerkraut to sandwiches, swap kefir for yogurt in smoothies, and use miso for savory sauces, dressings, and gravies.

Green Tea

Green tea's claim to fame is flavonoid compounds called catechins, the most famous of which being EGCG, or epigallocatechin-3-gallate.[1] EGCG has been widely studied for its role in cancer prevention and has been shown in the research to stimulate the production of IL-10, an anti-inflammatory cytokine.[1] Green tea has less caffeine than coffee and contains an amino acid, L-theanine, which helps to oppose caffeine's effects in the body for alertness without the jitters.

Easy ways to enjoy: Brew up a batch of strong green tea and keep in the fridge for a zero-sugar alternative to plain water, use as a novel base for a smoothie or sorbet, or replace some or all of your daily coffee with green tea for a milder stimulant effect.

Extra Virgin Olive Oil

Extra virgin olive oil is the best everyday oil for your anti-inflammatory kitchen. Its primary fat is oleic acid, a monounsaturated fat that does not promote inflammation in the body. In fact, some research suggests that oleic acid, an omega-9 fatty acid, has the ability to oppose the pro-inflammatory effects of saturated fats in the body.[25,26] Unfiltered (cloudy) extra virgin olive oil is also rich in anti-inflammatory plant compounds. Use the unfiltered oils only for finishing and salads; don't cook with them. Standard supermarket extra virgin olive oils are safe for cooking at medium-high heat on the stove and in the oven.

Easy ways to enjoy: Create salad dressings with unfiltered olive oil, sauté with half to one teaspoon of extra virgin olive oil per recipe serving, dip bread into olive oil instead of spreading with butter, or mix 50 percent softened butter with 50 percent oil to make a healthier spread.

Mushrooms

Wild and cultivated mushrooms, neither plant nor animal, are remarkable wonder foods worth a place in your anti-inflammatory kitchen. Mushrooms contain polysaccharides (that's a fancy term for a multisugar compound) that are known to modulate immune function and help squelch inflammation, along with a vitamin D precursor called vitamin D1 that contributes to their success. Lentinan, a polysaccharide compound in shiitake mushrooms, appears to support both cancer prevention and treatment.[21,22,23,24] Other beta glucan compounds in shitakes and crimini mushrooms support the immune system and heart health, and criminis are also a rich source of the antioxidant mineral, selenium. Do not eat mushrooms raw; they are best cooked.

Easy ways to enjoy: Sauté crimini or wild mushrooms instead of white buttons in stir fries and casseroles, roast them to top pizza and burgers, use them in large amounts to replace half the ground meat in your pasta sauce, or stir them into pilafs and risottos

Cooking Greens—Kale, Chard, Collards, Beet Greens

Greens are the queens of the vegetable world, as they are incredibly nutrient-dense and an important part of your daily diet. Regular consumption of green veggies is associated with better health outcomes over time.[27] In addition to being high in a number of vitamins and minerals, including antioxidant vitamin A and anti-inflammatory vitamin K, leafy green veggies are also potent sources of anti-inflammatory phytochemicals. Glucosinolates in greens are converted by enzymes in the raw leaves or by human intestinal bacteria to isothiocyanates, known to regulate inflammation and help prevent cancer formation in the body.[27,28] Indole-3-carbinol and sulforaphane, two of the best studied isothiocyanates found in this group, have the ability to down-regulate inflammation.[27,28] In addition, anti-inflammatory kaempferol, lutein, and quercetin are also particularly rich in these greens.

Easy ways to enjoy: Swap baby kale for lettuce in salads, add kale leaves to green or berry smoothies, sauté chard with garlic and olive oil for a delicious side dish, use trimmed collard leaves to create sandwich wraps, or add steamed beet greens to casseroles and stews.

Super Salads

It is time to abandon basic lettuce for good and instead look to the remarkable benefits of super salad greens. Parsley is more than just garnish;

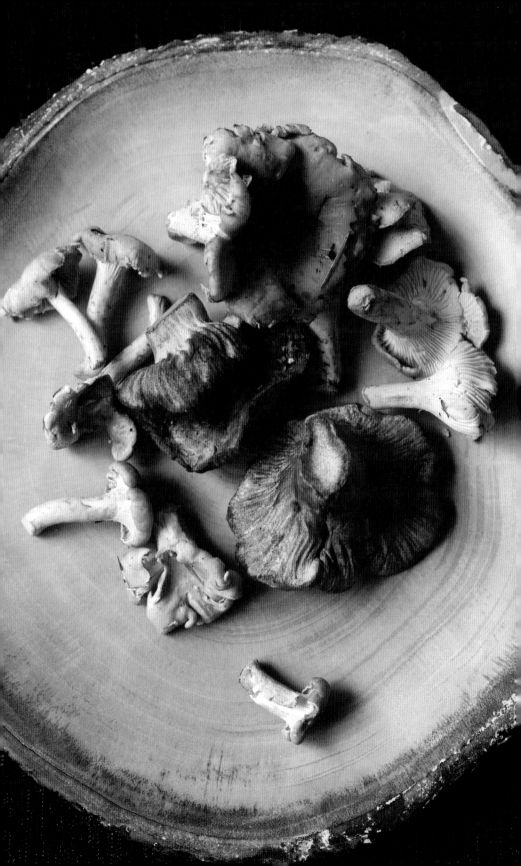

packed with anti-inflammatory chlorophyll, vitamin K, and flavonoids, it is worth putting more of this palate-cleansing green on your plate. Purslane and dandelion, otherwise known as weeds, are incredibly nutritious, too. Arugula is a green that has a peppery, slightly bitter flavor. All these greens contain chlorophyll, lutein, and zeaxanthin; purslane even contains omega-3 fatty acids.

Easy ways to enjoy: Toss in salads, sandwiches, smoothies, or blend into dips and pestos; mature purslane and dandelion leaves can be gently steamed if you wish.

Spinach

Spinach is well-known as a superfood and contains anti-inflammatory, bone-building, and immune-supporting vitamins K, A, and C. A relative of beets, spinach is also a source of betaine. Chlorophyll, the magnesium-rich pigment that gives spinach leaves their rich green color, is an anti-inflammatory force in its own right.[32] Rich in carotenoids, such as lutein and zeaxanthin, these compounds are both strong antioxidants and suppressors of pro-inflammatory pathways in body.[33]

Easy ways to enjoy: Toss baby spinach in salads or smoothies, add chopped wilted spinach to dips and casseroles, layer spinach in sandwiches, or sauté into pasta sauces.

Super Seeds

Everyone loves nuts because they are a convenient snack, but all too often, we forget about the remarkable power of seeds. Flax, chia, and hemp seeds all contain impressive amounts of omega-3 fatty acids, but each seed carries its own unique benefits. Ground flax is a source of lignans and flavonoids that also function as beneficial phytoestrogens; flax is also a great source of soluble and insoluble fiber. Chia seeds contain plenty of soluble fiber to soothe the digestive tract and keep blood sugars stable. Hemp seeds come packed with protein and lots of energizing manganese in addition to a special anti-inflammatory omega-6 fat called gamma linoleic acid (GLA).

Easy ways to enjoy: Sprinkle seeds on cereal, soups, or salads, add to smoothies, or bake into muffins, breads, and cereal bars.

Broccoli

Broccoli is one of the original superfoods; this bold member of the brassica family is filled with anti-inflammatory compounds, such as indole-3-carbinol and

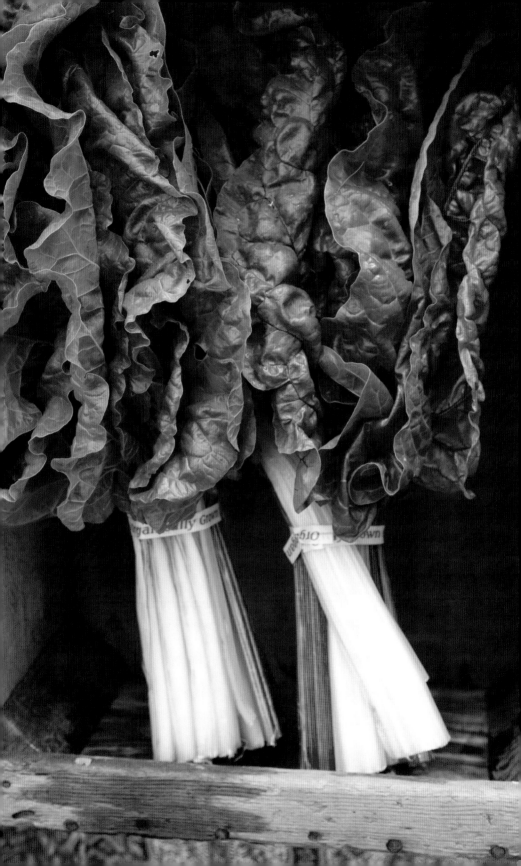

sulforaphane.[27,28] Sulforaphane appears to oppose inflammation in multiple ways, including blocking the pro-inflammatory effects of bacterial lipopolysaccharides.[34] For extra sulforaphane power, add broccoli sprouts into your broccoli rotation.

Easy ways to enjoy: Snack on raw broccoli, steam it as a side dish, toss it with pasta, add to stir fries, sautés, and casseroles, make a broccoli salad, or stuff sprouts into sandwiches and load onto salads.

Garlic

The sulfur compounds that give this earthly rose its stink are at the heart of its anti-inflammatory power. These compounds include alliin, 1,2-vinyldithiin, thiacremonone, and diallylsulfide.[35,36] Sulfur compounds have been shown to directly decrease inflammatory markers and cytokines[35,36] and are thought to be part of garlic's cancer-fighting power.[37] Crush garlic for best results, as these sulfur-containing compounds are transformed when precursor molecules are released from the cell walls.

Easy ways to enjoy: Add raw crushed garlic to dips and salad dressings, lightly sauté at the end of cooking in stir fries and vegetable dishes, or add garlic to soups and casseroles.

Beets

Sweet and jewel-toned, beets are an inexpensive and widely available ally in the inflammatory firefight. Both the root and the leaves are nutritious; the leaves share many of the same nutrients as the other cooking greens. The roots are incredibly nutrient-dense, containing a host of vitamins and minerals, including magnesium, manganese, and folate. However, there are a couple of unique anti-inflammatory treasures found in beets, too. Betalains, unique to beets and their relatives, chard and rhubarb, inhibit pro-inflammatory enzymes in the body.[29] Beets also contain betaine, which moderates inflammation via the nuclear factor kappa B (NF-κB) pathways, giving beets the potential to help slow cancer progression.[30,31]

Easy ways to enjoy: Grate beets into a slaw or salad, layer pickled beets into a sandwich or wrap, puree cooked beets with white beans and walnuts to make a nutritious dip, add chopped beets to smoothies, or roast for a delicious side dish.

Raw Nuts

Raw nuts help you win the inflammatory war in a few ways: packed with protein and healthy fats, they make a great low-glycemic substitute for

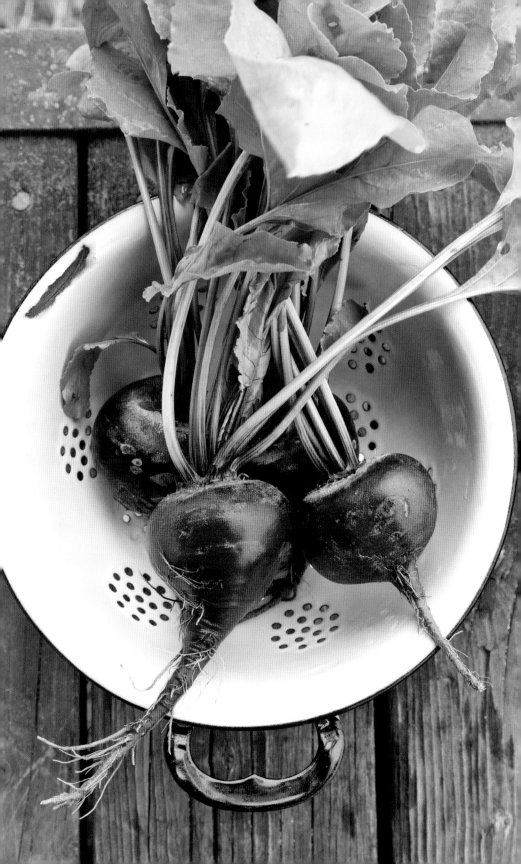

traditional pro-inflammatory snack foods. Nuts may assist with maintaining a healthy weight by keeping obesity-associated inflammation at bay.[38] Walnuts get a special mention because they are a source of anti-inflammatory omega-3 fatty acids. Choosing nuts raw helps preserve the integrity of their healthy fats.

Easy ways to enjoy: Snack on raw nuts on their own or with dried fruit, chop and add to salads or baking, use almond meal to replace some of the flour in recipes, use nut butters to spread, and blend soaked cashews to make a dairy-free cream substitute for dips and desserts.

Avocados

Avocados are luscious, creamy, and totally nutritious. Rich in anti-inflammatory oleic acid, avocados also boast four-and-a-half grams of fiber per half fruit. Avocados are a great option for replacing more inflammatory spreads for bread; the anti-inflammatory carotenoids lutein and zeaxanthin and catechins found in avocados bear their own potent benefits.

Easy ways to enjoy: Slice ripe avocado on whole grain toast as a snack, mash for a delicious dip or spread, slice into sandwiches, or whip as a creamy base for raw desserts.

Beans

Beans are a core component of an anti-inflammatory diet; they contain slowly digested carbohydrates and plant proteins for sustained energy and controlled blood sugars, in addition to cleansing fiber. The indigestible fibers support a healthy bacterial community and digestive tract. Black beans contain anti-inflammatory anthocyanin pigments, while chickpeas contain quercetin and kaempferol. Beans are also mineral-rich, providing valuable nutrition in plant-based diets. On their own or as part of a low-glycemic diet, beans have been found to lower inflammatory markers, such as IL-6 and TNF-α.[39,40]

Easy ways to enjoy: Roast chickpeas for a delicious snack, add rinsed canned beans to salads and soups to boost nutrition, mash white or black beans with your favorite seasonings for a delicious dip, add white beans to pasta dishes, or substitute lentils for ground meat in your favorite recipes.

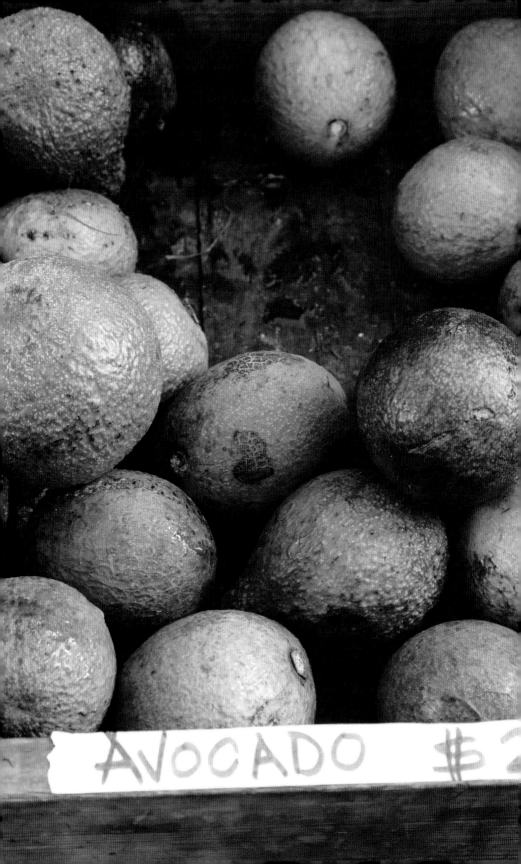

Cocoa

Chocolate is a tasty treat, but real cocoa is where the anti-inflammatory action is. Cocoa contains flavonoids that help moderate inflammatory pathways and lower inflammatory markers in the body.[41,42,43] Look for pure raw cacao beans, nibs, or powder, or non-Dutch process cocoa powder. Dutch processing can lower flavonoid levels. When enjoying chocolate, look for chocolate that is at least 80 percent cocoa solids for more cocoa power and less inflammatory sugar.

Easy ways to enjoy: Two squares of very dark chocolate make a satisfying anti-inflammatory treat, make your own hot cocoa with a nondairy milk and just a touch of honey, use cacao nibs in baking recipes, or use raw cacao powder to make delicious raw desserts.

Fresh Herbs

Don't think of herbs as seasoning . . . they are leafy green vegetables that just happen to be aromatic! Be generous with herbs, such as basil, dill, thyme, rosemary, and mint, as they contain plenty of health benefits. These herbs contain their own polyphenols, and many of them have anti-inflammatory effects related to their potent antioxidant potentials.

Easy ways to enjoy: Be generous when adding fresh herbs to soups, sauces, and stews, add basil and mint to salads, try mint in smoothies and sorbets, or add herbs to pestos.

Super Soluble Grains

Whole oats, steel-cut and thick-rolled oats, and whole barley are remarkable grains to add to an anti-inflammatory diet. In their least-processed forms, they are nutrient-dense and slowly digested for a moderate impact on blood sugars—contributing to an anti-inflammatory diet both directly and indirectly. The star here is the beta-glucan fiber that they contain, the same one found in shiitake mushrooms. These beta-glucans are an important anti-inflammatory soluble fiber that soothes the digestive tract and feeds the beneficial bacteria living there.[46] Beta-glucans also give these grains the amazing ability to lower cholesterol and keep blood sugar stable.[46] Eat these grains in their whole form, and you will see that a real whole grain is a thing to be appreciated.

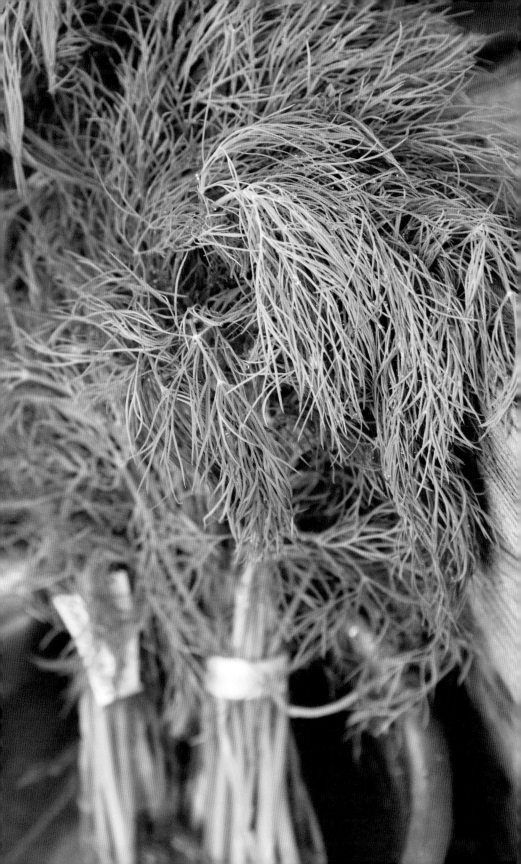

Easy ways to enjoy: Cook up oats for breakfast, use barley in risotto instead of rice, add whole oats or barley to soups or casseroles, or grind these grains into flour for a more nutritious alternative to all-purpose flour.

Sweet Potatoes

Potatoes get a bad rap; they certainly have a place in a healthy diet, but they don't quite measure up to the health appeal of sweet potatoes. The dark orange and purple varieties are great anti-inflammatory starches; in fact, anthocyanin pigments from purple sweet potatoes have been found to squelch inflammation caused by bacterial lipopolysaccharides (LPS) in an animal model.[49] Both purple and orange sweet potatoes have a more moderate impact on blood sugars than floury potatoes, such as russets, and they also contain greater levels of carotenoids.

Easy ways to enjoy: Boil, roast, or mash as a side dish, or use as a base for a low fat dip or in baking recipes.

Apples

An apple a day really does keep the doctor away! Eating apples has been associated in scientific literature with a lower risk of certain cancers, cardiovascular disease, and asthma.[44] These low-glycemic fruits contain soluble fiber to keep your gut healthy and anti-inflammatory and antioxidant compounds, such as quercetin, anthocyanins in red-skinned varieties, catechins, and chlorogenic acid.[45] The catechins in apples appear to be both antioxidants and directly anti-inflammatory; in one lab study, apple catechins were able to block the production of pro-inflammatory prostaglandins.[45]

Easy ways to enjoy: Eat raw as a snack, spread with nut butters, add to green smoothies, bake with cinnamon and walnuts for a healthy dessert, or chop into salads.

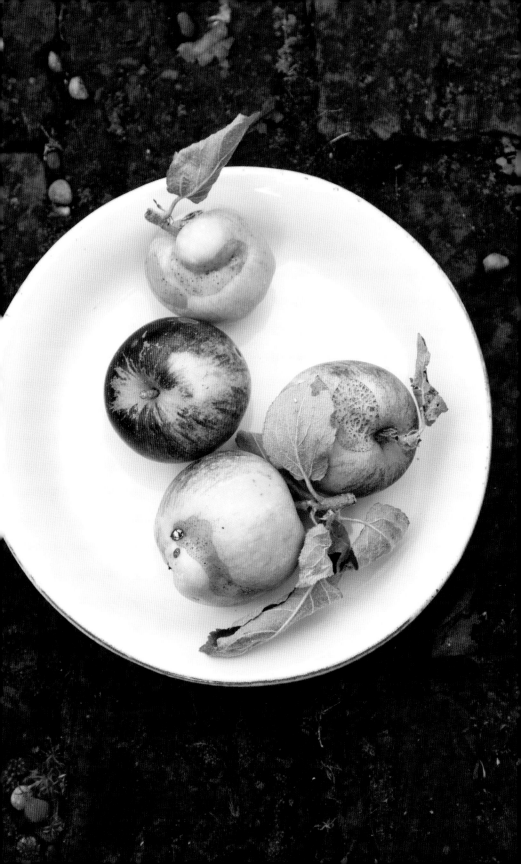

Cinnamon

Cinnamon is a powerful spice; not only does it have the ability to lower blood sugar levels, but it also is an anti-inflammatory in its own right.[47,48] Its use as an anti-inflammatory is both steeped in tradition and backed up by modern science; in one study, cinnamon was able to strongly block release of IL-6, a pro-inflammatory cytokine associated with damage from advanced glycation end products (AGEs).[48] Translation? Cinnamon is a great choice to help moderate blood sugars and the damage associated with them. Oh, and it tastes really nice in a cappuccino, too.

Easy ways to enjoy: Sprinkle cinnamon on cereal, yogurt, smoothies, stir into cocoa drinks and coffee beverages, or try Middle Eastern cuisines that feature a mixture of sweet and savory spices, including cinnamon.

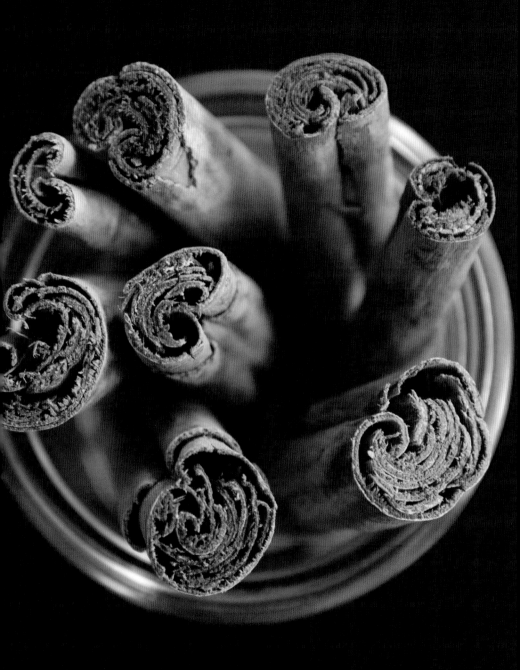

CHAPTER 7
START WHERE YOU ARE

"It is easier to change a man's religion than to change his diet." —Margaret Mead

Every January 2, people start following New Year's resolutions in the hopes that this will be the year they transform their lives for good. I say January 2 because who tries to transform their life with a hangover? And you know what goes well with a hangover? Brunch! And maybe a bit more champagne . . . so January 1 just won't work. The life makeover can always wait another day, can't it?

The trouble with this New Year's edition of extreme makeover is that by mid-February, most people have jumped off the transformation railway. Once-packed gyms are strewn with tumbleweeds. Fad diet books serve as coasters for margaritas. Flax seeds lurk, frostbitten, in the darkest corners of your freezer. This is the cycle so many of us fall into year after year. And it probably doesn't make us feel accomplished, strong, or energized. So, why do we allow it to happen?

If you ask me, it is because resolutions are often made with some vision of perfection that is incompatible with the way we actually live our lives. Love steak? Perhaps a six week vegan cleanse is not the right tool for you. Have trouble just carrying the groceries home? Maybe achieve some base-line fitness before throwing yourself into boot camp six days a week! This makes sense, right? So why do we torture ourselves in the pursuit of some unattainable and boring notion of perfection? Is it because we feel that we are somehow lacking? Remember—perfect isn't perfect. And chasing perfection can suck the joy out of living.

I don't know about you, but I have stopped making resolutions per se. I make a few goals for the year in terms of what I want to get accomplished, but I have stopped trying to jam this square peg into a round hole. For example, this year, one of my goals was to drink more green smoothies. I did it—and the goal was both easy to achieve and meaningful to my overall health values and lifestyle. All that extra greenery in my life is helping with my energy levels, my skin, and my digestion. That's how I get healthier now: with small, measurable, concrete changes. I am the world's worst candidate for a diet—believe me, I have tried most of them over the course of my adult eating life. After two days on a defined plan, I start getting restless. I quickly become bored and anxious, because as soon as I try to place my resistant brain into a series of absolute rules, it rebels faster than I can say chardonnay.

Sounding a little too loosey-goosey for ya? Don't mistake my realism for a carte blanche to eat whatever you want whenever you want. What kind of dietitian would I be? We all need to make at least some change to become healthier eaters; days filled with overprocessed junk food and a small side of iceberg lettuce won't cut it for long. We need to supercharge our diets with plant power—vital, living, and nutrient-dense foods to help us feel amazing. My point is that instead of launching into a doomed makeover plan for a new you, it is time to get real about who you are as an eater, what type of plan is going to work for you, and make concrete goals for positive change.

Change that accentuates the positive and affirms your desire for self-care.

Change that won't cause anxiety, shame, deprivation, or guilt.

Change that won't launch you into an all-out binge to get it out of your system . . . and your pantry before the real diet starts.

Ready? Sure you are . . . let's begin.

Know Thyself, Eater!

The first critical step in determining how best to clean up your nutritional act is to understand who you are as an eater. A great way to do this is to keep a food journal for a while; I would like you to record everything you eat and drink for at least a day or two so you can identify dietary patterns and habits. A week would be even better. The only rule here is no calorie counting. True health doesn't concern itself with calories—it revolves around eating good food. Quite frankly, the exact number of calories you need to maintain your weight is a moving target unless you can hook yourself up to a piece of machinery called a metabolic cart. Even the best research-based estimates of caloric needs are ballpark estimates. Fixating on calories will also tend to lead you toward a road of low-cal garbage, as opposed to worth every calorie whole foods.

No one has to see your journal but yes, it is important. In fact, research demonstrates that the simple act of food journaling can boast significant benefits in maintaining dietary change, particularly where weight loss is concerned.[1] Work through the food journal exercise as you read on; it won't impede your progress one bit, and, in fact, it will help to ensure your success.

When you can see in black and white what you actually eat on a daily basis, you will be better equipped to see the obvious places where you can easily make changes. That hazelnut mocha with whip? Lose the whip and the hazelnut syrup, and you could lose a pound or two by next month. You can even keep the mocha itself. Eat like a bird during the day and a gorilla at night? Maybe you can focus on eating a better lunch to keep the nighttime munchies at bay.

I have also created a little quiz to help you visualize who you are as an eater. Take the time to fill it out thoughtfully and without censorship. There are no right or wrong answers here! Let the headlines debate whether you should eat three square meals or six mini-meals a day. The better you understand yourself, the easier it is to determine your most successful path forward. All choices fit, in my opinion; the choices you make are the ones that have made sense for you and the way you live your life. And taking better care of yourself is all about worshipping at the temple of you, isn't it?

Today I Ate . . .

In this section, I want to show you how write down everything you eat or drink in your food journal. It doesn't have to be fancy; use scrap paper or keep it in a word document on your computer or smart phone. The important part is to go through this exercise, as journaling alone can be life changing for some people. Be totally honest . . . no one will see this but you! Note how hungry you were when you ate, what you were feeling, where you were, and what time it was. This exercise provides you with a snapshot of your typical eating day.

"But what if this was not a 'typical' day?" you ask. In fact, even if it seems out of the norm—a big party, a food you don't normally eat, a stressful or busy day—paper doesn't lie and usually reveals a lot about your eating habits. And dinners out or big doughnut-fuelled deadlines at the office happen more than we care to admit. If you like, photocopy this page and keep a record for three to seven consecutive days, including a weekend, and see what patterns emerge. Sometimes just writing down your food choices can change how you eat, so do your best to eat as you normally would during this time. No one will be grading this assignment but you! If you eat six cookies, write them down. If you skip breakfast, take note! You could even use this strategy as a check in once or twice a year to see how you are progressing down the road to a healthier you.

Date: _____

What I ate for breakfast:
Time:
Hunger (out of 10):
Mood:
Location:

What I ate for my a.m. snack:
Time:
Hunger (out of 10):
Mood:
Location:

What I ate for lunch:
Time:
Hunger (out of 10):
Mood:
Location:

What I ate for my p.m. snack:
Time:
Hunger (out of 10):
Mood:
Location:

What I ate for dinner:
Time:
Hunger (out of 10):
Mood:
Location:

What I ate for my evening snack:
Time:
Hunger (out of 10):
Mood:
Location:

Pop Quiz!

This quiz will help you discover your nutritional fingerprint so you can craft an eating plan that will fit you like a glove. What you learn here probably won't shock you, but the intention is to bring conscious awareness to who you are as an eater. You might not have given much thought to your eating personality, yet it will help determine what approach you should take to get healthier. Together with your food record, this exercise will provide a baseline picture of your current eating habits to help you do on your own what I do for my clients: identify opportunities for improvement.

Part One: All About ME! The Eater's Version.

1. The three foods/drinks I couldn't dream of living without are:

   a. What I love about them (taste? texture? smell? memories? culture?):

2. On the other hand, I could easily live without this food(s):

3. I would rather eat dirty socks than be forced to eat:

   a. I dislike this food because:

4. I like to eat:
   a. Three square meals a day. I hate eating all day long, but if I am hungry I might have a snack.
   b. Four to six mini-meals. The mini-meals keep my energy up, and I never feel too full.
   c. I am constantly eating something. A few carrots, candy, a half a sandwich. I love to munch!
   d. I have a big appetite—I can eat three good meals and have plenty of room for snacks.

5. Growing up, food *was/wasn't* an important part of my family's culture and my memories of being a child.

6. My parents or another family member taught me how to cook. *Yes/No*

7. I love to cook. *Yes/No*

8. If I had more time, I would cook every day. *Yes/No*

9. Cooking feels foreign to me and gets in the way of my healthy eating goals. *Yes/No*

10. I enjoy trying new recipes and would try more if I didn't have to think about where to find ones that fit my lifestyle. *Yes/No*

11. I have no trouble following defined meal plans. *Yes/No*

12. I dislike routine and have a hard time sticking to rigid plans. *Yes/No*

13. I have tried _____ diets in the past. _____ have worked. _____ haven't.

14. The diets that have worked worked because _____
    _____
    _____

15. The diets that didn't work failed because _____
    _____
    _____

16. I have lost _____ pounds and gained _____ in the past ten years.

17. When I am busy or stressed, I *often forget to eat/I overeat/nothing changes.*

18. I eat when I am (check all that apply):
    a. hungry
    b. craving something salty/sweet/crunchy
    c. bored
    d. sad
    e. stressed
    f. happy
    g. celebrating
    h. watching TV
    i. at my desk
    j. in the car
    k. in need of an energy boost

19. I often eat:

a. by myself
b. with my spouse
c. with my friends/roommate
d. with my family
e. in front of the TV/computer

20. I think I have an emotional attachment to food or eating. *Yes/No*

21. The idea of dieting creates feelings of (check all that apply):
    a. anxiety
    b. excitement
    c. hope
    d. self-love
    e. self-criticism
    f. desperation
    g. strength
    h. self-control
    i. motivation
    j. shame

22. I easily get consumed by new trends and change my diet, my fitness routine, and even my clothing style often. *Yes/No*

23. I eat *because I have to nourish my body/because food is so delicious*

24. To me, food is _____

This section is meant to help you understand yourself as an eater. Return to it when you are trying to decide which path of change to take. For example, don't take on the rigid meal plan if previous defined plans have failed in the past or the idea of dieting fills you with anxiety. Alternately, if structure makes you feel confident and in control of your health, maybe a meal plan system is for you!

Part Two: What's Your Food Philosophy?

1. Your idea of a cozy evening at home involves:
   a. Catching up with episodes of Nigella Lawson or reading *Bon Appetit*.
   b. Reading the health headlines on Huffington Post online.
   c. Watching your favorite show on TV with a bag of Cheetos.

2. At the grocery store:

a. You run to food that is handcrafted and in season, such as local goat chèvre or heirloom tomatoes.
b. You read nutrition labels religiously and are always on the lookout for foods with more fiber, omega-3s, or less salt.
c. You stock up on whatever is quick and easy and tastes good, such as frozen pizza, roast chicken, granola bars, and iced tea.

3. Your favorite place to buy fruits and vegetables is:
   a. The farmer's market or local green grocer.
   b. The organic section of the supermarket to avoid pesticides.
   c. Vegetables? I buy some frozen peas and corn and drink plenty of juice.

4. You think of diets as:
   a. Torture. A life without a little pinot noir and Serrano ham is not worth living.
   b. Confusing. It is hard to know who's right: the gluten-free folks, the paleo guys, or the vegans.
   c. Pretty pointless. After all, how bad can cola be?

5. Your favorite oil to cook with is:
   a. Organic butter.
   b. Canola oil, for the omega-3s.
   c. Whatever I have lying around.

6. How often do you cook dinner at home?
   a. Six nights a week. I love to cook and know how to create the flavors I crave.
   b. Most nights; sometimes I just grab a takeout salad from the grocery store.
   c. My roommate or spouse usually cooks or I get takeout.

7. I usually cook from:
   a. Cookbooks or recipes I find in magazines or online. I am always trying new flavors.
   b. I always have lots of healthy staples around, so I just throw something simple together.
   c. I don't really cook . . . I reheat or make reservations.

8. How much time do you have to get dinner on the table?
   a. You can't rush perfection.

b. Maybe thirty minutes (because I get home late/the kids are hungry).
c. If I can't eat it in five, what's the point?

9. Your dream getaway meal is:
   a. A leisurely tasting menu at the hottest restaurant in San Francisco, Vancouver, or Chicago.
   b. A gourmet lunch at a holistic destination spa.
   c. Taking down the quadruple bypass burger with flatliner fries in Vegas.

10. Breakfast is the most important meal of the day:
    a. I eat a hot breakfast or have homemade scones on hand for those days that I am busy.
    b. I start the day with a high-fiber breakfast cereal, fruit, and skim milk.
    c. A triple-shot mocha and a muffin . . . without coffee, I wouldn't function.

Your Approach to Food (the Super Scientific Results!):

Mostly As: The Foodie: You pore over food magazines, blogs, and cooking shows. You could wax lyrical about the majesty of bacon or kale for a half-hour. Food is art, food is pleasure, and life is too short for food to be boring.

Educating yourself about which healthy foods to stock your pantry with and gradually incorporating more healthy foods into your favorite recipes is likely a good bet for long-term change. This way, you can honor your love of food while adding more nutritious foods to your eating plan. A little kale here, a bit of quinoa there, and all of a sudden, you're not just a foodie . . . you're a superfoodie! Luckily, foodies often have the easiest time of healthy eating, as they have the skills and the passion to make any food taste delicious. Foodies really can have their cake and eat it, too . . . perhaps an olive oil and spiced orange cake made from almond meal more often than a cheesecake? Potential pitfalls here are torrid love affairs with bacon, butter, salt, or sugar.

Mostly Bs: The Food is Fuel Eater: You think about the benefits of the food (calories, antioxidants, fiber) usually over the food itself. You might be prone to nutritionism ("Now made with whole grains!" is a beacon for you) and are trying to do right in a busy life. So are we all!

Your approach to getting healthier might include getting the lowdown on nutrition in this book and studying the Supermarket Smarts chapter to help you resist the health-washing in the processed food aisles. Find the recipes in this book that can become your go-to for busy days, and if the meal plans work for your family, you won't ever ask yourself "What's for dinner?" again! Taking a food swaps approach will also give you the opportunity to create weekly food challenges for your family or friends so you can get healthier together. Potential pitfalls here are falling for hyper-processed foods masquerading as healthy choices or avoiding healthy whole foods because of their fat or carbohydrate count.

Mostly Cs: The Muncher: You need it cheap, fast, and tasty and aren't afraid to head to the corner store for a snack and count Olive Garden and The Cheesecake Factory as your favorite food haunts. Food is just . . . there . . . and you like eating it. And boy, it had better taste good.

Munchers can be of different stripes: some are truly junk food junkies and should absolutely take the slow baby steps approach to healthy eating to help their taste buds acclimatize to a new way of eating. Trying to abandon value meals overnight will just have you supersizing next week. And a kale salad could taste like sawdust to a bacon double cheeseburger palate. But some baby kale tucked inside a grilled cheese might just work!

Other munchers simply don't spend much time thinking about food and are fine eating just about anything. They eat the way they always have and the way their friends and family do. They would change if they felt it was important or if they knew how. If that is you and you really want to get healthy, why not follow the twenty-eight day meal plan so I can take the guesswork out of healthy eating for you? Or you can just start making the recipes from this book, getting used to one at time until eating well becomes your norm.

Part Three: The Edible Mirror

Here is the part where you take a look at your food journal and reflect on what you see. Consider the following questions . . .

1. What foods do you eat almost every day? Are they the same foods you listed as your favorites in part one? Why or why not?

2. Regarding the foods you decided you could live without in part one, do you see an opportunity to effortlessly cut back on nutrient-poor, high-calorie choices by eating fewer of them in your day-to-day life?

3. See anything that surprises you in your journal?

4. Name three things you think you do right—eating veggies, not eating while stressed, always having breakfast, etc.

5. Name three small things you think you could realistically and easily do to improve upon today, and for the long term.

6. Do your eating habits seem in harmony with your values on eating that you stated in parts one and two? If not, why? Is it time, money, habit? Do you think that your eating habits are a more clear statement of what you truly value and your stated values are in fact a projection of what you think is the right way to eat?

7. What has this exercise taught you that will make you a healthier eater? Has it illuminated any reasons why past healthy eating changes haven't been successful?

Know What You're Signing Up For (aka the Long Haul)

You might note that even though you have spent some time getting to know who you are as an eater, I haven't prescribed an exact solution for permanent change. No . . . it's not because I am avoiding you! It is because I don't think I can solve the world's eating issues with three prescribed personality types—there are as many food personalities as there are eaters! This exercise is intended to provide one more facet of self-awareness and help in the understanding that dietary changes need to speak to who you are as an eater or they will likely fail. All of those fad diets try to tell you that there is one way for you (and the whole world!) to eat—those plans leave you high and dry before you can say diet. This book is not about telling you what to do. You're a grown up . . . you get to choose.

Un-Junk Your Diet provides four plans of nutritional attack, from broad sweeps to the micromanaged, which you can follow to the letter or . . . you can mix and match to your heart's content what you mine from the nutritional gold in these pages. Want to go on a nutritional boot camp to motivate you for a year of slow and sustained change? Go for it! Gluten sensitive and need to alter my nutritional recommendations—of course! My only real rule is that you have to be realistic about what will work for you and NEVER give up because you ate a plate of nachos. A rigid all-or-nothing attitude will impede real progress.

Maybe you would like to be the person who simply follows the twenty-eight-day meal plan for life, but in reality you know that if you choose the food swaps option you will never need another diet again. In fact, I am describing myself here. That was the purpose of our little food quiz exercise. Your answers don't lie (unless you did, in which case—go back and be honest!). If you are uncertain about where to go, look back at your answers so you can start from exactly where you are. Then, as you read along in the book, allow that understanding to help you select a path forward that speaks to you. Each food plan will also begin with reminders on why you might like to choose that specific path.

Another question to ask yourself right about now is, how ready are you to change? If you are reading this book, you are likely open to the idea of change, but how much space do you have in your life for focusing on your health? If you are going through a particularly stressful or busy time, such as a divorce or loss of a loved one, a huge and critical project deadline at work, or recovering from an illness or injury, now might be the worst time (or the perfect time) for big change. For the time being, just playing with the twenty-five anti-inflammatory foods might be enough for you to explore healthier eating without the pressure of long-term change.

However, it's also important to remember that there might never be an ideal time . . . life is pretty demanding. You may relish being able to pour all of your negative energy into taking care of yourself to start getting your life back on track. If you feel like you are torn in a million different directions, perhaps just making a single food swap a week will be a small, doable, confidence-building option to get you through the rough patch. Keep it concrete by writing them in your smart phone calendar or placing photocopies of the 101 changes list on your fridge. You can tack on more challenges when you are ready.

A Word About Willpower . . . Maybe More Than a Word

Much is said about willpower and its place in dietary change. Willpower is necessary for resolutions. Willpower is critical for diets. Willpower also seems to be in dwindling reserve nowadays. Some of us appear to have it in spades, and others seem like they can never call on it when they need to. I feel like it takes tons of effort just to avoid checking my iPhone every five minutes! Maybe that's why I can barely remember what I had for breakfast yesterday or muster up the patience to tackle a closet clean out.

Willpower is a real phenomenon, and we have a set amount of it at any one time, which is why trying to change your eating habits when you are cramming for finals or training for your first marathon can be a bit tricky. That is also why it can be so difficult for average commuting/overworked/cleanthehouse/walkthedog/activitychauffeur parents to have the energy to clean up their diets.

Many of us expend superhuman amounts of energy and require heavy willpower just to live our high-octane lives. All the energy we need to get healthier (which, ironically, would help us feel more energetic and strengthen our resolve) is spent in the daily grind. Then, we berate ourselves for not being healthy, and we run to the nearest tub of Chubby Hubby for comfort. Sound familiar? Time to abandon the struggle against yourself. If you don't feel you have enough willpower for your chosen eating plan, you haven't chosen the right eating plan. Don't blame yourself for not having enough willpower. You probably have it in spades . . . so why not take it easy on yourself? One step forward is better than three steps back.

Willpower is also a muscle. Exert it, grow its strength, and new challenges will seem less, well, challenging. By gradually building food skills and confidence as a healthy eater, new changes will seem to take less effort. When you have already swapped your usual doughnut for a morning smoothie, it doesn't take much to start making green smoothies to get in some extra greens.

How is it possible to change your eating habits without using willpower? You have to circumvent the use of self-control and make eating well a habit. Habits are why you eat the way that you do now, and habits will be how you change those ways of eating for the better. The trick is getting to the habit part.

Pick and Mix: Ways of Creating New Healthy Habits

1. **Make a small change** (such as eating an apple a day) that is additive in nature—this is the rationale behind the food swaps approach in this book. Adding a new food doesn't take the self-control that avoiding a favorite food does, and eventually you just get used to eating an apple every day and don't have to think about it. When ready, you just move on to the next change. Because you have not deprived yourself of anything, you won't enter the deprivation-anxiety-craving-binge-shame cycle.

2. **Focus upstream.** Perhaps you eat too much fast food and know it is harming your health. Instead of banning it, ask yourself what encourages the behavior. If it is being hungry and pressed for time, why not start making a big batch meal on Sunday nights? Since you have to cook on Sunday anyway . . . make whatever you want as long as it makes enough servings so when you are stressed out with no time to cook midweek, you will have one meal taken care of that doesn't require the drive-through. Once this habit is set in stone, figure out another way to plan ahead and avoid the take out trap!

3. **Focus on the YUM.** Instead of worrying about what foods to eat or avoid, instead simply choose to make dinner twice a week using a recipe from this book. Forget about nutrition and enjoy the food. Pick up the ingredients on the weekend so the fridge is stocked and you are ready to hit the ground cooking when you get home! Eat however you like the rest of the week. All of the recipes in this book are created by yours truly to ensure they give you the nutrition you need, and they taste really good. When you are ready, choose a third dinner to make from the book or go crazy and try a breakfast! Focus on having fun in the kitchen; healthy eating will be the icing on the (carrot) cake.

4. **Enlist a partner-in-crime**. Find a friend or family member to join you on your healthy eating journey. Have fun with it. Announce it on Facebook and ask for your friends' support. One week, you could make a healthy dinner together, or you could challenge each other to food swaps for a month. A little healthy teamwork can go a long way!

Self-Responsibility Versus Self-Blame

Willpower is not the only hero of the personal growth story, and that is why a focus on weight as opposed to health can trip you up. Your body has strongly held mechanisms to maintain your weight within a comfortable set point for your metabolism. When you forcefully try to alter your weight below this set point, a host of biochemical changes will evoke feelings of hunger, lower your metabolism, and become incredibly thrifty with whatever nutritional scraps you throw its way.[2] So if you truly have been working hard at improving your diet but your weight doesn't budge, don't play the blame game.

Eating well is an act of self-love; don't let self-hatred creep in, because it will lead you headfirst into an unhealthy pattern. Having a big old burger, fries, and shake is not a failure . . . it's just food. This is why I am a fan of not focusing on weight, but on health. Weight is too charged a motivator and too easily overwhelms the eater. An appies and beers night can't erase all the good you did for your body over the past week unless all you care about is the number on the scale.

Instead of taking blame and inviting negativity, take responsibility. A less-than-healthy meal is not a big deal, it is simply your responsibility to ensure your next meal is amazing! If you have found yourself wading in the almond fudge crunch for a while, consider keeping a food journal for a week and compare your results to your healthy eating intentions. Whatever the outcome, do not stagnate in what has passed. Instead, remind yourself of how wonderful you feel when you are eating a nutrient-dense diet and how much you are worth taking care of. A few extra pounds is a distant second in importance to maintaining a healthy lifestyle that includes eating the right foods, being active, and keeping those all-important numbers, such as blood sugars, in check.

Getting Rid of What Gets in Your Own Way

The road to hell is paved with good intentions, as they say. While education, preparation, and planning can help set you up for success, there are a lot of ways that life and your brain tries to get in the way of living well. Let's talk about a few of them and how to push past the barriers standing between you and your best life.

An All-or-Nothing Approach

From a Cheetos-munching couch potato to a gluten-free vegan marathoner overnight? Don't think so, cowboy! What is it about our culture that loves extremes? I often think that the reason why dietitians sometimes fail to connect is that we love to preach moderation. It's just too sane for our crazy-making food world. We love black or white, bad or good, healthy or poison. That nutritional gray area is just too subtle.

Moderation isn't sexy, it doesn't promise you a beach body in thirty days, and it doesn't enlist the rule-bound soldier in the brain in a call to action against carbs. Heck, what does moderation even mean, anyways? My idea of moderation might be pizza three times a week while yours is pizza once a month. For the record, that is not my idea of moderation . . . it was just an example!

The all-or-nothing approach is great for motivating you, great for generating enthusiasm as you build up virtuous feelings of nutritional perfection, and great . . . for a couple of days. Maybe a few weeks at most. Then the weekend hits, and you are out at the big game when the trays of hot dogs and beer come around. You want to enjoy the experience, so you indulge. The moderation approach says, "Go for it! Have just one and eat something really healthy for dinner." The all-or-nothing approach inspires a backlash: "Why not follow it up with a huge steak dinner and a big greasy breakfast to chase the hangover tomorrow morning? Actually, you ruined your diet already, so just start again Monday, right?" The biggest problem with the all-or-nothing approach is that there is no wiggle room for real life. Fat is bad, carbs are bad, all of it is bad—so why not just resign yourself to the notion that it is too hard to eat healthfully?

A saner approach is one that leaves you 20 percent wiggle room for living. After work martinis, birthday cake, and Fun Food Fridays. So you can live well and still be healthy. This book is all about giving you the freedom to live while not letting up on this whole good nutrition business. Here, I try to quantify moderation by giving you rules, numbers, and plans that structure your eating plan so you feel supported swimming in the great big sea of moderation. This book is your moderation life raft. It takes maturity, patience, and trust to adopt a more rational approach to healthy eating change. You're up for it, I just know it!

Busy Bodies

We are too busy these days, we really are. I just can't for the life of me figure out how I am able to spend all this time on Facebook and still catch two hours of my favorite TV shows every night!

All kidding aside, for many of us, life is occurring at a breakneck pace. Between work, commuting, household responsibilities, family, and friends, it can be hard to have a minute to yourself. Forget eight hours of sleep a night! Living like this can make it seem ridiculous to spend time actually preparing food. This is about getting clear about your priorities; we won't survive eighty years on this planet if we don't prioritize food in our day. The crazy thing is, once we decide to eat well and make it a priority, it actually doesn't take up a lot of time. In fact, it can save us time. Going to the grocery store once a week instead of a few times plus a few runs for takeout will save you time and money. Prepping a lunch the night before will mean you actually have thirty minutes to eat it (and maybe check your Facebook page), instead of wasting twenty minutes picking something up.

For parents, the cinq à sept routine can be maddening. Where there used to be after-work drinks and a fun saunter home, there is now the rush to the bedtime finish line. How do you get dinner on the table, spend time with the kids, clean up, get them to bed, and make lunches all before 10 p.m.? Having a meal plan helps. Enlisting the kids to help is critical if they are old enough. Take it step by step. Planning is the key to success here, too. Having an arsenal of recipes that can be prepped in thirty minutes and ensuring a kitchen full of supplies will make meal prep simpler so your family can eat well and stay sane.

Get Your Kids in the Kitchen!

Think the only thing your kids can make is a mess? Well, I can't say it won't get messy, but the more you engage kids in food preparation, the better they will get—and the better they will eat. Eventually, it will make meal prep quicker, too. Here are some examples of age-appropriate kitchen tasks for the kiddos.

Preschoolers: Mixing ingredients, tearing salad leaves, washing produce, peeling eggs.

Early Grade Schoolers: Cutting soft foods (such as bananas) with a butter knife, setting the table, measuring ingredients, helping to plan meals.

Tweens/Preteens: Fully assist with the oven duties and cutting jobs (under supervision), making basics such as salad, packing their own lunch.

Teens: Consider them your sous-chef . . . they can even take over once in a while so you can take a night off!

The Enablers

You know who they are . . . those pesky enablers! The ones that just had to bring that flat of doughnuts into the office, like they do every week. The people who call out the healthy eaters at the table when they refuse dessert, "Wait! Don't tell me you are on a diet, are you?" The people that always mention how just one wouldn't hurt (and they say it every single day!).

Enablers are the trolls waiting under the bridge for you to fall off the wagon or sometimes preferring to push you off themselves. Some enablers are well-meaning; often they have learned to love others through food and they want to show you love. A refusal of food is seen as a refusal of their love. Others enable because they don't want to be bad alone, and it makes them uncomfortable to see others making better choices. Others share food freely so that they themselves eat less of a food.

Honesty really is the best policy here. People who love you will hopefully support your journey to healthy eating; people who don't, well . . . at the end of the day only you are accountable for your choices. So when you are trying to make better choices, just let the enablers know that you are thankful for the offer but you would rather decline. It's okay to say no if you really mean it. If the enablers press, tell them that you would love their support as you are trying to improve your health by eating a bit better. Also, don't forget that since a grounded approach to healthy eating means never having to say never, if someone offers you something really special and you want to eat it

. . . eat it. Never mind with the usual low-quality junk food, but something homemade and fancy, enjoy! Talk about a radical concept!

It's Not Just Food . . . It's Everything That Food Means to You

Except for the rare birds among us, most of us eat not just to service our hunger but our souls (what did you write on your quiz?). For me in particular, food is a huge part of my culture and my childhood memories; it is my passion, my profession, and even my hobby now! Food is an important part of our daily lives, our celebrations, and our cultural or religious mores.

As a dietitian, I never try to place eaters into my perfect diet box. At the end of the day, all foods can be made to fit into a truly healthy eating plan. So whatever your nonnegotiables are, figure out a way to make them part of your lifestyle in a healthy way. I have a friend who won't eat brown rice because white rice was a particular cornerstone of his food culture. Cutting out red meat entirely will probably not work for someone who grew up in cattle country. And try telling a French gourmand to abandon butter! In North America, our love of more makes a diet that relies on eating a lot less next to impossible to honor.

That is why a focus on more . . . of the good stuff . . . is such a winning strategy in the war against a junk food culture. Eat more kale! Eat more apples! Revel in the rich flavor of a ripe tomato with just a crush of sea salt on a hot summer's day! Yes, I really do geek out that much about food. I could stare at beautiful food photos all day long.

There is another group of eaters who have an alternate problem. The more they read, the more they learn about food and nutrition, they more they cut out of their diet until there is almost nothing left but organic kale and triple filtered water. This approach brings with it a new set of concerns: the potential for malnutrition, the potential for social isolation, and the potential loss of food love. When eating well means avoiding every single food that has ever been called out on a blog post, there is a good chance that food will no longer bring you joy. Food will be seen as a thing to be feared, not as a thing to be celebrated. So in our earnest attempt to find better health, we need to find a middle path. It takes openness, honesty, love, and responsibility for our choices.

How Did This Bag of Chips Disappear? I Couldn't Have Eaten It All

Think you love food and eating? How often are you actually present when you eat? Do you taste your food or simply ingest it? I used to be famous for eating a whole bag of ripple chips in front of the TV. Now, more than a small bowl makes me feel like garbage. Yes, dietitians eat potato chips—although not nearly as often as I used to when I was a kid.

How long does it take you to finish dinner? Five minutes? Ten? Has the dinner hour become the dinner pause? This is a big problem, because mindless munching is inherently unsatisfying, and when you eat quickly, you are able to eat a lot before your brain has even registered that food is present. So you honestly don't feel like you have overeaten, but that button on your jeans is getting farther away from the buttonhole. Even worse, most snack foods are designed to be eaten quickly, providing nary a seed or hunk of protein to even require chewing. That's why it is so easy for an otherwise sane person to eat a 1200-calorie bag of chips; try eating 1200 calories of broccoli . . . I think your stomach will rebel before you get to 400.

Mindful Eating Exercise

Truly enjoying food and creating nourishing eating opportunities requires that you be mindful of the eating experience. Ready for what? For some, this might feel like an exercise in torture. Grab a piece of (preferably) dark chocolate and let's begin.

Sit in a comfortable chair. Have a look at that piece of chocolate. What color is it? Is it shiny? Does it look smooth or granular? Really take in its appearance and then close your eyes.

Take a sniff. What does it smell like? Yes, it smells like chocolate, smart aleck. But, anything else? Cinnamon? Hazelnut? Vanilla?

Now place it on your tongue. Keep your eyes closed. Let it melt. Don't chew, just let it melt. Note how badly your brain wants you to crush through it. Ignore that impulse and really taste the chocolate. What kind of flavors are you experiencing? Do you actually like the taste, or has it always been about the sugar high for you? Given all that mouth exposure . . . is it now too sweet? Does it have any off flavors? What is the texture like? Does it melt well? Is it creamy? Does it linger or does it dissolve?

When was the last time it took you three minutes to eat a single piece of chocolate? Do you normally eat a whole bar in the same timespan?

If you found this interesting, you can also try the classic Buddhist exercise of trying to slow down eating a single raisin for as long as humanly possible. If you, like me, tend to crunch through hard candies . . . that raisin can teach you a lot about patience!

You might be surprised that if you slow down and truly experience many of your indulgence foods, they either become far more satisfying in smaller doses or you realize that they don't actually taste that good. Many typical junk foods affect me in that way. I can taste off tastes brought about by fake flavor enhancers, and those once desirable foods no longer seduce me. So tune in, enjoy eating, and let's move along the path to a healthier, better nourished you.

Don't Punish Yourself . . . Nourish Your Body

Start from where you are . . . it is as good a place as any.

Don't dwell on eating a bad diet or being overweight . . . like attracts like, and focusing on the negative will draw you toward the negative.

Engage in self-love by honoring your body with a commitment to eating healthier foods.

Don't fall into the all-or-nothing trap; ruining your diet because you ate a cheeseburger is akin to smashing your cell phone to pieces with your foot because you already dropped it.

It's all about progress; instead of bemoaning the triple chocolate milkshake, celebrate the week of healthy eating you had leading up to it.

PART TWO:

Un-Junk Your Diet Eating Plans

CHAPTER 8

101 FOOD SWAPS AND EASY ADDITIONS TO MAKE YOU HEALTHIER FOREVER!

The second day of a diet is always easier than the first. By the second day, you're off it. —Jackie Gleason

Welcome to option one of the *Un-Junk Your Diet* plan. It is the gentlest, most gradual, and most forgiving option in the book, because it will never ask you to give up anything you already eat . . . if you don't want to. You hold the keys, and you choose your path down the highway o' health! Having nachos after work? No problem—just ask for a small spinach salad so you can get your daily spinach in. Sounds painless, right? That's the point.

It is a great option for those who are sick of diets and just want to clean up their diet to get healthier for life. As I mentioned, my own eating journey has been a continuous progression from a child who snuck ice cream and chips for breakfast to the largely plant-powered gal I am now. When I was a teenager, I thought being a vegetarian was about eating mac and cheese daily. Now, I buy enough beans and barley to run my own bulk foods shop!

This gradual approach is also useful in times of stress or massive life change (divorce/house renovations/grieving/work troubles) because it will allow you to transform your relationship with food in a way that builds on positive choices and small successes over time. When you need all of your willpower to overcome a difficult life stage, it is not the time to frustrate yourself with some dramatic diet overhaul. There is only so much of you (and your willpower) to go around—don't wear yourself out trying to eat a certain way.

Please don't underestimate the power of small changes. This is, in fact, my favorite change strategy in this book—this is how I transformed my own diet when I finally got tired of following fads. There are 101 changes to try here, and while you might have already made some on your healthy eating journey, if you followed every single one of them, in less than two years you will have largely madeover your diet. Your reward? You will eat healthier than the majority of the North American population, and you will have also initiated behaviors that are proven to lower your risk of chronic disease and maintain a healthy weight. All without breaking a sweat.

Wait—I just said two years . . . seems slow, doesn't it? You are in the driver's seat here: you can speed up the process if you really want to, but some of these changes are so powerful that you will feel better quickly. You don't have to wait for two years to see and feel results. These swaps are designed to improve your fiber intake, boost potent disease-busting nutrition through powerful plant foods, clean up your food quality, and even help you indulge guilt-free. You will eat healthier fats, keep that protein lean and green, and along the way you might even lose a pound or two. Your body will benefit greatly from the flood of nutrition that these swaps are designed to provide (along with cleaning up a lot of gunk out of your current eating plan).

Many of the most successful weight loss stories start with just a few simple changes that gave the eaters the energy and confidence to make even more. This is important stuff: fad diets typically undermine confidence because the eater thinks that there must be something wrong with them if they are unable to stick with the diet. It's not you . . . it's the crappy diet plan! Unfortunately, this frustration and shame usually leads the eater to seek comfort . . . that he or she finds in the doughy arms of a loaf of garlic bread. The rationale behind a food swap plan is that instead of triggering the deprivation/craving/anxiety/binge/guilt madness that most diets do, your brain will never hear the word no. Instead, we will gradually and painlessly nudge our minds and our bodies toward health. "An apple a day? Why not? I can eat it after the mac and cheese." See . . . that wasn't so hard now, was it?

How do you make this section work for you? Choose one change (Right now! Don't wait until Monday!) to initiate, and follow it daily until it is an effortless part of your life. Choose the swaps that appeal to you, don't bother with the ones that don't. The key here is to continue the change forever, plus or minus a day or two. It's okay if you run out of apples one day and miss a serving—the idea is that the choice becomes as effortless and habitual as brushing your teeth. So if there is a change you don't think works for you right now, don't initiate it! Make one change, ten changes, or all 101 changes. Each one is a step to a healthier you. Not as dramatic as losing fifty pounds in time for Labor Day or a three-week vegan detox, but when you consider that a year from now, any progress made on a fad plan will probably have relapsed, you might agree that slow and steady really does win the race.

Remember, the only rule here is to choose one swap and do it every day until it feels like a normal part of your diet, from three to twenty-one days. An easy rule of thumb is to add a new habit each week, so you can simply choose a change day and stick with it. You might be super excited and want to try two or three at a time, but instead, simply build new habits faster. Remember, you are trying to sneak your way into health, past your pesky rationalizations and meddling emotions. As you transform your diet, your skin should become clearer, you should have more energy, and you should feel healthier and happier. Because eating well is just that powerful . . . and feeling good is addictive.

Because the gradual plan doesn't come with a lot of fanfare, you might want to help yourself out with some visuals. Why not photocopy the list and place it on your fridge? That way, you can see how far you have come as you tick off the changes. Rewards are always nice, too—how about treating yourself to fancy bath salts after three changes or your dream chef's knife after eight? Six months' worth of positive change might even be worth a guy's getaway to see the big game.

Here are some other options for simple rewards to help keep you motivated:

—A night out at the movies

—A new pair of shoes (if they are athletic shoes, all the better!)

—A relaxing and muscle-melting massage

—A new book or magazine

—A new kitchen gadget

—A fine scotch or bottle of wine

—An investment in your favorite hobby, from new fishing tackle to fine yarns or paintbrushes

—A day off work to lie on the beach or go for a hike

—New music for your iPod

—Tickets to a music or sporting event

If you are wondering where you should start, start at whichever change appeals to you right now because it looks easy, tasty, or just because it is labeled with the number one! If you need some suggestions, there are a few swaps/additions that I find particularly powerful . . . and I have marked them with an acorn!

Remember, this book is about choosing your own nutrition adventure, so if two years of changes seems like a bit of a yawn, you could always kick off the 101 swaps plan with the two week kick start in Chapter 9 to flood your body with feel-good nutrition that should motivate you for the long term. Or, if you want to work up to trying the full 80/20 lifestyle featured in Chapter 10, you could plan twelve weeks of simple swaps as a warm up before going full anti-inflammatory.

101 Fabulous Food Swaps and Tasty Additions

Get with the Grain

1. Switch from white bread to 100 percent whole grain bread for everyday use.
   White bread is nonfood. All that is good is stripped from the grain. Whole grain bread keeps much of the original fiber and vitamins intact.
   I tried it! Starting _____ (date)

2. Switch from 100 percent whole grain bread to 100 percent sprouted grain bread.
   Many whole grain breads are still processed in a way that makes them super squishy, and they raise blood sugars too quickly. Sprouted grain bread is made from the whole wheat kernel, and it provides more protein and fiber.
   I tried it! Starting _____ (date)

3. Cook your pasta until its al dente, not soft.
   Cooking pasta until al dente (firm) will keep it from raising blood sugars too quickly to keep your energy stable.
   I tried it! Starting _____ (date)

4. Choose 100 percent whole grain pasta and cook it al dente.
   Because whole grain is always more nutritious . . . try thin varieties, such as spaghettini or spaghetti for a better, less mealy texture.
   I tried it! Starting _____ (date)

5. Add 1/3 cup All Bran Buds, Nature's Path Smart Bran (organic), or Enjoy Life Crunchy Flax (gluten free) to your breakfast cereal, salad, or yogurt daily. Be sure to drink plenty of water so the fiber can do its work.
   This is a dietitian's secret fiber weapon. Add a good fourth to half your daily fiber to your diet just by sprinkling some on! Oh, and drink the water. . . or the fiber will act like a plug instead of a broom in your digestive tract. Consider yourself warned!
   I tried it! Starting _____ (date)

6. Switch from a bagel or scone to two pieces of whole grain toast.
   Many bagels can be the starchy equivalent of three to six pieces of bread! Keep the carb-loading at bay by switching to toast.
   I tried it! Starting _____ (date)

7. Look for a breakfast cereal that has fewer than eight grams of sugar per serving (or zero added sugar) and at least five grams of fiber per serving. *Most breakfast cereals are candy with a little fiber sprinkled in. If cold cereal works for your busy life, get cozy in the cereal aisle and read those labels.* I tried it! Starting _____ (date)

8. Swap your instant oats for slow-cooking or steel-cut oats: Make a big batch Sunday night, package in single servings, top with your favorite toppings, then just heat and eat in the mornings. *Instant oats raise your blood sugar more quickly than slow-cooking varieties and can be loaded with sugar. But slow oats are slow to cook! So whip up a little breakfast assembly line. In thirty minutes, you can have all your breakfasts prepped for the week and streamline your mornings.* I tried it! Starting _____ (date)

9. Switch your usual crackers to 100 percent whole grain crackers. *If you can devour a whole box of crackers, you're eating the wrong ones! Look to varieties that are made with 100 percent whole grain to provide a bit more nutrition.* I tried it! Starting _____ (date)

10. Upgrade your whole grain crackers to a natural whole rye or whole wheat version. *The healthiest mass-market crackers are those lovely crisp ones, like Ryvita, Wasa, or Mary's Organic Crackers because they have no garbage in them to make them irresistible. They beg to be covered in a healthy toppings, such as nut butter or mashed avocado.* I tried it! Starting _____ (date)

11. Make your own muffins using whole wheat flour instead of purchasing them. *Most commercial muffins are more like eating three cupcakes, nutritionally speaking. Too big, too much sugar, and not enough good stuff. Make them yourself with whole grain flours, and enjoy a healthier snack.* I tried it! Starting _____ (date)

Rethink Your Drink

12. Swap one soda per day for sparkling water or seltzer. Swap another, if you dare, until you are down to one (or none) a day. Consider each swap its own change.

Drinking soda is associated with weaker bones, crazy blood sugars, and weight gain (even the fake sugar kinds!). Drinking even one fewer will do you good.

I tried it! Starting _____ (date)

13. Swap your energy drink for a cup of coffee or all-natural cola.

    Yes, you read that right: I would rather you drink a mocha or a cola than a bloody energy drink. They are that bad for you—don't fall for the marketing.

    I tried it! Starting _____ (date)

14. Switch your soda to an all-natural, fruit-juice-based soda.

    The sugar is one thing . . . but all the metabolism-destroying garbage they put in soda is another thing entirely. See the resources sections for recommendations.

    I tried it! Starting _____ (date)

15. Switch your usual fruit drink/juice to 100 percent not-from-concentrate juice.

    Are you drinking juice or orange drink? Look for the words 100 percent not-from-concentrate on the label. Prepare to be shocked at how many juices aren't the real deal . . .

    I tried it! Starting _____ (date)

16. Cut your juice with half sparkling water or seltzer.

    Let's work on cutting the sugar load . . . juice and fruit are not equally healthy. This makes a lovely soda pop substitute, too. Depending on how large your glass is, you might be saving yourself one hundred sugary calories a day with this swap . . . potentially leading to a significant weight loss in a year.

    I tried it! Starting _____ (date)

17. Enjoy sparkling or plain water with fresh fruit, such as berries, lemons, or limes, instead of pop.

    This is a great option when you get tired of plain water. Store plain water (not sparkling) in a jug in the fridge, as the longer the fruit steeps, the tastier it gets.

    I tried it! Starting _____ (date)

18. Get your coffee drink half-sweet.

    There can easily be four teaspoons of sugar in your coffee. You don't need 'em . . . but your taste buds are used to them. For the first little while, your drink won't taste like much, then magically, your taste buds will start working again, and you can tease out that mocha or caramel flavor!

    I tried it! Starting _____ (date)

19. Downsize your coffee drink to a tall/regular.

    That's all you need . . . I kid you not. Most regular sized drinks are almost 500 ml! That's a lot of sugar and/or caffeine. If you can't live without your large drink, get your regular drink in a large cup topped up with decaf plain coffee.

    I tried it! Starting _____ (date)

20. Switch your half-sweetened drink to a plain latte.

    That's right . . . don't give up your coffee but ditch the sugar. As your taste buds acclimate, you might note that milk is naturally sweet. Now you can have your latte and drink it (guilt free), too!

    I tried it! Starting _____ (date)

21. Swap one cup of coffee for a cup of green or black tea.

    Coffee is not bad for you . . . unless it's in excess. Try swapping one (probably not the first of the morning) for a cup of tea. See how you feel with this lower caffeine drink. Tea (especially green tea) is also packed with potent antioxidants.

    I tried it! Starting _____ (date)

22. Drink one to two cups of green tea (caffeinated or decaf) daily.

    A good addition to any diet. Green tea contains EGCG, a potent antioxidant that helps protect your skin from UV damage and might help prevent cancer growth (albeit when consumed at much higher doses than a cup a day . . . still good for ya, though!).

    I tried it! Starting _____ (date)

23. Keep a one-liter (one-quart) water bottle at your desk and drink its contents before the end of the day.

    Our bodies desperately need the stuff to thrive and drinking out of piddly little cups won't work. Fill once or twice, drink all day!

    I tried it! Starting _____ (date)

Protein on the Prowl

24. Cut your ground beef with ground turkey, 50/50, in your recipes.

    Red meat, particularly typical supermarket meat, is not a great option for your health. Too much inflammatory saturated and omega-6 fat and too much heme iron that can contribute to colon cancer. Lighten it up!

    I tried it! Starting _____ (date)

25. Cut your ground meat with cooked lentils, 50/50, in your recipes.
    Go the extra mile by packing your ground with extra fiber and vital minerals, such as magnesium and veggie iron.
    I tried it! Starting _____ (date)

26. Swap ground meat for 100 percent cooked lentils or crumbled firm tofu in an appropriate recipe once a week.
    You don't have to be vegetarian to go meatless once in a while! More fiber, less fat, and more vital nutrients.
    I tried it! Starting _____ (date)

27. Eat fish twice a week.
    Sustainably caught fish are fairly gentle on the planet and a lean source of protein. Get extra points for choosing omega-3-rich fish, such as wild salmon, black cod or sablefish, barramundi, herring, mackerel, and sardines.
    I tried it! Starting _____ (date)

28. Switch your usual sliced sandwich meats for an all-natural version.
    Sliced sandwich meat is laced with fillers, carcinogenic nitrates, and tons of salt. Take a step in the right direction by choosing natural, good quality (no added nitrates) meats.
    I tried it! Starting _____ (date)

29. Cook extra meat at mealtimes and use in place of deli meats.
    The best sandwich meat? Real meat! Just buy larger portions of meat; you will save money over buying deli meats and get better quality protein.
    I tried it! Starting _____ (date)

30. Snack on cottage cheese with crackers (savory) or Greek yogurt with fresh fruit and honey (sweet) for a high-protein snack instead of pastries.
    We have a tendency to choose nutrient-poor carbs at snack time. Protein helps keep you energized! Cottage cheese and Greek yogurt are packed with satisfying protein.
    I tried it! Starting _____ (date)

31. Choose to eat red meat only once per week, eating fish, chicken, or beans on the other days.
    If you love red meat, you probably don't want to say goodbye forever. If you can find/afford grass-fed beef, even better! So choose one night a week, indulge, and feel good about it—knowing that the rest of the week you make super-healthy protein choices.
    I tried it! Starting _____ (date)

32. Join the Meatless Monday crew: go without meat for a whole day each week.

Could you go for one day without meat? Try tofu scrambles, lentils in vegetarian moussaka, or a salad packed with chickpeas. Feel awesome.

I tried it! Starting _____ (date)

33. Buy organic and/or humanely raised eggs.

Eggs are an economical source of clean protein, but factory farming is horrible. If budget is an issue, eat fewer meat products to afford better eggs. Or, go super local and see if your town allows backyard chickens and rescue a pair. Sell the egg overstock to your neighbors.

I tried it! Starting _____ (date)

Get Vegucated

34. Eat an apple (or pear) a day.

Why an apple? It is usually affordable, widely available and, in fact, nutritious. One of the higher-fiber fruits, it has a moderate blood sugar impact and those brightly colored skins have antioxidants to help you get your glow on.

I tried it! Starting _____ (date)

35. Add a half-cup of blueberries or other berries (fresh or frozen, thawed) to your breakfast.

Berries are a real-world superfood. Packed with anti-inflammatory, antioxidant phytochemicals to help boost your brain, get you glowing, and fight off stress.

I tried it! Starting _____ (date)

36. Buy prewashed baby spinach and eat a big handful daily: in your smoothie, a soup or sauté recipe, or as a simple side salad.

No time to prep veggies? No excuses! Baby spinach is ready to go when you are. Eat a massive handful of this antioxidant- and mineral-rich goodie daily.

I tried it! Starting _____ (date)

37. Ensure that there are two different vegetables served as a side/salad or mixed into your dish at every dinner.

More veg! Whether you are eating pasta, meat and sides, or a casserole, make every recipe with two different vegetables.

I tried it! Starting _____ (date)

38. Ensure that there are two different vegetables served as a side/salad or mixed into your dish at every lunch.

    The more veggies you eat, the healthier you will be . . . you will also stay fuller longer, and maybe you won't fall asleep at your desk at 2 p.m.!

    I tried it! Starting _____ (date)

39. Eat hummus with sliced veggies as a snack three times a week.

    Snack time doesn't mean snack foods; get your real food fix! Hummus and veggies gives you that magic protein and produce mix that will keep you well-nourished and lets you have fun munching.

    I tried it! Starting _____ (date)

40. Eat a piece of fruit with or after each meal (for a total of three pieces a day).

    Most of us are preconditioned to want a sweet after a meal. Get that sweet working for you and magically get three of your ten servings of produce for brilliant health.

    I tried it! Starting _____ (date)

41. Eat yam fries instead of regular fries.

    Just because it's a treat doesn't mean you can't make it work for you with a little extra nutrition!

    I tried it! Starting _____ (date)

42. Get side salads instead of fries with your entrée at restaurants.

    Ditto. Enjoy the burger/beef dip/egg salad sandwich, but round it out with a salad.

    I tried it! Starting _____ (date)

43. Go (dark) green.

    Swap your usual lettuce for baby kale, romaine, baby chard, or baby spinach. Iceberg and butter lettuces have little to offer nutritionally speaking. Make that rabbit food work for you!

    I tried it! Starting _____ (date)

44. Start your day with a smoothie.

    This is one of the easiest ways to get more produce into your life. In go the berries, the spinach, and some protein in the form of Greek yogurt or silken organic tofu. Just ensure that there is at least one-and-a-half cups of produce in there. Some of my favorite smoothie recipes are included in this book.

    I tried it! Starting _____ (date)

Better Bone Builders

45. Buy plain yogurt and mix it 50/50 with your usual sweetened variety.

    A lot of yogurts are just health-washed candy—way too much sugar! Ease your taste buds into health with a 50/50 mix.

    I tried it! Starting _____ (date)

46. Eat plain yogurt, and add your own honey or maple syrup.

    It is unlikely you will add as much sweetener as the manufacturers do.

    I tried it! Starting _____ (date)

47. Eat plain yogurt with chopped up fruit. Thawed blueberries make for a particularly saucy and sweet mix.

    Make that sweet stuff a healthy choice! Now we're talking . . .

    I tried it! Starting _____ (date)

48. Switch to low fat/1 percent milk.

    Skip the animal fat where you won't really miss it . . . so you can save it for a more interesting splurge.

    I tried it! Starting _____ (date)

49. Switch from margarine to butter.

    You got that right—get the garbage fats out of your system, and switch to real dairy butter. Just don't overdo it!

    I tried it! Starting _____ (date)

50. Spread sandwiches with hummus, mustard, natural mayo, nut butters, coconut butter, or mashed avocado instead of butter or margarine.

    Clean up the fats on everyday items with these options for healthy plant fats. Don't butter your sandwiches or fry in it . . . save that butter for Sunday morning muffins.

    I tried it! Starting _____ (date)

51. Switch to milk from grass-fed cows if it is available.

    Grass-fed cows produce milk with less saturated fat, more omega-3 fat, and fewer inflammatory substances. Happy cows=healthier milk!

    I tried it! Starting _____ (date)

52. Swap milk for your favorite veggie milk.

    This is an easy place to go plant-based because there is a veggie milk for every taste! Experiment with quinoa, organic soy, hemp, almond, and more; just be sure it contains calcium and choose an unsweetened variety.

    I tried it! Starting _____ (date)

53. Buy real cheese.

You may be shocked to learn that much of the cheese we are buying is not made from 100 percent fresh fluid milk. Read ingredients: if there are modified milk ingredients or milk protein concentrates, give it a pass.

I tried it! Starting _____ (date)

54. Try replacing 50 percent vegan cheese in recipes that call for grated cheese.

Going 50/50 will help reduce your intake of saturated fat and helps your taste buds get used to the change. Find my favorites in the resources section.

I tried it! Starting _____ (date)

Health Boosters

55. Add three tablespoons of hemp hearts to your breakfast cereal/smoothie, salad, or soup each day.

Hemp seeds are rich in protein, omega-3 fatty acids, a special anti-inflammatory fat called GLA, calming magnesium, and energizing manganese. Eat daily . . . feel good.

I tried it! Starting _____ (date)

56. Every time you eat a meal or snack, ensure that your plate is 50 percent covered in fruits and/or vegetables.

This is the easiest way to ensure you are healthy for life. It works with any meal or snack. Just up the veg, shrink the other stuff. If you followed no other diet change for life, this would be the one!

I tried it! Starting _____ (date)

57. Eat at least one fermented food daily.

Fermented foods are critical for increasing the live bacteria in your diet and promoting digestive health. Eat yogurt, kefir, live kombucha, kimchi, live sauerkraut, or miso daily.

I tried it! Starting _____ (date)

58. Take 1000 IU of vitamin D3 daily.

Vitamin D3 is critical to bone health and studies suggest it could even help strengthen the immune system and help prevent cancer. 1000 IU is probably much more than you are already getting, but it is safe enough for every man and woman.

I tried it! Starting _____ (date)

59. Take a good-quality probiotic daily.

Fermented foods provide a community of innocent bystanders to your daily diet. A high-potency probiotic is like flooding that community with Rhodes Scholars to ensure everything works in harmony. Probiotics support digestive, immune, and nervous system health. Get at least 10 billion CFU (colony forming units, aka live and active cells) per day.

I tried it! Starting _____ (date)

60. Take omega-3 DHA daily.

Found in cold-water fish and algae, a supplement with at least 200 milligrams of DHA is a smart bet for every man and woman. DHA supports brain health, healthy fetal development, and a healthy heart. If you are on blood thinners, talk to your doc first.

I tried it! Starting _____ (date)

61. Consider making a green smoothie or juice a daily habit.

The easiest way to get extra greens is to drink them! If you are new to green juice, start slow . . . maybe try the smoothie in tip 44 and start scaling up the greens as you get used to it. If you have a high-powered blender, such as Vitamix or Blendtec, you will get the consistency of juice with all of the natural fiber—the best of both worlds! Cucumbers, celery, kale, spinach, and romaine lettuce are all great mix-ins.

I tried it! Starting _____ (date)

62. Sleep at least seven hours per night.

Why is Ms. Dietitian poking her nose in your bedroom? Because if you don't sleep enough, you won't eat well. You will drink too many sugary, caffeinated drinks and not have the energy to stick to a healthy eating plan.

I tried it! Starting _____ (date)

Shop Smart

63. Read ingredients and refuse to buy anything that contains an ingredient you wouldn't find in a healthy kitchen.

That's all you need to know. A healthy body starts with quality, real food ingredients.

I tried it! Starting _____ (date)

64. Start your shopping trip at the produce department, and fill your basket or cart at least one-third full with produce before moving on.

Produce is the foundation of a healthy diet; you can't buy a few bananas and a head of broccoli and feed yourself well for the week! Buy a lot. Force yourself to use it. Just think, if you adopt that three fruit a day habit, it works out to twenty-one pieces of fruit a week just for you!

I tried it! Starting _____ (date)

65. Try one new fruit or veggie each week, and if you don't know how to use it, Google it!

Healthy eating isn't boring . . . we are! Bust ruts by stepping outside of your produce box. The miracle of the Internet will ensure you find something tasty to do with it. This is a great activity for families to encourage broader taste buds.

I tried it! Starting _____ (date)

66. Shop with a grocery list . . . and stick with it.

A grocery list saves you time and money by ensuring you buy only what you need without forgetting anything. No wasting time with midweek trips to the store!

I tried it! Starting _____ (date)

67. Plan out your dinners for the week.

The easiest way to avoid the takeout trap is to plan and shop for a week's worth of dinners. You always know what's for dinner, and you can plan recipes that are quick and easy for a busy life.

I tried it! Starting _____ (date)

Snack Smart

68. Swap your granola bar for a small handful of raw almonds and a piece of fruit.

Most granola bars are little more than candy bars with a few puffy grains thrown in. Stop the sugary madness with a nourishing snack of fruit, protein, and fiber.

I tried it! Starting _____ (date)

69. Switch from salted, sweetened trail mixes to unsweetened raw mixes.

Roasted trail mixes can harm the nutrient quality of raw ingredients, and seasoned varieties incite overeating. Go au naturel.

I tried it! Starting _____ (date)

70. Portion out snack foods into a small bowl, put the bag away, and eat out of the bowl. Refill the bowl if necessary.
Because we often snack mindlessly, we will finish whatever portion is in front of us. Having to get up to refill a bowl will help us become more conscious of how much we are really eating.
I tried it! Starting _____ (date)

71. Try eating only one small bowl of snack foods at a time. Savor them.
The way to have your cake and eat it, too, is to not eat the whole cake. Serve yourself a small portion of snack foods.
I tried it! Starting _____ (date)

72. Try eating only one serving of your usual cookies. If it doesn't satisfy, the next time you shop, look for a cookie with better ingredients, such as real butter, so you can enjoy eating just one serving.
This is where the low-fat/low-carb/low-sugar monster comes back to bite you. They don't satisfy . . . and you end up eating the whole package. Go for the real deal and savor it.
I tried it! Starting _____ (date)

73. Switch from your typical ice cream to an all-natural version.
Most ice creams aren't real ice cream anymore . . . or even made with 100 percent cream! If you are going to indulge, do it right.
I tried it! Starting _____ (date)

74. Switch from your ice cream to an all-natural, coconut- or almond-based frozen dessert.
A delicious place to go plant-based to avoid overdoing it on dairy: the new frozen coconut desserts usually have simple, quality ingredients and a healthier, plant-based fat.
I tried it! Starting _____ (date)

75. Look for a milk chocolate that has at least 35 percent cacao solids and real ingredients.
Even if it's milk chocolate, you deserve one made with real cacao, not fillers.
I tried it! Starting _____ (date)

76. Switch to a dark chocolate with at least 50 percent cacao solids.
The more cacao bean in the chocolate, the more healthy plant nutrients it contains.
I tried it! Starting _____ (date)

77. Upgrade your dark chocolate to one with at least 80 percent cacao solids.
    Now you're speaking my nutrient-dense language! These are chocolates to savor, not chew. Usually just a square or two satisfies.
    I tried it! Starting _____ (date)

78. Swap chips or microwave popcorn for an air popper or make popcorn in a pot on the stove.
    Popcorn is a healthy snack, but microwave popcorn is filled with garbage. Unearth the old air popper or try this: in a pasta pot over medium-high heat, add two tablespoons olive or coconut oil and a half-cup of organic popcorn kernels. Place a lid and using oven mitts, watch closely, shaking side to side occasionally until the popping seriously slows (just like in the microwave).
    I tried it! Starting _____ (date)

79. Don't fall for the muffin myth—at a café, choose a small pastry over an oversized muffin.
    See change 12. A mini cookie is usually a better option—unless your café is run by hemp seed-loving hippies—then go for the hemp and bran-laden muffin!
    I tried it! Starting _____ (date)

The Healthy Pantry

80. Choose only organic and/or certified non-GMO soy foods, such as tofu, tempeh, hot dogs, and soy milk. 🌰
    Genetically engineered foods, or GMOs, have no place in our healthy food supply and most soybeans are GMO; in addition, nonorganic soy products are treated with nasty hexane. Read your labels.
    I tried it! Starting _____ (date)

81. Choose only organic and/or certified non-GMO corn products, such as breakfast cereals, tortillas, tortilla chips, crackers, and cooking oils. 🌰
    Ditto.
    I tried it! Starting _____ (date)

82. Choose only organic and/or certified non-GMO canola oils and products made with them. 🌰
    GMOs suck.
    I tried it! Starting _____ (date)

83. Switch your usual cooking oil to extra virgin olive oil.

    Extra virgin olive oil is the last uncontroversial fat, because it is naturally anti-inflammatory, antioxidant-rich, and contains primarily monounsaturated fats, which won't raise cholesterol levels.

    I tried it! Starting _____ (date)

84. Switch your high heat cooking oil to almond, avocado, or coconut oil.

    You can take extra virgin olive oil to medium-high heat. For occasional frying, you need a more stable oil.

    I tried it! Starting _____ (date)

85. Switch to low sodium cooking broth or stock.

    Get less salt with no effort.

    I tried it! Starting _____ (date)

86. Switch from your typical peanut butter to a natural, unsweetened one.

    A lot of peanut butter varieties are essentially peanut flavored icing. Peanuts and salt . . . nothing else: that's real peanut butter.

    I tried it! Starting _____ (date)

87. Switch your usual jam to an all fruit, low sugar (no artificial sweetener) variety.

    Fruit should be the first ingredient; compare labels for the one with the least sugars per tablespoon—without resorting to fake sugar.

    I tried it! Starting _____ (date)

88. Make better butter: let butter come to room temperature and mix it 50/50 with extra virgin olive oil for use as a spread.

    Margarine doesn't stand a chance; real butter mixed with super-healthy EVOO is a dream.

    I tried it! Starting _____ (date)

89. Clean up the sugar drawer.

    Use up or donate your existing sweeteners and replace with pure honey, pure maple syrup, and real (Fair Trade if you can find and afford it) sugar. Zero low calorie sweeteners allowed, except for a bit of real stevia if you really love it.

    I tried it! Starting _____ (date)

90. Buy canned goods with no added salt.

    An easy way to clear the artery-hardening sodium out of your pantry.

    I tried it! Starting _____ (date)

Creating a Healthier Eater

91. Downsize your plate to downsize *you.*

    Research shows that we eat less off smaller plates. You can still have seconds, but if you are looking to eat less, eat your meals off of side plates instead of giant dinner plates.

    I tried it! Starting _____ (date)

92. Stop eating in front of a screen.

    When we are distracted by a screen, we are less conscious of how much we are eating. We derive less pleasure from our food . . . which leads to more pleasure seeking (aka overeating). Eat meals without TV, smart phones, or your computer. Even if all you can take is ten minutes at work. Try it!

    I tried it! Starting _____ (date)

93. Chew each bite twenty-five times (or try to).

    People who chew less have a tendency to eat more in less time, robbing your body of the opportunity to tell you you're full. Not thoroughly chewing your food can also exacerbate digestive issues, such as gas, bloating, and IBS. This could have an illuminating effect on your eating habits.

    I tried it! Starting _____ (date)

94. Never finish your child's meal.

    Don't eat just because the food is there. If you are worried about waste, pack it up for a snack later or as your child's lunch.

    I tried it! Starting _____ (date)

95. Stop drinking your calories.

    If you drink a lot of juice, soda, iced tea, and coffee drinks, you could still be getting a lot of extra energy your body doesn't really need—even if you make healthier choices. Consider scaling back to plain coffee, tea, and waters when you're ready.

    I tried it! Starting _____ (date)

96. Eat Breakfast.

    You can't run your tank on empty and expect to feel amazing. If you are out of the habit, start with something small, such as a piece of fruit or a hard-boiled egg. Work your way up to a proper meal over time.

    I tried it! Starting _____ (date)

97. Buy yourself a new healthy cookbook and try a recipe each week.

The best way to eat well? Cook well! Look for a book that features Mediterranean cuisine, whole food vegan choices, seafood, or one that focuses on innovative vegetable dishes, and enjoy deliciously good health.

I tried it! Starting _____ (date)

98. Makeover a favorite dish.

Take a lazy afternoon and figure out how to make a family favorite healthier, using the swaps in this book or resources on the Internet. Swap in healthier fats, add vegetables, change the protein up...make it all your own!

I tried it! Starting _____ (date)

99. Bring your own lunch to work.

Eating take out usually leads to less healthy choices (or at least a lighter wallet!). Commit to packing your own lunch and use all that money you save to treat yourself to a healthy reward!

I tried it! Starting _____ (date)

100. Don't eat when you are sad . . . well, not all the time.

While food can provide the sensation of comfort, eating will not ease sadness or anger. If emotions are getting the best of you, take a bath, a nap, or a walk or call your best friend. Eat only when you are feeling better. Work through the emotion; then eat to nourish the body. If you feel that you have use food as a coping tool for larger emotional issues, get the help you need to truly treat the root cause instead of masking emotions with eating.

I tried it! Starting _____ (date)

101. Enjoy eating.

Food is a pleasure, but poor-quality foods are not rewards. Get reconnected with food by sharing it with friends, grow herbs in a windowsill, or plant a garden. Bring more positive relationships with food into your life, and respect your body and your taste buds with quality food that is prepared simply and with love.

I tried it! Starting _____ (date)

CHAPTER 9

LEAVING ROOM FOR CHOCOLATE: THE 80/20 APPROACH

"I never worry about diets. The only carrots that interest me are the number you get in a diamond." —Mae West

My core eating strategy is living by the 80/20 rule: 80 percent of the time, I eat really well. Not just Special K and fat-free ice cream well—kale quinoa, and lentils well! That leaves 20 percent wiggle room for whatever is turning my foodie crank that week—be it homemade lemon curd, a nice malbec, or a wedge of manchego cheese. I don't worry about what I am eating, because treats make up a small enough portion of my diet as to not make too much of a dent—particularly because the rest of my diet is so nourishing.

I wish I could take credit for such sane, reasonable nutrition advice, but a long line of health professionals have touted the 80/20 philosophy before me. What makes my approach a bit different? A stricter definition of the foods that should make up your 80 percent. You see, as a whole food loving, plant-strong kind of dietitian, sugary yogurts and standard brown bread covered in margarine don't meet my standard of truly healing, nutrient-dense food. To truly fortify your anti-inflammatory defense system, you have to dig a little deeper into the garden.

Powerful Foods for a Healthy Life

My goal is to supercharge your system with truly anti-inflammatory, nutrient-filled foods that give more than they take. Plenty of phytochemicals, few calories. Lots of fiber, not a lot of artery-clogging animal fats. Energizing protein, no sugar crashes. You get the picture!

Your body is designed to deal with a little bit of less-than-perfect living—otherwise our species would not have survived the industrial revolution intact. Your body has elaborate systems for creating antioxidants, cleansing the blood, and healing DNA damage. But those systems only work well if you give them what they need: lots of good food, clean water, rest, and movement. The trouble is, we have been so twisted around by food marketing that what we have been taught to consider good food is candy disguised as breakfast cereal and Kool-Aid disguised as a vitamin drink.

A diet filled with overprocessed foods and lacking in fresh plant foods diminishes your healing capacity; inflammation, fatigue, and ill-health result. It's not that a doughnut or slice of deep dish pizza every now and then will kill you—of course that is not the case, it's just food. The trouble is, a life filled with those foods instead of nourishing plant foods is like a chronic poison. Each day, you become a little less nourished, a little less able to heal, and a little more broken down.

Deciding if 80/20 is Right for You

The 80/20 approach is the loosest and easiest to follow, yet potentially the most challenging and transformative of the four plans I will outline here. Loose, because I won't tell you how to eat, what meals to make, or quantities to choose. Easiest to follow, because you have the ultimate freedom to eat in a way that suits your taste buds and lifestyle. From grazing to three squares, gourmet to simply heat and eat, you can do it 80/20 style. Transformative, because once you walk over to the light side of anti-inflammatory eating, your body will be flooded with nutrients the likes of which it may have not seen before, and the most challenging because hey, without strict rules . . . it can be easy to slide. Twenty percent becomes 30 becomes 60 . . .

I think at this point it is a good idea to take a step back and discuss what it means to eat well and what it looks like over the course of, well, forever. Before I became interested in healthy eating, my diet probably looked like a 40/60 plan. When I became a vegetarian as a teenager, I probably drifted between 100/0 and 0/100, each extreme usually as a backlash to the other. Then I seemed to stabilize myself at 50/50 and started clawing my way on up as I studied nutrition and refined my own eating habits. Sometimes, I look closer to a 90/10 plan. I tend to dip lowest to a 70/30 plan, and this all seems to average out around the ol' 80/20 ideal. It took me fifteen years to get here. You can do it in fewer . . . but perhaps trying to do it in fifteen days isn't realistic.

If you are new to anti-inflammatory eating, this plan might look nothing like how you eat now and you will need a roadmap and perhaps some baby steps to transition. In fact, this way of eating is the destination you get close to after taking the 101 steps outlined in the previous chapter. Why not craft a path that leads you here? Make baby steps for three, six, or twelve months with the 80/20 approach as your destination.

Reality Check

As you get all juiced up about anti-inflammatory eating, beware the desire for overnight success. I hold the 80/20 approach as the ultimate in anti-inflammatory eating. It is the closest to perfection you can get as an anti-inflammatory eater. If your diet looks more like 30/70, getting to 60/40 will place you in the really healthy eater category. Heck, maybe that is where your own individual goal should lie! If you feel amazing simply living 60/40, I would call that a success. For me, I know that my body leans towards a more inflammatory state, and 80/20 is necessary for me to be in tip-top health. Remember, trying to dramatically makeover your life overnight can lead to hardship and rebound.

If you need more clear-cut guidance, I would recommend adopting one of the other three plans in this book. This plan is destined for the don't-fence-me-in type; you simply fill your kitchen with the 80 percent foods and get eating. However, while simple to say, it's not always easy to do. This kind of eating is swimming upstream from our crappy food culture. Knowing this, if you are looking at that list of 80 percent foods and thinking to yourself, "I can do this!"—let's get started!

Living the 80/20 Life

It's simple—what follows is a list of foods to eat 80 percent of the time and a selection that falls into the 20 percent category. Eighty/20 is the anti-inflammatory goal; don't expect to get here overnight.

To achieve greater success, a kitchen clean out helps. Take the weekend and survey your kitchen according to the list. Finish up or remove most of the foods that don't fall into the 80 percent category. Don't go crazy here—don't throw out all of your baking supplies if they could be used to make good cookies that can be frozen for a 20 percent treat when you want it. However, remove those foods that will make it tougher to reach your goals—give the snack foods and sodas away to a hungry college kid, and get rid of unhealthful cooking oils, deli meats, and baked goods. Donate whatever is unopened, and try not to be too wasteful. Eat it up . . . then move on.

Then, you are going to need to plan out what you will actually eat and go grocery shopping! Flip through the recipes to find some easy meal and snack ideas. Write them on your calendar so you know what you're making. If you need a little help navigating food choices, I have also created an anti-inflammatory grocery list in the Supermarket Smarts chapter to make it easy.

You can keep a food journal if you feel you need it to keep on track. It can be helpful with a more unstructured plan because the journal keeps you honest and the act of journaling connects you to your intentions on a regular basis. Perhaps start your journal with three intentions for your eating transition so you can refer back to them as you journal. Keep the journal until this way of eating feels intuitive or the process of journaling starts to feel too much like a chore. Or, you could keep a journal for a week out of every month as a way of reconnecting to your goal. And repeat after me, "Progress . . . not perfection." That bag of chips is not a failure. It's a bag of chips. Chase it with a tofu and bok choy stir-fry.

Creating Structure Where None Exists

Staring into the 80/20 void can feel a bit vast . . . particularly if you aren't there yet. What does keeping to 80/20 even look like in real terms? You can define it for yourself, but it certainly helps to go through the work of defining it; that definition can become your anchor in the moderation storm. Here are some examples:

1. If you eat three square meals a day, you eat twenty-one meals a week—giving you three meals a week to fill the 20 percent category. This is a great approach for those who like to dine out a lot; however, don't fall into the cheat meal mentality. If you hunker down for three super decadent three-course meals during the week, chased by bottles of wine, you probably aren't keeping to the 20 percent rule. Which is fine, but be honest with yourself about it. Keep 20 percent meals moderate in portion and be sure to eat some veggies alongside that linguine, too.

2. If you like to eat five mini meals a day, you have up to seven opportunities for the 20 percent.

   Remember that if you fully utilize those seven opportunities, those other twenty-eight should look darn close to 100 percent anti-inflammatory foods if you are going for the 80/20 balance.

3. If you love to have a little something every day, give yourself two food choices a day out of the 20 percent category—perhaps a glass or two of merlot and a small dessert when you go for an otherwise healthy dinner.

Feast Your Eyes on a Feast for Your Cells . . . the 80/20 List

Anti-Inflammatory Foods for 80 Percent of the Time	Potentially Pro-Inflammatory Foods for 20 Percent of the Time
All fruits and vegetables in their whole, unseasoned forms: —fresh fruits and vegetables —frozen, unflavored fruits and vegetables —unsweetened dried fruit *This is the nutritional mother lode: vitamins, minerals, fiber, and phytochemicals without too many calories. This is the foundation of an anti-inflammatory life.*	**Alcohol in all its forms . . .** *Alcohol is great (and delicious!) in small amounts but troublesome for waistlines, livers, cancer risk, and inhibitions in large amounts.*
Raw, unsalted nuts and seeds *Nuts and seeds provide protein, healthy fats, and minerals. Great for snacks and recipes.*	**Baked goods, such as cookies, muffins, scones, cakes, and pastries (other than those you make from healthy ingredients at home)** *Our overconsumption of baked goods bites us in the butt every single time since they're easy to overeat, blood sugar spiking, and devoid of most nutrition. Choose nuts, fruit, and veggies over baking at snack time.*
Beans and lentils, dried or canned *Legumes are a critical daily food—packed with protein, vitamins and minerals, and fiber. Keeps blood sugars balanced and the healthy bacteria in your gut well-fed.*	**Dairy foods other than plain yogurt and kefir** —Cheese —Milk —Butter —Ice cream

Dairy foods don't fall into the anti-inflammatory realm, but if you love them, they can fit into an anti-inflammatory life in small amounts.

Quality counts: choose dairy foods with real ingredients, growth-hormone-free, made from fresh fluid milk, and organic when you can. European cheeses tend to be made from grass-fed milk and are a better choice.

All meats other than fish

Meats have a nutrient profile that is more inflammatory than not. Poultry is a best runner up to fish, and pork and beef should be consumed squarely in the 20 percent category. Eggs are another runner up and can be consumed moderately on an anti-inflammatory plan instead of meat.

Whole, intact grains
—**steel-cut oats**
—**wheat, spelt, or einkorn berries**
—**whole barley**
—**whole rye kernels**
—**quinoa**
—**brown, black, or red rice**
—**amaranth**
—**buckwheat groats**

Don't be fooled by "made with whole grain"; these are the real whole and intact grains. You find them in the bulk bins, without fancy cartoon characters on them. Cook as porridge, side dishes, or add to soups and casseroles. Keeping grains intact will keep them filling and less trouble for your blood sugars. Grains are rich in fiber, protein, and minerals.

Minimally processed grains

—100 percent sprouted grain bread and tortillas
—100 percent whole wheat or other whole grain pasta
—unseasoned hard rye or 100 percent whole grain crackers
—select whole grain breakfast cereals (see resources)

These are the convenient and common grain staples, made better by being totally whole grain without additives and better for blood sugars. Don't let this group crowd out other whole foods though.

Minimally processed, whole organic soy foods

—organic tofu or tempeh
—organic edamame (green soybeans)
—organic miso, soy sauce, tamari
—organic soy milk made from the whole soybean

Unless you are allergic or intolerant to soy, whole soy foods are protein and mineral rich and help round out a protein-packed diet that is easy on the waistline and the planet. Most meat analogues made from soy aren't the best choices.

Healthy Fats

—olives
—avocados
—nuts
—extra virgin olive oil or avocado oil
—virgin coconut oil (small amounts)
—expeller pressed almond oil (for high heat)
—flavoring oils: walnut, hazelnut
—superfood oils: hemp, chia, flax

Healthy fats are your friend; just don't go overboard if you are weight-conscious. Choose whole food sources of fats, such as nuts and avocados, most often. Don't cook with flavoring oils or superfood oils—drizzle them on at the table.

Chocolate, candy, and desserts

This one is pretty self-explanatory, but I have to say that 85 percent dark chocolate is essentially cocoa, so enjoy in small amounts on the 80 percent side!

Fast food

Yes . . . pretty much all standard fast food. Even the wraps with tomatoes in them. Of course, if you are lucky enough to live by a truly healthy quick service place (such as a juice bar or salad bar), just because you can get it fast doesn't make it fast food. I am talking pizza-burgers-burritos here.

Processed grain foods, such as most breakfast cereals, crackers, granola bars, and breads

This is where many unhealthy foods masquerade as healthy foods.

These are unsatisfying and devoid of nutrients. Stick to the grain choices on the 80 percent side of the list . . . use your 20 percent for way more interesting choices, such as cheese, beer, or chocolate.

Optional: Sustainably caught fish and seafood, ethically raised

If you eat fish, it is the sole animal protein that is totally anti-inflammatory. Low in calories and artery clogging fats.

Fermented Foods

—**Plain, unsweetened yogurt**
—**Plain, unsweetened kefir**
—**Low sugar kombucha**
—**Unpasteurized sauerkraut**
—**Unpasteurized kimchi**

Fermented foods keep your belly happy and promote the anti-inflammatory love. Eat daily.

Nutrient-dense flavorings

—**fresh and dried herbs**
—**fresh and dried spices**
—**raw and/or unsweetened cocoa powder**
—**ginger, garlic, turmeric**

Get used to flavor! Don't sprinkle herbs and spices, luxuriate in them.

Plain coffee and black, green, and herbal tea

These beverages are essentially plant extracts and all are antioxidant-rich. Watch the caffeine if you tend to be a bit coffee crazy; drink tea more often.

Unsweetened, calcium-fortified vegetarian milk alternatives

—**almond, rice, hemp, quinoa**

Get the calcium, avoid the animal fat. Watch sugar as many can be overly sweet; most brands offer unsweetened varieties. Note that only soy milk is high in protein; if using other varieties, get your protein elsewhere.

>>

Eat to Live . . . and Enjoy Every Bite!

—*Living 80/20 will help fight inflammation and heal your body while still allowing you some wiggle room for the fun stuff.*

—*Eighty percent of the time, your diet should be filled with unprocessed or minimally processed plant foods.*

—*The framework is 80/20 living; if all you need to feel phenomenally better is 60/40 living, go for it!*

—*All real foods fit in a healthy diet, it is how they dominate our eating pattern that can make them bad for us.*

CHAPTER 10

STUCK IN THE MUCK?: A FOURTEEN-DAY KICK-START

"When diet is wrong, medicine is of no use. When diet is correct, medicine is of no need." —Ayurvedic Proverb

For Those Whose Butts Need Kicking

Feeling particularly wretched these days? Does it take seven presses of the snooze button before you can drown your sorrows in a pot of coffee? Does lacing up your walking shoes seem like more effort than you can muster? Can't remember the last time you ate a home-cooked meal? Wish there was some way to start feeling amazing again? Need a strong nutritional approach to get you motivated? (Sick of reading these questions yet?) Well, you have found your solution. I have created a fourteen-day nutritional reboot to get you back on your energetic feet again.

It's not a diet. But you might lose a little weight. You might not. I don't want you going hungry over the two weeks. Eat until you are satisfied but not stuffed. Because stuffing yourself is a habit that needs to be unlearned anyway.

It's not a detox. But the plan will support your body's natural cleansing mechanisms. It is essentially a 99/1 anti-inflammatory plan, so there is nothing to junk up your pipes and plenty of nourishment to support healing and restore energy levels.

So why do I insist on calling it a kick-start? Because intention is everything. The intention here is to give yourself two weeks to show your body what healthy can feel like. I want to create a space where you can flood your body with good, nourishing food and realize that, hey . . . this is an awesome place to be! To really help give you a fresh start and begin reclaiming your health, I have provided some basic suggestions for working through other areas of your lifestyle over these two weeks to better support your healthy eating work.

It's Like Speed-Dating for Healthy Eating

My intention behind including this option in the book is twofold: sometimes you need a heavy dose of nourishment to begin to correct your current health picture and get yourself on the right path, physically and mentally. If you have been going through a tough year of work, terrible eating, or poor sleeping, your body needs some heavy-handed nutrition to lift you out of your inflammatory funk. Spending a finite amount of time on a structured plan will help you focus on getting healthier and more energetic so you can have the motivation to make long-term change.

In addition, because many of us get antsy waiting for the long-term benefits of a slower healthy eating transition, it can be easy to lose focus in the face of a jalapeño popper or twelve. This is a plan that is relatively dramatic and will have you feeling good so quickly that it should hopefully motivate you to continue on the 80/20 path. It is dramatic because you will be feasting on so many nutrient-dense, nourishing whole foods that your cells are going to jump up and dance a jig. There will be no more clawing your way out of bed or staring trance-like into a chocolate bar at 3 p.m. This plan gives you a big nutrition to jumpstart your engine.

Of course, I can imagine that some of you reading this might want to use it as a diet to slim down for a trip to Bermuda; well . . . at least it is a healthier approach than diet-in-a-can. This plan was not designed for weight loss, but depending where you are starting out, it might help you reach your goals—but the minute you return to your old patterns of eating the weight will likely come back. Lasting change requires . . . making lasting change! So I hope that if you are interested in the two week kick-start, you will take all this healthy eating stuff to heart and continue down the anti-inflammatory path for life. The whole intention of this book is to remove dieting from your vocabulary and help you learn to live in the deliciously grey area of healthy eating that still lets you live a little.

Junk-Free Living

One of the major differences between a traditional cleansing program and what I have described here is that my two-week program is not everything-free.

This is not intended as an allergy management diet, which I recommend you do only under the guidance of a skilled dietitian with food allergy experience. It is low-gluten but not gluten-free—although if you are gluten-free, you can easily modify it to be gluten-free. It is void of overprocessed grains, so you can keep blood sugars balanced and try a few awesome grains that you might not have in your current rotation. Many of us eat standard wheat flour three to six times a day, and it crowds out the nourishing variety of plant foods we need to help us feel great.

The plan isn't strictly vegan, but it is largely plant-based; a savvy vegan could swap vegan proteins for the animal-based ones shown. It is dairy-free, because we could all stand to experiment with how we feel without dairy for a little while; this is particularly true because dairy falls into the 20 percent foods category, and we tend go a bit overboard with all the processed foods that have cheap dairy ingredients added to them.

What this meal plan was designed to be was junk-free—few added sweeteners, only the highest quality fats, and ridiculous amounts of plant foods to get those engines running at high speed. The idea is that you focus on eating super-nourishing food for two weeks and see how it changes your body and mind. Then you can choose to carry on with whichever meals and habits serve you in your daily life long term.

Uncovering Food Sensitivities with the Kick-Start

As I described earlier in the book, the interplay between inflammation, a leaky gut, and food sensitivities can become a self-sustaining firefight. Identifying food sensitivities can help stop the cycle. An elimination diet and challenge program is an effective way of determining what your food sensitivities might be. If you feel dramatically better on the kick-start, consider keeping a food journal as you reintroduce your usual diet and note if any symptoms come back. If you suspect that food sensitivity is leading to symptoms, talk to a dietitian about designing a proper elimination and challenge. The kick-start can easily be modified with a few simple swaps to make it free of the foods that commonly are associated with food sensitivities, such as gluten and soy. However, I strongly recommend that you work with a health professional during this time because there can be other mitigating factors that you might not uncover on your own, such as stress, caffeine use, medications, or other lifestyle factors contributing to your digestive troubles. It can also be easy to confuse a true food sensitivity with feeling terrible because of food quality—like that time you ate a giant double bacon cheeseburger that tied your stomach in a knot.

How to Use the Kick-Start

First, you must plan. Without a plan, you can't stick to the plan! Run out of food midweek, have a late meeting, and suddenly you don't have time to run to the supermarket and cook your intended meal. Oh well, might as well just stop for some pizza, right? Totally fine with me, except that you might miss out on some of the dramatic benefits you were hoping for on the kick-start. You will still get a lot of good into that body of yours, as long as one meal doesn't turn into ten.

If you are looking to truly commit, plan ahead. Use the grocery list to buy everything you need for the seven day menu (which you will cycle through a second time). On the weekend, prepare the make-aheads for the week so midweek eating goes by smoothly; this kick-start was designed for real people with real jobs! You are going to have to commit some time to food preparation, but none of the recipes are complex or time-consuming. Then, simply enjoy the food and feel the good.

Optimizing the Kick-Start

To reap the most of this healing plan, it makes sense to pay attention to other areas of your life that might be breaking you down. Turn off the TV, put down the smart phone, make sleep a priority. Treat yourself to a few yoga classes. Go for a gentle hike or walk on the beach.

Sleep needs to be a priority to help restore your health and your energy levels. Try to carve out seven to eight hours each night for the next two weeks; in addition, choose a bedtime and a wake up time and stick with them. Schedule bedtime and wake time alarms in your phone as reminders if you have to. Your body loves routine—it is calming and reassuring to those cells of yours. Sleep is the time when the body rests, restores, and heals, and lack of sleep can lead to poor choices and health behaviors. You can think of sleep as the time when all your good lifestyle work really knits itself together.

You also have to make time to move your body. Exercise helps move lymphatic fluid through the body to help the body cleanse and restore as intended. Sweat is a great cleanser for both body and mind—that pumping heart helps bust the cobwebs out of the brain, as well as the muscles. Exercise is also a positive stress that in moderate amounts ensures the body is strong, supple, and resilient. Choose whichever activity you love the most—from swimming to walking, basketball to shadow boxing. Your chosen activity doesn't have to be strenuous—even going for a daily thirty minute walk will help get that blood pumping and focus your mind. The only real requirement is that you commit to breaking a real sweat daily.

Speaking of clearing your mind, the thoughts in your head can sometimes be as integral to healing as the food on your plate. Try to avoid particularly contentious situations for a couple of weeks if you can—you might not be able to take vacation, but you can try to avoid that crabby colleague for a while. Take note of negative self-talk and let it go. Actively try to focus on positive thoughts and feelings. Repeat a positive mantra or watch a hilarious clip during your coffee break. Do something daily to relieve stress, whether it is the square breathing exercise on page 101, a hot bath, taking a walk in nature, or reading a good book.

Try to limit alcohol and coffee during this time, and really let your body fly solo without stimulants or depressants. If you get caffeine withdrawal headaches, you might just want to have a small cup of coffee in the morning to avoid the pain. If allergies or food preferences get in the way, of course feel free to modify the recipes. The only real rule here is to keep it totally anti-inflammatory; keep dairy, added sugars, processed grains, and meat out of the equation. Eat as much as you need to be full and satisfied. Shall I say this again? You are not on a diet. You are committing to nourishment, for body and soul. Hunger drives feelings of anxiety and craving and derails healthy eating intentions. The optional snacks are there to keep your belly happy, as much as you need them.

Taming a Rumbly Tummy

If you are used to a far richer diet, you may have a hard time feeling satisfied on this plan, as your body isn't getting the calorie bombs it is used to—you are literally not reaching that salt/sugar/fat high that restaurant meals and hyper-processed foods provide. Don't give up; instead, fill up! To help keep you full, make sure to eat plenty of healthy snacks, and don't skimp on protein portions at mealtime—double up if you have to. Protein and fiber are filling and will help keep you energized. Keep with it, and try not to get discouraged. These two weeks will be like real food rehab for your taste buds. The more you lay off the crutches of sugar, fat, and salt, the more your taste buds can wake up and start tasting the diverse flavors of real food.

On the other end of the spectrum are the rumbles that come from further on down . . . if your baseline diet isn't that high in fiber, you will have to come to a newfound understanding with your bowels. They might complain a bit now, but they will thank you for it later.

Repeat After Me: Everybody Toots

Increased bathroom trips and flatulence are to be expected as your body adjusts to processing all this extra plant matter. Doing the kick-start with your significant other or roomie is a good idea so you are both on the same digestive page, if you know what I mean! Buy the extra soft bathroom tissue for once.

To make the transition easier, drink plenty of fluid to help the fiber do its good work. Gentle exercise will keep everything moving. Chew your food thoroughly—this is so important to help your body effectively breakdown the plant matter—and eat slowly to allow your body time to process all of this newfound roughage.

Get Mindful as You Fill Your Belly

Over the course of this two-week health kick-start, you may notice something you didn't expect. You may feel some anxiety at the thought of not having your morning doughnut. You may feel sad and find yourself wanting to run to mac and cheese for comfort. As you quiet your mind and release the nutritional garbage, you may find that some emotional garbage starts bubbling to the surface.

For some of us, food can be a way of numbing thoughts, feelings, and heartache. When we remove that mindless eating reaction from our arsenal, we can be left with some pretty raw mental states. Acknowledge it, and let this be the opportunity to care for your emotional self as well as you are trying to care for your physical self. Should these situations occur for you, talk to someone that you deeply trust to help you work through the situation. Depending on your needs or inclination, it could be a spouse, a friend, or a counselor.

Getting Down to Business: The Seven-Day Menu

Here it is, without further ado . . . your seven day menu plan! You will cycle through this plan a second time for a total of fourteen days on the kick-start. All the recipes you need are included in the recipe section of this book. Feast your eyes on this feast for your cells!

You can start this plan any day of the week, but I encourage you to start on a Sunday, leaving Saturday for shopping and Saturday and Sunday for some prep cooking that will allow the week to breeze by.

Weekend Prep Kitchen

Prepare these goodies on the weekend to breeze through the weeks of healthy eating. You will thank me later, I promise! The freezer is your friend when it comes to stocking up for busier times. No time for breaky? Grab a breakfast bar out of the freezer and enjoy with an almond milk latte. Done.

—One batch of breakfast bars for the two weeks (freeze them)

—One batch of trail mix for the two weeks

—One batch of little gems for the two weeks (freeze them)

—One batch of white bean dip each week

—Chop some snacking veggies each week and store in an airtight container in the fridge for quick snacks

—If you want to work with dried beans, now is the time to soak, cook, and store them for the weekly recipes

---

Sunday	Monday	Tuesday	Wednesday	Thursday	Friday	Saturday
Say Yes to Salad for Breakfast	Liquid Gold Smoothie + protein choice: On the side: ½ cup almonds OR 2 egg whites + 1 egg scramble. Blended in: 1 serving vegan protein powder.	It's Easy Being Green Smoothie + protein choice: On the side: ½ cup almonds OR 2 egg whites + 1 egg scramble. Blended in: 1 serving vegan protein powder.	Liquid Gold Smoothie + protein choice: On the side: ½ cup almonds OR 2 egg whites + 1 egg scramble. Blended in: 1 serving vegan protein powder.	It's Easy Being Green Smoothie + protein choice: On the side: ½ cup almonds OR 2 egg whites + 1 egg scramble. Blended in: 1 serving vegan protein powder.	Liquid Gold Smoothie + protein choice: On the side: ½ cup almonds OR 2 egg whites + 1 egg scramble. Blended in: 1 serving vegan protein powder.	It's Easy Being Green Smoothie + protein choice: On the side: ½ cup almonds OR 2 egg whites + 1 egg scramble. Blended in: 1 serving vegan protein powder.
¼–½ cup Energy to Spare Trail Mix	Chopped veggies with ½ cup spiced white bean dip	One piece of fruit: apple/pear/berries + 2 Little Gems	One piece of fruit: apple/pear/berries + 2 Little Gems	Chopped veggies with ½ cup spiced white bean dip	One piece of fruit: apple/pear/berries + 2 Little Gems	Brilliant Breakfast Bar
Broccoli Crunch Salad	Cauliflower Tabbouleh with Baked Sesame Tofu	Kale and Avo Salad with ¾ cup chickpeas or ½ can tuna	Leftover Edible Medicine Soup	Kale and Avo Salad with ¾ cup chickpeas or ½ can tuna	Leftover Tempeh Tacos	Broccoli Crunch Salad
Kombucha Break Have 1-2 cups kombucha with a snack if you are hungry	Kombucha Break	Kombucha Break	Kombucha Break	Kombucha Break	Kombucha Break	Kombucha Break
Cauliflower Tabbouleh with Baked Sesame Tofu	Miso Ginger Salmon Collard Pockets, served with ½–1 cup cooked quinoa	Edible Medicine Soup	Portuguese Baked Beans, Weekday Style served with leafy greens of your choice	Tempeh Tacos, served with brown rice or quinoa (optional)	Spicy Tomato Soup	Herb crusted tofu or halibut, served with whole wheat pasta tossed in olive oil and a Black Bean Brownie

A Word About Snacking

This kick-start is about lavishing your body with nourishing food, not weight loss. Eat as much of the recommended foods as you need to feel full and satisfied. Focus on proteins, such as tofu, fish, and beans, if appetites are high. On the flip side, don't feel like you have to eat all the recommended food either. If you have a smaller body size, are sedentary, or you are getting too full, don't force it. Tune into your own body and your true hunger to drive your portion size choices.

Making it Easy. . .Your Shopping List

Just to make things even simpler, I have compiled a shopping list for the seven day menu. Photocopy it and check it against the recipe variations you want to make and what you already have in your kitchen. Then go shopping. You're welcome.

Complete Shopping List for Your Seven Day Anti-Inflammatory Kick-Start!		
Grains	*Fruits*	*Veggies*
¾ cup large flake oats	6 lemons	2 bunches parsley
1 cup large flake oats	4 red apples	6 large crimini mushrooms + 1 pound mixed mushrooms
quinoa	1 cup purple grapes	large bunch of broccoli
brown rice	5 bananas	cauliflower
whole wheat pasta	1½ cup not-from-concentrate orange juice	5 oz. clamshell each of baby spinach, arugula
	1 lime	2 cucumbers
	8 medjool (large) dates	fresh mint
	Plus 3–5 pieces of fruit for snacking: apple, pear, berries, summer fruit	pint of cherry tomatoes
		1 garlic bulb
		3 small golden beets
		3 small carrots
		fresh turmeric (if available)

>>

Grains	Fruits	Veggies
		fresh thyme
		large bunch of collard greens (at least 8 leaves)
		2–4 green onions
		fresh ginger
		large bunch curly kale, large bunch black kale
		1 avocado
		2 bell peppers
		4 yellow onions
		1 small bunch cilantro
		Snacking veggies

Proteins	Condiments	Extras
1 package tempeh bacon or smoked tofu	real mayonnaise or Veg-enaise	2 cups raw almonds
turkey bacon	seeded + Dijon mustards	1⅓ cup raw pumpkin seeds
dozen eggs	white wine or apple cider vinegar	1 cup shaved coconut
vegan protein powder	honey	½ cup dried golden berries
4 x 15 oz. cans white beans	extra virgin olive oil	¼ cup cacao nibs
2 packages extra firm tofu	cumin, powdered and seeds	½ cup sesame seeds
4 pieces halibut	allspice	Kombucha 2 liters (~67 ounces)
4 pieces wild salmon	salt and pepper	green tea bags
15 oz. can chickpeas	red pepper flakes	ground flax
1 can light tuna	cinnamon	hemp hearts
2 x 19 oz. cans kidney beans	vanilla extract	¼ cup raw walnuts
2 packages tempeh	soy sauce	½ cup dried apricots
15 oz. black beans	toasted sesame oil	tomato paste
	rice vinegar	100g bar of 85 percent cacao dark chocolate

Proteins	Condiments	Extras
	maple syrup	unsweetened chocolate almond milk
	chili powder	⅓ cup almond meal
	½ cup passata (strained) tomato sauce	28 oz. can of whole plum tomatoes
	oregano	white wine
	coriander	
	cayenne pepper	
	salsa	
	1 cup + 1 quart vegetable stock	
	natural peanut butter	
	harissa spice paste	

You really can start to change your life in two weeks . . .

—Getting healthy is more about what you choose to eat than what you don't eat. Don't assume that everything is bad for you just because you read it on a blog.

—You don't have to get strict to get well, but a two-week break in nutritionland can really set a new lifestyle in perspective.

—Nourishing your mind is just as important as feeding your belly; take care of your body and your mind in equal measure to help you feel amazing.

CHAPTER 11

A TWENTY-EIGHT DAY ANTI-INFLAMMATORY MENU PLAN TO MAKE YOUR LIFE SIMPLE

"One cannot think well, love well, sleep well, if one has not dined well."
—Virginia Woolf

Some of my clients just want to keep it simple: they want to know exactly what they should eat, and they are happy to do the work. So I created this twenty-eight-day meal plan for them. It is my 80/20 approach made deliciously simple . . . eat the food, feel the good!

That is the beauty of us humans as eaters; I personally can't follow meal plans, but I know that others can and, in fact, prefer the clarity and structure of them. If that is you, know that I have created this meal plan to get you through four weeks of deliciously healthy eating. There is no cheating to worry about—don't like a meal? Change it! Going out for dinner? Enjoy! The structure is there for those who want to make it easy to know what to eat—not because this is a perfect plan that is set in stone. For those who love food and can't stand getting caught up in the minutiae of nutrition, I do the thinking . . . you do the cooking and eating. No fuss, no muss—all good.

The meal plan is an 80/20 anti-inflammatory pattern but it is 100 percent healthy. There are no unhealthy, hyper-processed foods on the menu; however, there are weekly freebie meals so if you really need some nachos or a steak, you can eat them worry-free and enjoy. I have designed this meal plan to be chock-a-block full of nutrient-dense foods in a ratio that will help soothe inflammation, but if high levels of inflammation are not a worry for you right now, you can easily swap out some more meals as you wish and still feel healthy and vibrant.

Of course, if the idea of having to shop for and prepare all these meals turns your feet cold, this is not the plan for you. As I mentioned, my favorite plan in the whole book is the food swaps—don't think that because this meal plan is the most elaborate and structured it is somehow better. It is best for those who are drawn to it . . . terrible for those who aren't. There is no one right way to eat. There are right patterns of eating . . . and a million different ways to get there. This is just one option, offered for the structured, unemotional eater to get on with it—healthfully!

Getting Started

All the recipes you need are found within this book, and the meal plan includes some prepared foods and no-cook items too. Some of the meals also call for simple foods that don't really require a recipe. Simply do your weekly shop, photocopy the plan and throw it on the fridge, and enjoy!

In planning your shopping and managing your food inventory, think critically as you scan the week's menu and recipes. If you are just cooking for one and a recipe makes four servings, do you need an extra for lunch the next day? If so, you can opt to cut the recipe in half or make the full portion and freeze the other half for later on so you won't have to cook. This kind of task is perfect for Sunday mornings as you sit with a cup of tea. Take your time, think about what you need and the rest of the week will go smoothly—the last thing you want is to be at the grocery store every night, or to have a fridge full of leftovers going to waste.

Twenty-Eight Days of 80/20 Anti-Inflammatory Living

Week One	Week Two	Week Three	Week Four
Sunday	**Sunday**	**Sunday**	**Sunday**
Breakfast: It's Easy Being Green Smoothie— (page 231)	Breakfast: Two eggs, poached over a bed of wilted spinach (start with about 6 cups of spinach, sautéed with olive oil, salt and pepper, and served with one or two pieces of sprouted grain toast, spread with a little bit of butter.	Breakfast: Avocado toast: top two slices of toasted sprouted grain bread with a ¼ ripe avocado each. Top with salt, freshly cracked pepper, and some pumpkin seeds for crunch.	Breakfast: It's Easy Being Green Smoothie (page 231)
Snack: Apple with ¼ cup raw almonds			Snack: Apple spread with 2 tablespoons almond butter
Lunch: Almost instant spinach salad (page 237)		Snack: ½ cup plain greek yogurt, sprinkled with cinnamon and topped with ¼ chopped walnuts and 1 diced date	Lunch: Grown Up Lunch Box (page 237)
Snack: ½ cup spiced white bean dip (page 259) with 1 cup sliced veggies	Snack: One apple, spread with 1 tablespoon natural, unsweetened peanut butter	Lunch: Grown Up Lunch Box (page 237)	Snack: Black Bean Brownie (page 264)
Dinner: Grilled salmon with roasted veggies and cooked quinoa	Lunch: Lunch out: salad with beans, chicken, or fish	Snack: ½ cup pink dip (page 262) with 1 cup sliced veggies	Dinner: Mediterranean tofu scramble: crumble extra firm tofu and sauté with olive oil, garlic, cherry tomatoes, olives, diced zucchini and shredded kale; season and serve on a bed of quinoa.
	Snack: 2 slices aged white cheddar, 2 hard rye crackers, and a pear	Dinner: Herb crusted tofu (page 255) and colorful winter slaw (page 247)	
	Dinner: Grilled chicken with cauliflower tabbouleh (page 242)		
Monday	**Monday**	**Monday**	**Monday**
Breakfast: Cocoaberry Smoothie (page 229)	Breakfast: Liquid Gold Smoothie (page 229)	Breakfast: It's Easy Being Green smoothie (page 231)	Breakfast: It's Easy Being Green smoothie (page 231)
Snack: ¼–½ cup Energy to Spare Trail Mix (page 260)	Snack: ¼–½ cup Energy to Spare Trail Mix (page 260)	Snack: One apple, spread with 2 tablespoons natural, unsweetened peanut butter	Snack: One apple, spread with 2 tablespoons natural, unsweetened peanut butter
Lunch: Grown Up Lunch Box (page 237)	Lunch: Leftover grilled chicken and cauliflower tabbouleh	Lunch: Leftover colorful winter slaw and sliced turkey	Lunch: salad bar lunch, don't forget the protein!
Snack: ½ cup spiced white bean dip (page 259) with 1 cup sliced veggies	Snack: Pink Dip (page 262) and 1 cup of sliced veggies	Snack: Brilliant Breakfast Bar (page 232) and a pear	Snack: 2 slices aged white cheddar and 2 hard rye crackers and a pear
Dinner: Portuguese Baked Beans, weekday style (page 250) served	Dinner: Eat Your Greens frittata (page 248) and roasted baby red potatoes	Dinner: Dinner Out	Dinner: Grilled chicken with

Week One	Week Two	Week Three	Week Four
Tuesday	**Tuesday**	**Tuesday**	**Tuesday**
Breakfast: ¾ cup plain greek yogurt, layered with ¼ cup chopped walnuts, 1 cup thawed or fresh blueberries, 1 tablespoon dried tart cherries, 1 tablespoon hemp hearts, sprinkled with cinnamon and cardamom	Breakfast: Avocado toast: top two slices of toasted sprouted grain bread with a ¼ ripe avocado each. Top with salt, freshly cracked pepper and some pumpkin seeds for crunch.	Breakfast: ¾ cup plain greek yogurt parfait, layered with ¼ cup chopped walnuts, 1 cup thawed or fresh blueberries, 1 tablespoon dried tart cherries, 1 tablespoon hemp hearts and sprinkled with cinnamon and cardamom.	Breakfast: ¾ cup plain greek yogurt parfait, layered with ¼ cup chopped walnuts, 1 cup thawed or fresh blueberries, 1 tablespoon dried tart cherries, 1 tablespoon hemp hearts and sprinkled with cinnamon and cardamom.
Snack: 1 pear with ¼ cup raw pecans	Snack: Apple spread with 2 tablespoons almond butter	Snack: 1 pear with ¼ cup raw pecans (page 237)	Snack: One apple, spread with 2 tablespoons natural, unsweetened peanut butter
Lunch: Leftover Portuguese Baked Beans with veggies	Lunch: Kale and avo salad with ¾ cup white beans (page 244)	Lunch: Almost instant spinach salad (page 264)	Lunch: Leftover grilled chicken and cauliflower tabbouleh
Snack: ½–1 c Amazing Roasted Chick Peas (page 263)	Snack: Banana sushi (page 261)	Snack: Black bean brownie (page 264)	Snack: a whole food bar
Dinner: Roasted Veg and Barley Salad (page 241)	Dinner: Spiced Tomato Soup (page 245)	Dinner: Greens and Beans Casserole (page 258)	Dinner: Tempeh Tacos (page 252)
Wednesday	**Wednesday**	**Wednesday**	**Wednesday**
Breakfast: Easy Being Green Smoothie (page 231)	Breakfast: Cocoaberry Smoothie (page 229)	Breakfast: Two eggs, poached over a bed of wilted spinach (start with about 6 cups fresh), sautéed with olive oil, salt and pepper and served with one or two pieces of sprouted grain toast, spread with a little bit of butter.	Breakfast: Liquid Gold Smoothie (page 229)
Snack: Apple with ¼ cup raw almonds	Snack: 1 slice sprouted grain toast spread with almond butter	Snack: Amazing Roasted Chick Peas (page 263)	Snack: Energy to Spare Trail Mix (page 260)
Lunch: Leftover Roasted Veg and Barley Salad	Lunch: leftover spicy tomato soup with 3 hard rye crackers spread with olive tapenade and topped with ¼ cup of crumbled feta cheese		Lunch: Leftover tempeh tacos (page 252)
Snack: ½ cup plain greek yogurt, sprinkled with cinnamon and topped with ¼ chopped walnuts and 1 diced date	Snack: 1 pear with ¼ cup raw pecans		Snack: 2 little gems (page 262) and a pear
			Dinner: Stir-fried or roasted veggies and tofu

>>

Column 1	Column 2	Column 3	Column 4
Dinner: Turmeric Chicken Bake (page 257) and a baby greens salad	Dinner: Tofu sesame "steaks" (page 243), served over soba noodles tossed with 1 cup grated veggies and a splash of soy sauce and seasoned rice vinegar	Lunch: Broccoli crunch salad (page 240) with candied salmon or chopped turkey Snack: fruit salad sprinkled with energy to spare trail mix (page 260) Dinner: Edible Medicine Soup (page 246)	
Thursday Breakfast: ¾ cup plain greek yogurt, layered with ¼ cup chopped walnuts, 1 cup thawed or fresh blueberries, 1 tablespoon dried tart cherries, 1 tablespoon hemp hearts and sprinkled with cinnamon and cardamom Lunch: Almost instant spinach salad (page 237) Snack: 2 little gems (page 262) and a pear Dinner: Mediterranean tofu scramble: crumble extra firm tofu and sauté with olive oil, garlic, cherry tomatoes, olives, diced zucchini and shredded kale; season and serve on a bed of quinoa.	**Thursday** Breakfast: Slow cooked oatmeal topped with 3 tablespoons hemp seeds, ½ cup berries and ¼ cup raw sunflower seeds Snack: ½ cup plain greek yogurt, sprinkled with cinnamon and topped with ¼ chopped walnuts and 1 diced date Lunch: Broccoli crunch salad (page 240) served with a leftover tofu sesame "steak" Snack: Rice crackers and ½ cup pink dip (page 262) Dinner: Colorful spiced chicken lettuce cups (page 254)	**Thursday** Breakfast: Cocoaberry Smoothie (page 229) Snack: ½ cup Energy to Spare trail mix (page 260) Lunch: Kale and avo salad, (page 244) with ¾ cup chickpeas Snack: ½ cup plain greek yogurt, sprinkled with cinnamon and topped with ¼ chopped walnuts and 1 diced date Dinner: Baked Mexican Dip (page 260), served with chopped veggies and organic corn tortilla chips	**Thursday** Breakfast: It's Easy Being Green Smoothie (page 231) Snack: Amazing Roasted Chick Peas (page 263) Lunch: Almost instant spinach salad (page 237) Snack: Rice crackers and ½ cup pink dip (page 262) Dinner: "Fish and Chips": 1 cup baked sweet potato fries, served with grilled or herb crusted halibut or sable fish (page 255) and a ½ cup of colorful winter slaw (page 247).

Week One	Week Two	Week Three	Week Four
Friday	**Friday**	**Friday**	**Friday**
Breakfast: Feel Good Pancakes (page 234) and fresh fruit	Breakfast: South of the Border tofu scramble (page 232)	Breakfast: Say "Yes!" to salad for breakfast (page 235)	Breakfast: Slow cooked oatmeal topped with 3 tablespoons hemp seeds, ½ cup berries and ¼ cup raw sunflower seeds
Snack: ½ recipe Cocoaberry Smoothie (page 229)	Snack: The Real Muffin (page 230) and a piece of fruit	Snack: Brilliant Breakfast bar (page 232)	Snack: ½ recipe Cocoaberry Smoothie (page 229)
Lunch: Spicy Korean Sandwich (page 238)	Lunch: Grown Up Lunch Box (page 237)	Lunch: Spicy Korean Sandwich (page 238)	Lunch: Kale and avo salad, with ¾ cup chickpeas (page 244)
Snack: 2 little gems (page 262) and a pear	Snack: 2 little gems (page 262) and a peach	Snack: your favorite smoothie	Snack: 2 hard rye crackers spread with almond butter and honey
Dinner: Arugula Blackberry Salad (page 247) and grilled halibut	Dinner: Sweet potato and Chick Pea curry (page 249) served over ½–1 cup of your favorite grain	Dinner: Comforting Sweet Potatoes (page 253)	Dinner: Dinner Out
Snack: Berry Frozen Yogurt (page 265)	Snack: Black Bean Brownie		
Saturday	**Saturday**	**Saturday**	**Saturday**
Breakfast: The Real Muffin (page 230), with fresh fruit	Breakfast: Brilliant Breakfast Bars (page 232) and fresh fruit	Breakfast: Feel Good Pancakes (page 234) and fresh fruit	Breakfast: Baked Apple Oat Pudding (page 266)
Snack: Cherry tomatoes and raw walnuts	Snack: ½ recipe It's Easy Being Green Smoothie (page 231)	Snack: ½–1 Whole Food bar	Snack: 1 pear with ¼ cup raw pecans
Lunch: Lentil and Veggie Soup, with carrot sticks and hard rye crackers, spread with spiced white bean dip (page 259)	Lunch: Lunch out	Lunch: Arugula Blackberry salad (page 247) with a hardboiled egg	Lunch: Spiced Tomato Soup (page 245)
Snack: ½–1 whole food bar (see resources for suggestions)	Snack: 2 little gems (page 262) and a piece of fruit	Snack: ½ cup Amazing Chickpeas (page 263)	Snack: Spiced white bean dip (page 259) and 1 c chopped veggies
Dinner: Dinner out	Dinner: Leftover sweet potato and chick pea curry and grain (page 249)	Dinner: Chipotle Maple Baked Beans (page 251) and a green salad	Dinner: Broccoli crunch salad (page 240) with turmeric chicken skillet (page 257)

Eat the food, feel the good . . .

—A meal plan can be the perfect solution for those who don't want to think about what's for dinner . . . but it is not the only road to good health.

—Don't think that a meal plan is set in stone, if you don't like something, change it up!

—Watch food waste; it is better to eat (or freeze) leftovers rather than make a new recipe. Your wallet and your conscience will thank you.

CHAPTER 12
SUPERMARKET SMARTS

"The odds of going to the store for a loaf of bread and coming out with only a loaf of bread are three billion to one." —Erma Bombeck

If you are an anti-inflammatory warrior, the grocery store is your battleground. Don't underestimate the power of shopping—the foods that fill your buggy are the foods that you will cook and eat and create new cells from. You can't live an anti-inflammatory life if you fill your buggy with granola bars, frozen pizza, and bacon. Building energized, functional cells that defend you against modern living requires vital, nourishing foods that only nature can design. Factory foods are a distant second to the wisdom of unprocessed eating.

You are going to need a strategy to help you navigate the minefield of unhealthy foods on offer at the average supermarket. It is in the aisle where you decide if your diet will look more like 80/20 thriving or 20/80 coping.

Basic Training

To be a savvy shopper, you need to start with the basics—the rules of grocery engagement, as it were. These are tips like, "Don't shop on an empty stomach unless you are planning on loading your cart with chocolate and nachos." Another golden rule that is often overlooked is to make a shopping list and to stick to it—with few exceptions. Am I sounding like a broken record yet? If you are busy, planning out your meals for the week will necessitate using a shopping list and it will streamline your eating life. After all, it is the cooking and the eating that is fun—not the schlepping! Making a plan and a list keeps your chore score at a minimum. Even if you don't meal plan, an intelligent shopping list will ensure you always have the basics for a multitude of meals when you open the fridge and wonder . . . what's for dinner?

Shopping at the same store each week also makes the shopping faster; when you know where everything is, you can zoom around in no time. I can be in and out of my favorite store in twenty-two minutes with a week's worth of groceries. Of course, you may find that as you change your eating habits, it takes a bit longer to shop, as you are reading labels and finding new healthy favorites. Your old stomping grounds might not even cut it any longer and you might find yourself looking for a new supermarket. What you see is what you eat, so if you are able to switch to a store that carries healthier food, you are more likely to make better choices. You don't necessarily have to shop at a fancy health food or gourmet store; depending on your neighborhood, ethnic stores such as Korean, Greek, or Iranian greengrocers can be a treasure trove of healthy and affordable food. At a typical supermarket, you can absolutely find the ingredients for a healthy life; you will just have to work a little harder to avoid all of the pitfalls of factory foods.

Another golden-oldie rule is to shop the perimeter of the grocery store, as that is where the fresh departments are usually found. A modern refinement of that rule is to always start with the produce section. Take that empty cart and fill it up with plants! Make your next stop bulk foods—consider it the produce section for dried goods. This is where you will find all of your raw nuts, seeds, legumes, and intact whole grains to create a truly anti-inflammatory pantry. Make a quick pit stop in the refrigerated section for kefir, eggs, and some almond milk. Stop for dairy, poultry, and fish if they are on your list and when you finally wind your way into the inner aisles for a few staples, such as whole wheat pasta and canned tomatoes, your cart will already be too full for that tub of Chubby Hubby.

Desiree's Old-Timey Rules for Healthier Grocery Shopping

1. Make a list and stick with it, unless one of your pantry staples is on sale. In that case, stock up.
2. Shop the perimeter of the store first, starting with the produce section.
3. Don't shop hungry; buy a snack and eat it first if you have to.
4. The healthiest picks are always the ones without fancy boxes or packages.
5. If you can't understand the ingredients label, give the product a pass.
6. That warehouse pack is not a good deal if it goes bad before you can eat it . . . or it doesn't pass the ingredients test. A giant bag of chips is usually not a good idea.

Mastering the Nutrition Label

If you have made it this far, you know that the healthiest foods in the store are the simplest choices. The fruit, veggies, bulk nuts, seeds, legumes and grains, and fresh proteins, such as fish and tofu, earn top spots in an anti-inflammatory cart.

Once you leave the clear skies of whole food, you will find yourself wading into murky, hostile territory—food that does come in fancy packages. How to choose? Which ones are friends and which ones are foes . . . because they all claim to be good for you. The front of food packages look like billboards for whatever nutrition concerns are trending right now: Sugar free? High fiber? Protein? Hemp seeds? All your favorite claims are there, right on the ice cream and toaster pastries.

The first place you need to look to determine if a packaged food is a healthy one is the ingredients list. Generally speaking, the fewer the ingredients, the better. Apple = one ingredient = good! Super cookie fudge crunch avalanche frozen dessert = thirty-seven ingredients = not so good.

Next, if you cannot understand an ingredient on the list, move on. You should not require a degree in chemistry to understand your food. Salt, I getcha . . . polysorbate 80, not so much. Another way of saying this is, if a food contains ingredients that you would not find in your anti-inflammatory kitchen, you should not buy it and place it in your anti-inflammatory kitchen. You would be surprised how many of the 38,000 foods in your supermarket this rules out. This ingredient test is all about determining food quality. Pasta sauce should be made of tomatoes, olive oil, and spices—there is no need for glucose-fructose, lecithin, and hydrolyzed plant protein. Those ingredients are your first clue that the manufacturer is more worried about their profit margin than your health.

Next, if a food passes your anti-inflammatory ingredients test, you might want to look at the nutrition facts just to make sure nothing jumps out at you as being out of sync. Does it have a reasonable serving size or does the manufacturer expect you to make a breakfast of one-fourth of a cup of cereal? Make sure the food doesn't have too much sodium, sugar, or saturated fat or see if it gives you some extra fiber or protein. A little salt is fine within the context of a healthy diet, but you might not want to consume a whole day's worth of salt in a single serving of soup. Just sayin', because I am a dietitian, et cetera . . . and I care about that stuff.

But then comes the question, how much is enough . . . or too much?

Glad you asked!

The biggest difficulty in interpreting nutrition facts panels is placing that information into context. Yes, you want to lower salt, but if sodium-laden soy sauce only serves to brighten up a plate full of naturally low sodium whole foods, doesn't that balance everything out? It does, in my book. I think where the real power lies is in understanding that soy sauce is a salt bomb and that just a little will do the trick. Or that if you are going to indulge in a sugary treat you will want to ensure that the rest of your food choices that day are supercharged with nutrition and unsweetened. This is where the good and bad lines blur. And why focusing solely on nutrition facts can lead to nutrition confusion.

Food choice is crystal clear. Apple, good! Processed cocoa cookie snack, not so good. Is a cookie snack better when it is lower in sodium and saturated fat? No—it is merely less detrimental to your health. Removing something from a more inflammatory food choice doesn't magically make it anti-inflammatory and nourishing.

I want you to be armed with all the information you can absorb, so here is what you need to help you place those little black and white nutrition panels into the grey area of living and eating. What follows is my take on current nutrient guidelines; it is a blend of evidence-based official recommendations and expert consensus. In the absence of a clear evidence-based guideline, I have chosen the expert recommendation I agree with most—and you can check out which one I chose in the references for this chapter.

Nutrient	Recommended Daily Intake
Sodium *Otherwise known as half of the compound called table salt, sodium chloride.* *Why should you care?* While research debates the direct correlation of high sodium intake to high blood pressure—What about genetics? What about total diet? What about chloride?—there is still a large volume of evidence that links high-sodium diets to higher blood pressure.[2]	Try to stick to no more than 2300 mg per day.[1]
Saturated Fat (preferably veggie-based) *Why should you care?* Saturated fat has long been the enemy number one in the war against heart disease, and while the face of the evidence is changing,[4] there is still a link between animal-based saturated fats and inflammation.[5,6] However, my biggest concern is that a dietary pattern that contains lots of animal-based saturated fats is likely an unhealthy one.	No more than 10 percent of your daily calories, which is between 22–33 g per day for most.[3] *Yes, this is a bit unhelpful, but the research on requirements is scant. Bottom line? If a dessert contains 15 g of saturated fat, that is your signal that it shouldn't be a daily treat.*

Sugars (added . . . not naturally occurring)	No more than 25 g (women) or 37 g (men) per day.[7]
Why should you care? Well, added sugars are unnecessary to the human body. And they provide empty calories that spike blood sugars and stoke the fires of inflammation. (See Chapter 5).	
Fiber	At least 25 (women) and 38 g (men) a day.[8]
Why should you care? Fiber is a feast for all those wonderful bacteria in your colon and is like a personal trainer for your digestive tract. In addition, a high fiber diet pattern is one that contains all those wonderful plant foods I am trying to get you to eat.	

Think of those numbers associated with nutrients as a nutritional budget. If a packaged food has 1200 milligrams of sodium in a single serving, you are spending more than half your day's sodium budget on that food. Is it worth it? Can you make up for it with unprocessed, low-sodium choices the rest of the day? Then go for it . . . just don't make it a daily habit.

The sugar one is a toughie because the nutrition facts panel doesn't discern between added and naturally occurring sugars. A good rule of thumb is that if a food (such as an apple) has no nutrition facts . . . then you don't have to worry about it, unless you are an insulin-dependent diabetic.

If the food does have a nutrition facts panel, the number on the nutrition facts panel is really high, and there isn't actual fruit on the ingredients label, give it a pass. If sugar appears in the first three ingredients of a food, give it a pass—unless it's actually a bottle of honey or maple syrup. If sugars show up four or five times on an ingredients label, give it a pass.

Then, of course, there are all the hyper-processed starches that hit your bloodstream almost as quickly as sugar does—such as white wheat or rice flour. You won't find those starches mentioned anywhere in a nutrition panel, but seeing refined flours and starches will give you the hint that something is up (like your blood sugar if you eat those foods!).

You are going to get really good at saying no to hyper-processed food.

Be a Sugar Sleuth!

O sugar, where art thou? Everywhere!
Here are just some of the ingredients that are sources of added sugars on a label

Agave nectar, brown rice syrup, brown sugar, cane crystals, cane sugar, corn sweetener, corn syrup, corn sugar, crystalline fructose, dextrose, evaporated cane juice, fructose, fruit juice concentrates, glucose, glucose-fructose, high-fructose corn syrup, honey, invert sugar, lactose, maltose, malt syrup, maple syrup, molasses, raw sugar, sucrose, sugar, syrup, treacle . . .

Tiptoe Through the Grocery Aisles

Concrete rules are great . . . but isn't this book all about living in the grey area? It's not like you can't have a scoop of good quality triple fudge chunk or a handful of tortilla chips once in a while. The trick is to get your diet to an ultra-clean 80 percent so you can enjoy the 20 percent foods without guilt or ill-health. Since we have the basics out of the way, it is time to delve deeper into the supermarket aisles and learn how to make the best choices as you shop. I started my career giving grocery store nutrition tours, and now it's time for your own personal virtual tour! Join me as we wander through the aisles and I give you my favorite tips and tricks for getting the most out of your grocery shop.

The Produce Section: Ground Zero for Healthy Eating

—This section is all about buying large! Buy about a half-pound of vegetables per person, per day. That's three-and-a-half pounds a week for each of you! Buy three pieces of fruit per person, per day—or twenty-one pieces a week. You have probably never purchased that much produce in one go . . . and it can change your life.

—If you are cooking for one and are worried about food waste, plan purchases carefully with a meal plan. Another way to lower food waste is to purchase both fresh and frozen. Focus on munching the most perishable items, such as leafy greens first, transition through the week to hardier items like apples and carrots, and boost your intake with always-ready frozen items.

—Choose locally grown produce whenever possible; less travel time usually means riper, tastier (and more nutritious) produce and fewer chemicals needed to keep them fresh during travel and storage. Locally grown produce is often more affordable at the peak of the season.

—Organic is great when it is available and affordable. Prioritize leafy greens, apples, and berries. Learn more about the Dirty Dozen to help you prioritize your organics spend. If you can't afford organic, don't stop eating fruits and veggies! Paradoxically, the more you eat, the more you will expose yourself to the beneficial plant compounds that will help protect you from environmental assault.

—Don't be afraid to try something new! Throw shiitake mushrooms on a pizza, scoop up white bean dip with kohlrabi chips, or add pizzazz to a salad with watermelon radish. This is especially fun to help kids grow their veggie repertoire. Have them choose something they haven't tried, Google the recipe information, and try it out.

—Produce is about color—your shopping buggy should look like a rainbow; each color (even brown and white) has its own unique properties. Don't get stuck in peas and carrots land.

Bulk Foods: Not Just for Hippies Anymore

—Buy your bulk foods from a store that has high turnover. The bins should look clean and dry goods should smell fresh—no off scent.

—Buy large in the bulk section, these dry goods keep for a long time. Store in clear jars in a dark and cool place in your pantry for easy access. Maintaining a good selection of beans, nuts, dried fruits, seeds, and grains at home makes for easy meal planning. Nuts and seeds are best kept in the freezer unless you go through them quickly.

—Buy only raw nuts and seeds to reduce damage to healthy fats during processing and storage. If you like them toasted, toast them in small batches yourself.

—To streamline home cooking from scratch, batch cook. Cook up a few varieties of grains and beans, then cool and package into freezer bags in single recipe-sized servings. Now, you can have healthy meals in fifteen minutes instead of more than an hour. You can prep cook while you watch a movie or do the laundry . . . it is the ultimate healthy multitasking.

—Less exotic grains will be less expensive and just as healthy as trendier varieties! Try wheat berries, buckwheat, barley, and rye kernels as chewy, tasty substitutes for quinoa, black rice, or amaranth when they are pricey.

—Some people are surprised to know that couscous isn't a unique grain . . . it's a wheat pasta. Better to eat actual pasta, as couscous' tiny puffs can send blood sugars soaring.

—If you don't have a lot of time to be soaking beans, eat more lentils—they can cook up without a soak.

—Look for dried fruit and trail mixes without added sugars.
—Unfortunately, if you have severe food allergies or intolerances, steer clear of the bulk section—there is too much potential for cross-contamination.

The Butcher Case: Keep it Light on the Planet and the Waistline

—If you eat meat, buy your meat from a store with a knowledgeable meat cutter; ask them where they source their meat and how it was raised. There can be dramatic differences in the ethical, health, and environmental impact of meats that look virtually indistinguishable from one another.
—Buy better quality meat and just eat less of it—it will keep your meat costs the same. Meat should be considered more of a garnish, not the anchor of most meals.
—Make the majority of your butcher spend fish, with a bit of poultry thrown in. Purchase 100 percent grass-fed beef if available; keep beef as an occasional choice, once every week or two. Choose specialty, humanely raised poultry and pork whenever possible. If you can afford organic, go for it.
—Use a sustainable seafood app (see resources) to help you choose environmentally friendly seafood; generally speaking, the smaller the fish, the fewer the accumulated toxins. If you are pregnant or planning to become pregnant, get to know your low-mercury choices for a healthy pregnancy.
—Place fresh meat in a separate plastic bag and store it in the fridge on a lower shelf for immediate use or have the meat cutter wrap it up for freezer storage.

Refrigerator Case: Look for the Nutritional Diamonds in the Hyper-Processed Rough

—Buy only growth hormone (rBGH)–free milk and products made from it (such as butter), organic and grass-fed when available and affordable. All Canadian milk is rBGH-free.
—Buy unsweetened, non-GMO vegetarian milk substitutes as an affordable and healthy everyday option. Soy and almond milks tend to be the crowd pleasers. Know that usually only soymilk contains protein on par with dairy milk. If you prefer other varieties, be mindful of including protein from other sources into your day.
—Buy plain yogurt that contains only milk and cultures. No gelatin, no emulsifiers, no garbage. Add your own fruit and honey if you need a little more

flavor. Many popular yogurts are closer to dessert than health food.

—Buy organic or at least humanely raised free-range eggs. Look for the ASP-CA seal—it is worth the price in terms of ethical standards.

—Be aware that many vegetarian meat substitutes are highly processed and laden with salt and additives. Check ingredients thoroughly if you enjoy these foods; use them to help you adjust to a lower meat diet or as an occasional treat.

—Look for organic and non-GMO tofu and tempeh. Extra firm tofu is the most versatile for cooking and pressed tofu makes for great kebabs or burger substitutes, as it contains less moisture.

—Buy butter or coconut oil spreads for occasional use. Avoid soy oil spreads. See the resources section for my picks.

—Ensure that cheese has pure ingredients—100 percent fresh milk and cultures. European cheeses are typically made from high-quality milk and are well-aged—they make a better choice and can be quite affordable at warehouse stores (just freeze extra so it doesn't spoil).

Cereals and Breads: From Grainy Goodness to Sugary Smackdown

—The closer that cereal comes to the original grains they were made from, the better. Look for breakfast cereals that contain at least five grams of fiber per serving and fewer than eight grams of sugars (or no added sugar).

—Old-fashioned European style grain mueslis are a great choice as are the new super seed cereals.

—The best way to sneak more fiber into your diet is a high fiber cereal—these typically have more than ten grams of fiber per serving. Keep them in the pantry for those days you feel your diet needs a fiber boost.

—Look for breads and wraps that are 100 percent sprouted grain—sometimes these are in the freezer section. They should have at least four grams of fiber per slice.

—Beware the multigrain trap! Multigrain breads are often white breads with seeds sprinkled in. Read those ingredients lists.

—Need to grab and go? Generally speaking, the heavier a bread is, the better quality. Also, if you can squish it easily . . . move along. Squishy breads = spiky sugars. Grainy breads are usually dense and heavy.

—Unsweetened instant oatmeal is a great emergency food for the office or travelling. Carry a package of mix-ins, such as dried fruit and seeds, with you for more flavor and nutrition.

—The difference between instant, quick, slow, and steel-cut oats? Beyond the time it takes to cook them, the difference is how quickly they raise blood sugars. All plain oats are a good choice but slow and steel-cut are a little more stick to your ribs. Cook up a weekly batch or try overnight oats to make mornings a breeze.

Bakery: Where Dough Conditioners, Sugar, and Cheap Fats Love to Bask in the Warmth

—Generally a section to skip unless your local store makes excellent, from-scratch items for a treat or high-quality traditional breads, such as 100 percent sourdough rye. Watch ingredients and if they don't pass your anti-inflammatory kitchen test, pass on them!

Crackers and Snacks: More the 20 than the 80

—Most crackers don't pass the healthy kitchen test and are way too over-eat-able, thanks to tons of salt, flavoring agents, and fat. Look for simple rye and 100 percent whole grain crackers without seasonings. See the resources section for my favorites.

—Give blended trail mixes a pass unless you are in a rush and need a healthy snack. You can customize your own for less using bulk foods. Ensure trail mixes are raw and unsweetened.

—Yes, chocolate can have a modest place in a healthy diet! Chocolate bars should contain at least 70 percent cocoa solids for a more nourishing, lower sugar treat.

—Fruit snacks are more honestly considered fruit candy. They are a 20 percent food; you are better off giving the kids real fruit or homemade fruit leather.

—Most granola bars are sugar bombs in disguise. Look for ones with pro-nounceable ingredients and watch the sugar content; the chewier they are, the more sugar syrups hold them together. Crunchy ones without added soy protein are usually better. Homemade is best!

—Save money and eat healthier by popping your own organic popping corn. It is mere pennies a serving; dust off that old air popper or pop in a large heavy pot with some coconut, olive, or avocado oil.

—Even in the chip aisle, choose the best quality snack for your 20 percent treat. Avoid unrecognizable ingredients, going for natural brands with sim-ple ingredients. Those all-dressed-hot-wing-explosion chips are filled with chemicals to keep your taste buds hooked and your teeth munching.

—Above all else, remember that plant foods make a better snack 80 percent of the time. Best not to load up your kitchen with foods from this section.

Canned Goods: Yes, You Can

—Yes, canned goods can be an important part of an anti-inflammatory pantry. Load up on beans, organic corn, sustainable fish, and tomatoes canned without salt.

—Look for cans without BPA in the can lining if you can find them; BPA is a known endocrine disruptor.

—The healthiest soups contain lots of veggies and beans in a broth or blended base—and usually come in a tetra pak carton. Find your favorites and keep them on hand for emergency meals.

—Canned refried beans often aren't fried. Shocker! They make great, nutritious fillings for quesadillas, sandwiches, casseroles, and dips.

—Brown baked beans are another surprisingly good-for-you food, provided you skip the ones with heaps of sugar and chunks of pork fat. Beans on sprouted grain toast with a side of baby spinach is my kind of instant-but-healthy meal.

Baking and Condiments: The Spice of Whole Food Life

—Don't worry about low-salt condiments unless you have a medical reason to do so. Be aware that condiments, such as soy sauce and ketchup, are salty and use sparingly. Keep ingredient quality high instead. No high fructose corn syrup, thanks!

—A great way to save money (and avoid gnarly ingredients) is to stop buying salad dressings; it takes just a minute to shake up some oil, lemon juice, salt, and pepper.

—Choose 100 percent whole grain flours for baking; whole wheat pastry flour is very fine and bakes up almost exactly like white flour. Spelt or Einkorn flours are great options to try. Add in other flours like almond, quinoa, oat, and barley for nutrition and flavor when you bake.

—If baking gluten-free, look for flour mixes that contain bean flours, sorghum, and gluten-free oats for better nutrition than plain ol' white rice flour.

—Keep honey and maple syrup on hand as your go-to sweeteners. For those times when only sugar will do, try a less-processed turbinado sugar. If you have the budget for fair trade, go for it.

—Be bold with spices! Keep small amounts in the drawer so they are always fresh, and use a diverse spice palette to enliven healthy dishes. To save money, buy larger formats of spices you use regularly and keep them in the freezer. Ethnic grocers are a great place to buy spices—don't pay eight dollars for a tiny container of paprika!

Master Class: Your Anti-Inflammatory Shopping List!

Now that your head is swimming with shopping advice, you might be wondering how you will remember it all. The easiest way to ensure a healthy shop is to focus on the simple foods—and use my shopping list. Here it is . . . everything you need to have a kitchen full of anti-inflammatory foods!

How to use this list? Use it as a reminder before you shop. Alternately, you could photocopy and place the list on your fridge as a running inventory. When you run out of something, circle it or write it down. Then, when it comes time for the weekly shop, add the specific items you want for this week's meals, and then you are off to the races!

So there you have it: the ins and outs of making the right choices when you shop. If you are what you eat, then you truly are the contents of your grocery cart. Make it lush, colorful, and fresh instead of dull and lifeless!

Real Food Doesn't Hide Behind a Fancy Cartoon Character . . .

—Fill that cart with whole plant foods first.

—Once 80 percent of your cart is full of wholesome anti-inflammatory foods, add in the little extras that make your heart (and your tummy) sing.

—Ingredient quality matters more than nutrient counts, but when choosing processed foods, know that fat, sodium, and too much sugar can't hide from the nutrition facts panel.

—Beware of health-washing; all of that front of package nutrition information is more accurately described as marketing tactics.

Shop the Perimeter	Pantry Staples	Add Flavor
Buy 3½ lb. of veggies per person per week and twenty-one pieces of fruit per person per week		

Fruit and Veggies I need:	Sweeteners:	❑ Mustards: Dijon, grainy, hot
❑	❑ Honey	❑ Soy sauce or gluten free tamari
❑	❑ Maple syrup	❑ Mayo, regular or vegan
❑	❑ Unrefined sugars	Hot sauces:
❑	❑	❑
❑	Raw nuts and seeds:	❑ Tahini
❑	❑	❑ Cooking oils: extra virgin olive oil, coconut oil, avocado oil, almond oil
❑	❑	Dried herbs:
❑	❑	❑
Keep these staples on hand!	Nut butters:	Dried spices:
❑ garlic, onions, leeks, shallots	❑	❑
❑ fresh herbs	Dried fruit:	Curry paste
❑ frozen veggies	❑	❑
Healthy Proteins:	Teas:	Salts
❑ Organic extra firm, smoked, or pressed tofu	❑	❑
❑ Organic tempeh	Canned Coconut Milk	❑
Fish:	❑	
❑	Grains:	
Poultry:	❑ Steel-cut or rolled oats	
❑	❑ Whole wheat or gluten free pasta	
❑ Greek yogurt or cottage cheese	❑ Wheat or rye berries	
	❑ Quinoa	
❑ Eggs	❑ Farro	
Bean dips:	❑ Barley	
❑	❑ Amaranth	
Cheese:	❑ Buckwheat	
❑	Whole grain flours:	
Milk or vegetarian milks:	❑	
❑	❑ Sprouted Grain Bread	
❑ butter	❑ Sprouted Grain Wraps	
	❑ 100 percent Corn Tortillas	
Fermented Foods:	❑ No salt added tomatoes	
❑ kimchi	Canned beans:	
❑ kombucha	❑	
❑ miso	❑	
❑ sauerkraut	❑ Good quality pasta sauce	

CHAPTER 13
WHOLE FOODS FOR LIFE

After the Honeymoon Ends . . .

Forever is a long time . . . which is why fad diets end up being just that, a fad.

Eventually you get tired of the rules or the deprivation, and you let it all hang out, nutritionally speaking. Even on a sensible plan, there will be times in your life where things go astray—perhaps your diet is looking like a 50/50 plan instead of 80/20 after taking a new job or the busy holiday season. That's okay; you can always reconnect with your goals and get back on the healthy eating wagon. You haven't ruined anything—that is the whole point of a saner approach to healthy eating. It's for life, minus a few days here and there.

Ironically, it is the strict regime or the all or nothing approach that keeps us from maintaining this 80/20 life over time. A few days of less healthy eating sends the rigid eater into a binge/shame spiral that involves inhuman amounts of stout and double cheeseburgers. The healthy for life eater instead views a vacation in Treatsville as something to enjoy while it lasts and then he moves on to really healthy food to help his body recalibrate and get re-energized. Over time, the peaks and valleys become less pronounced and you become even healthier as the years pass, instead of less healthy. Yes, really. Lose the nutritional baggage and it will be smooth sailing down the highway of health. This chapter is all about how to navigate those challenges with your good healthy eating name intact.

Plan, Plan, and Plan Again

A failure to plan is a plan for failure? Yes, generally speaking. The necessity to plan for success depends on both who you are as an eater and your life circumstance. When I was in my mid-twenties, it was no big deal to linger at the grocery store after work deciding on a healthy meal. I had both plenty of energy and plenty of time. Now that I am a decade older with a more demanding career and a preschooler in tow, spending a single second extra in the chore of shopping is frustrating. I don't want to have to think about what to make for dinner. I just want to know . . . and have the supplies at the ready. For me, a meal plan makes for a simple and stress-free week of healthy eating.

The weeks that I don't meal plan, preparing dinners feels like a chore. Which is usually about the time you pick up the phone and order pizza, right?

The benefits of a meal plan are many: save time, save money, free up your mind for more pressing concerns, and eat better with less waste. However, if the confines of a meal plan make you feel claustrophobic, perhaps ensuring you have a hefty pantry of staples will give you the freedom to shop fresh when you are inspired and make do with the pantry when you aren't. No time to shop? Whip up a pasta with frozen rapini, store-bought sauce, and crumbled tofu. Feel like something special? Find a recipe on your lunch break and shop after work. The idea here is to plan your pantry but free-flow during the week as time and inclination allows.

Of course, if time, energy, and inspiration are in plentiful supply, planning might not be necessary for your life stage. If you eat out a lot as a circumstance of your lifestyle, food rotting in the refrigerator might be equally frustrating. Enjoy the ride . . . make the best choices you can at each meal and know that when the time comes, you have the tools right here in this book to streamline your food life.

Getting Social

One of the great challenges on a healthy eating plan is socializing. You might find it easy to get plant-powered at home, but what about at a sports bar? Or girl's night out? The healthiest thing on the menu might be Belgian ale, with a side of celery. The moment of truth is here: are you going to starve or pig out? That is what the all-or-nothing approach would get you. A bunch of anxiety with a tequila and crab dip chaser.

In an alternate scenario, there could be some sad, lifeless "health food" on the menu. Are you worried about how it will look to order the flimsy salad when everyone else is having wings? There is a better way: preparing yourself for these situations is where the rubber really meets the road. What are your healthy eating intentions? Do you want the healthy food but feel awkward ordering it? Or, do you really want to eat what everyone else is eating?

This is where 80/20 living comes in handy. As long as you aren't eating out three nights a week, you can feel good about eating whatever you truly crave when you go out. The key here is not to let one indulgence snowball into ten (margaritas!). If you do tend to socialize over food a lot, then you are going to need to be mindful. You could eat really clean the rest of the time and leave these meals for your 20 percent budget. You could also determine when the indulgence is really going to be worth it.

Ways to Have Your Fun and Eat Healthier, Too!

Breaking bread with friends and family is a cornerstone of what makes us human; it is important not to let healthy eating intentions sideline you from the fun. Here are a few ways to navigate social eating that will help you feel confident, enjoy eating, and feel good the next day!

—Choose restaurants where the healthy options are actually tasty. So many restaurants offer their sad, token salad but it is obvious that they don't really care about healthy food. There is a new breed of food-forward, healthy, and even specifically plant-based restaurants where eating well is truly an art form, particularly in major cities. You pick the restaurant, you control the menu!

—Review menus before you go out (and before you are starving) to choose the healthiest meal so that when it comes time to order, you are prepped to do the healthy thing. Most often, this is a protein and produce combo, such as salmon with veggies or an entrée salad.

—Share a variety of appetizers with friends and order a veggie-full starter salad for yourself. Eat the salad first to fill up and then enjoy a few bites of each appy.

—If eating out is a once a week treat, order whatever you like and just don't overstuff yourself. At many restaurants, portion size is so huge that half a plate might suffice. Share dessert with the table and have a pint of beer or a glass of wine. When the rest of the week is filled with healthy food, you most definitely have room for a bit of indulgence.

Have a Healthy Holiday . . . No Really!

Oh the "holidays . . ." By my television and shopping observations, the holiday season starts mid-October and ends at Easter. If you succumb to the temptations at the grocery store, you pretty much have a reason to celebrate for six months of the year. Of course, the period in-between is known as "fad diet—bikini" fest. It is a futile, crazymaking cycle. You can have your cake (turkey, matzo, pumpkin pie, chocolate eggs) and eat it, too. The trick is not to abandon carrots, lentils, and oats for half the year.

You need to keep feasting in its place. In an 80/20 life, there is room for a couple of feast days every once in a while. In fact, 20 percent of a year is seventy-three days. So in theory, if you could go 100 percent anti-inflammatory the rest of the year, you would have a ridiculous amount of feast days to play with. The trouble is that it is really tough to go 100 percent for so long—best instead to keep the feasting short. The worst offender is of course the last six or so weeks of the year, otherwise known as elastic waist and puffy jackets season. What could be a harmless two to three days—heck, even a week—of feasting typically ends up being a two month free-for-all, leaving us with indigestion, sore joints, and tight pants come January 2. It doesn't have to be that way.

Choose Your 80/20 Holiday Adventure

The sanity of the 80/20 approach is that it works during a feast period, too. You simply decide how to honor it. For example, if you want a long weekend of eating with abandon at the folks, the holiday goodies cannot be welcome in your home the week before or after the holidays. Or, if you like a little holiday cheer every day, you get to fit in a daily 20 percent with an ultra-healthy 80 percent. You will also notice that the more you clean up your diet, the less all of this stuff becomes a temptation. Seriously. The better you feel, the more wary you are of the stuff that will junk up your pipes. It took me a good long time but I can actually look at a box of cookies and not care one single bit. A bar of chocolate lasts at least a week in my house.

Five Ways to Survive a Holiday Season with Your Buttons Intact

1. **Be choosy.** Don't eat every cheap and chemical-laden candy, cookie, and sheet cake that drifts past your nose. They aren't really that tasty and they are about as inflammatory as a snack can be. That doesn't mean you can't have a treat, just be choosy. Keep your diet clean and plant-powered, so when someone brings in your favorite type of chocolate or you want to make your favorite childhood holiday treat, you have room for it.

2. **Navigate buffets like a pro.** The first rule of holiday buffets? Do not socialize next to them. Ever. The second? Make your first plate load strictly fruits and vegetables and gobble them with a glass of water. That way, your belly will be full and you will be far more discerning about your next choices. The third? Know that for each cocktail you

consume, you will probably eat another plate of food. Alcohol lowers inhibitions and not just when it comes to dancing on the photocopier; it works for food intake, too.

3. **Create a virtual wall around the feasting.** Enjoy chocolates on Valentine's Day, not every day of the week. Freeze leftovers so you don't feel you need to gobble them up before they go bad. During the holidays, don't eat treats on days when there is no holiday party or special event. Eat really well leading up to celebrations so you can enjoy the treats on offer knowing how healthy you have been eating that week. Remember, Thanksgiving is one calendar day, not a weeklong event. Okay, if you are going home to your parents' house, it might be a three day event—but that's it!

4. **Keep working out, no matter what.** Fitness builds self-confidence and makes you wary of tanking your energy and ruining your good vibes with too much junk food. Keeping active will help you to feel energized, happy, and powerful and you will make food choices accordingly.

5. **Enjoy the holidays.** Feasting is a joyful event. If you follow the first four rules, stop worrying about calorie counts during a holiday meal. We share food as an act of celebration, community, and love. Do right the rest of the time and make special occasions special.

Healthy Travel

Healthy bodies love routine and travel can stress your body and lead you astray from good eating habits. Staying healthy as you travel doesn't have to be a challenge, but certain situations can definitely make it harder to stay well. Travel once a year and it probably won't make a dent, but what if you travel more? Remember, it is the patterns you live that make your health. If you travel at least every couple of months, altering your healthy habits on the road will have a real impact on your life over time. So let's pack our bags for a healthy getaway, no matter how you travel or where you are headed!

The Resort: Booze, Brunch, and Bacon

In a fast paced life, who doesn't love a resort vacation? All you have to do is lie in the sun, read, swim, and sip umbrella drinks. Except that when you pack away your flowing sundresses and elasticized swim trunks, you notice that your suit is tighter and you are sleepier than before you went on holiday.

The Resort Trap: All-Inclusive Treats
The solution: choose your indulgence wisely, you 80/20 maven

Humans are hardwired to make the most of times of plenty to survive the lean times. That's what all those fat cells are supposed to be for—lean times. Trouble is, most of us live in a time of plenty 365 days a year, and an all-inclusive environment simply puts it all on display! If you are offered seven days of all you can eat food, you're going to need to pace yourself. Seven days of Belgian waffles, whipped cream, and burgers is not a good idea. You go on vacation to feel good, and about three days into a nonstop feast you are not going to feel good. Frankly, the food won't even taste that exciting after a while. And your sluggishness will leave you wishing you had more time to sleep it off.

Vacations are all about a little indulgence, you just need to put some structure in place to help you enjoy it and feel awesome. A good rule of thumb is that at least one meal each day should be totally healthy. Think protein, fruits, and veggies. Next up, no matter what you are planning to eat, you must eat your fruits and veggies. Don't double down on indulgence by robbing your body of the food it needs to bounce back. If meals are buffet style, always start with a plate of fruits and vegetables. Only when you finish that can you go back for more; then enjoy whatever strikes your fancy. Not only will this help you to eat fewer of the rich foods, if all goes to pot during the week, at least you can say you still got all your veggies in!

You will also need a beverage strategy. Many people really overdo it on alcohol on vacation; at the very least, commit to drinking large amounts of water and alternating two glasses of water for each alcoholic beverage. Especially on beach vacations! Best yet, try to limit yourself to evening drinks with dinner. Lunchtime cocktails are a quick ticket to an afternoon of snoozing and sunburns.

The Road Trip: Fast Food, Boredom, and Gas Station Snacks

I have fond memories of road trips as a child; I would create a fort in the back seat with pillows, blankets, toys, and treats. I could just sit back and enjoy the ride . . . fast forward a few decades and now road trips often mean traffic, deadlines, and boredom. You know the perfect antidote to boredom? Something to keep your taste buds entertained. Just what you need when you are locked in a car, expending practically no energy!

Family road trips can come with their own challenges: our ever-entertained kids now have difficulty surviving a journey without some sort of technology, and you just want to get to your destination as quickly as possible.

Living in a country as large as Canada or the United States, a trip to the relatives can be a ten-hour journey, and usually, the only food found along the way is filled with grease and sugar.

The Trap: Fake Food Fallout
The solution: pack an extra bag . . . of healthy food!
Navigating healthy eating on the road is the easiest thing in the world; simply pack a cooler of healthy snacks to help you avoid the gas station snack raids. If travelling with a family, have each family member nominate one to two of their favorite snacks so that everyone is kept happy on the road. Prepare for all taste whims: salty, sweet, crunchy, and creamy. Pack one cooler with snacks and another with healthy beverages. Think water, club soda, individual servings of chocolate soy milk or organic milk, or make your own healthy sodas by mixing one-fourth of a cup of fruit juice with club soda.

Packable Snacks for the Anti-Inflammatory Road Trip
1. Roasted chickpeas, salty or sweet
2. Whole grain crackers for crunch
3. Chopped veggies for something refreshing
4. Dark chocolate for a sweet
5. Unsweetened dried fruit in place of candy
6. Sliced chicken, turkey, or tofu sticks
7. Sliced cheese
8. Apples for crunch, bananas for something creamy
9. Baked chips to appease the junk food craving
10. Healthy sandwiches or salads for the lunch stop

Work Travel: Wining, Dining, and Indigestion
Travelling for work always seems like such a perk until it becomes how you live your life. Constant travel is hard on your digestive system, your immune system, and your nerves. Food becomes the ultimate comfort when away from home but making the wrong selections too often can leave you vulnerable to catching whatever little travel bugs come your way. Remember, you are your patterns and if frequent work travel is a way of life, you need to rethink how you treat your body on the road.

The trap: Eating whatever is around . . . and having another round.

The solution: When eating out isn't a special occasion, don't view it as a treat.

When you travel, the easiest way to keep energized is to pack along the right foods. I always travel with an assortment of easy-to-pack staples like apples and instant oatmeal. I also carry an empty water bottle that I fill as soon as I am through security, so I can stay hydrated without the use of those tiny water cups on the plane. I call those cups tiny gulps, because a gulp is all it takes to drain them.

Choosing food in airports is totally hit or miss. Some airports have plenty of healthy options. Smoothies, salads, and trail mixes abound. Others hold you nutritional hostage with nothing but a Burger King if you end up in the wrong terminal. Generally speaking, I try to eat a meal before I head to the airport. I also carry a whole food snack bar and a piece of hard fruit in my bag so that if there is nothing else to eat I can make a meal-on-the-go with a latte. If you are forced to eat in an airport without a healthy option, you will have to get creative. The first option: eat what you want, just don't pig out. The second option? Look for protein-rich foods and just eat around all the extra junky carbs. Stir-fries, fish (with not too many chips), or burritos served in a bowl, without the extra rice and tortilla wrap, will all get you through to your next good meal.

Desiree's Favorite Healthy Packables

As a fairly frequent flier, I am starting to get my packing routine down to a science. I always pack food, even if I am only traveling overnight. Sometimes I find myself in a hotel with no healthy eating options before I have to speak or meet with a client and I get hangry without breakfast! Here are some of my favorites to help keep it healthy on the road.

1. Plain instant oatmeal—can be prepped in a hotel room with hot water.
2. Dried fruit and nuts—add to your oatmeal or eat as a healthy snack.
3. High quality protein shake and a plastic shaker cup—breakfast with just cold water!
4. Apples—they pack quite well, but you can't bring them across borders.
5. Whole food meal bars—fits in your carry on and can ease a sweet craving.
6. Vitamin C drink powder—because planes are filled with germs!

>>

7. Probiotics—to keep your tummy tamed on the road.
8. Dark chocolate—so I can succumb to a treat craving with good quality food.
9. Tea—often picked up from hotels along the way!
10. Roasted chickpeas—for a salty and filling snack.

Another hurdle is finding the right restaurants. If entertaining clients, you are usually at indulgent restaurants where an extra-large steak and a bottle of red are the order of the day. Remember the rule, an indulgence only flies if it is occasional business. If business travel is a part of your life, you need to treat restaurants as your private healthy chef. Think salads. Fish. Fruit for dessert.

Sometimes, simply knowing the best places to go in a new city can be the challenge. Here is where the Internet can be a remarkable tool. Simply search "healthy restaurant or vegetarian restaurant in City X" and see what happens.

Anti-Inflammatory Families

What's that you say? Kids don't eat spinach? Well, now is as good a time as any to help them start! That goes for husbands, wives, grandparents . . . the whole family.

I've got a bit of a (vegetarian) bone to pick here: the notion of kid food. You know how kids learn to love grilled cheese, juice, chicken fingers, and ham and swiss on white? Because adults serve it to them. Cementing certain foods in our culinary histories can have enormous effects on how we eat as adults and what we run to as comfort foods later on. Now, I know that the only thing more personal than what we feed ourselves is what we feed our kids, but hear me out for a minute.

Children come into this world hardwired to eat what their body needs to survive. They eat when they are hungry and stop when they are full. They also don't know that junk food exists until we, the adults, provide it. So why do we feel we need to introduce them to incredibly bland, lifeless food? The first foods my child ate were fruits and veggies. He wrinkled up his nose (which I could have interpreted as dislike) and then . . . he ate like crazy. The only thing that didn't connect immediately was the kale I tried to hide in applesauce. As parents, we assume that if a child doesn't love something immediately, they don't like it at all—and they never will. In fact, that couldn't be further from the truth.

Children's preferences are as changeable as the weather. My son used to love cheese; now it depends on the day. Some days he gobbles, other days it comes back in his lunchbox uneaten. So if the first introduction of kidney beans was a massive fail, try again in a week or so! It is true that my preschooler still doesn't eat much spinach salad; he prefers to feed the leaves to his dinosaurs. He will, however, eat spinach chopped into a tomato sauce or layered in a casserole. If I let him, he would eat a whole package of tofu plain. He snacks on cucumber and raw almonds. From his earliest food experiences, I have been training his taste buds to appreciate the foods we eat as a family. Kale took a couple years. Beans, tofu, and pickled ginger were easy wins.

Now that he is in preschool, he knows the mysteries of red Jell-O. And sugary cupcakes. But those early years gave me the opportunity to hone his taste buds so that he will still accept all of this healthy food mom lays on the table. Children's bodies are pretty adaptable, and they can tolerate a bit of junk, but what is difficult to overcome is a taste bud that has been trained in the ways of white flour, sugar, salt, and fat. I have parents ask me all the time about how to get their kids to eat veggies. My next question is always, "Well, what do they eat now?" Invariably it is cheese, flour, and sugar. You can't blame a kid (or an adult, for that matter) on this kind of diet to think that green veggies are gross. They are totally foreign flavors!

If you have a family with different taste buds, you are going to have to wean them onto new tastes. It can take as many as ten to twenty offerings of a new food before it is fully accepted. Keep at it . . . and they will come around!

Desiree's Secret for Speeding Up Acceptance

Introduce a new food in a family favorite. Friday night noodle casserole? Sauté some grated kohlrabi into it. Stir white beans into an old standby soup. Make a smoothie with kale. This essentially tricks the brain into associating the new food with something they already love. Here are some ideas to get you going:

Family Standard: Spaghetti and Tomato Sauce
What to Add: Ground chicken or crumbled tofu instead of beef, veggies—such as bell peppers, spinach, or cauliflower (pureed into the sauce if need be for picky eaters).

Family Standard: Nachos
What to Add: Black beans, vegan cheese (Substitute 50/50 with real cheese), diced veggies, greek yogurt in place of sour cream.

Family Standard: Meatloaf
What to Add: Lentils (Substitute 50/50 with ground meat), greens, pureed squash, or sweet potato.

Family Standard: Chicken Noodle Soup
What to Add: White beans such as cannellini or navy, diced or grated kohlrabi for crunch, plenty of garlic, whole wheat or quinoa noodles.

Family Standard: Pizza
What to Add: Whole grain thin crust and extra veggies; smoked tofu is great, too. Try herb pesto as a sauce; spread with white bean dips for creaminess without the cheese.

Family Standard: Tacos
What to Add: Substitute beans or crumbled tofu for meat, add shredded cabbage, kohlrabi, or broccoli and other veggies, use plain greek yogurt in place of sour cream; eat on 100 percent corn tortillas.

Family Standard: Chili
What to Add: Substitute beans and crumbled tofu for meat, double the veggies: use plenty of carrots, onions, and celery as a base and even chop up some steamed greens to stir in.

> Family Standard: Pot Pie
> What to Add: Change up the oils on the crust or buy or make a whole grain crust, double the veggies, add beans in place of half the meat, go for miso-based gravies.

Life is a highway . . . keep your sights on the anti-inflammatory destination.

—Remember that your health reflects your patterns over time; if travel or feasting becomes a regular occurrence, inflammation will creep up on you.

—Plan ahead and pack healthy staples to get some more nutrition while on the road.

—Life is a buffet these days . . . don't treat an actual food buffet like your last chance at a meal unless it actually is.

—Start kids young on the right nutrition path; that way, when they become surly junk-food-munching teenagers, you know that you started them off right.

PART THREE:

The Recipes

CHAPTER 14

LET'S EAT! WHOLE FOOD, PLANT-STRONG RECIPES FOR LIFE

This is it . . . you have climbed the nutritional mountain, now you are ready for the celebratory feast! The recipes on these pages have been created with love by my partner-in-food, Heather McColl RD, and me. She is the foodie yin to my plant-powered yang, and these delectable dishes wouldn't be the same without her. Our goal with these recipes is to create food that you actually want to eat—and just happens to be amazing for you. These recipes feature whole foods, lovingly prepared; they are incredibly nutritious, delicious, and designed to fit into real life.

What's missing? The calorie counts. Why? Because I want you to focus on the food; if there is fat in a recipe, it is there because it is good for you. I don't want you getting scared away by a number. A little salt makes whole foods pop—and by avoiding packaged goods, you will be eating a lot less salt overall and will have room in your sodium budget for a bit of fairy dust. Focus on good food choices, not fat grams or calories. It is the pattern of anti-inflammatory eating that will protect you over time, not niggling for one hundred calories here or there.

Heather and I hope that you will take the time to make high-quality meals for yourself and for your family; this time is just as important to your longevity and vitality as exercising or sleeping well.

To your health!

Desiree and Heather

Morning Glories

Liquid Gold Smoothie

Hello sunshine! This is the perfect way to brighten up a dull day. Turmeric sets the stage for a golden anti-inflammatory feast that will energize your cells. The sweetness of this smoothie will vary with the sweetness of your veggies; if they aren't sweet enough to counteract the natural bitterness of turmeric, consider substituting more orange juice for water or adding ¼ cup of frozen mango to suit your taste buds.

Makes one breakfast or two snack smoothies

1 small golden beet, peeled and chopped
1 carrot, scrubbed and chopped
½ inch piece fresh turmeric, peeled and sliced or ¼ teaspoon ground turmeric
½ cup not-from-concentrate orange juice
½ cup water
¼ lemon, peeled and most of white pith removed

Place everything in a high-powered blender and use the smoothie setting.

If using a standard blender, add the beet and carrot first and use the ice crusher setting to break them up. Add the orange juice to liquefy more smoothly. Add remaining ingredients and blend until it is as smooth as possible. You may want to strain out some of the pulp or simply chew through your smoothie for better health! All of that fiber is good for you.

Tip: If you like to juice, add the veggies to your juicer and swap two small mandarins for the orange juice. Sip slowly to lower the sugar load on your body.

Cocoaberry Smoothie

Yes, chocolate has its place in a healthy diet—even at breakfast! This smoothie, with all of its cocoa and berry polyphenols, is like a love letter for your heart and your soul. Because the way to a (healthy) heart really is through your stomach.

Makes one breakfast or two snack smoothies

1 cup berries or cherries, fresh or frozen
½ banana, fresh or frozen
1 cup unsweetened chocolate almond milk

1 scoop berry-, vanilla- or chocolate-flavored vegan protein powder
1 tablespoon raw cacao or cocoa powder

Place everything in a blender and blend until smooth. For extra anti-inflammatory benefits, drizzle in 1 teaspoon of your favorite omega-3 oil, such as hemp oil.

Tip: Raw cacao powder has the highest phytochemical levels because it hasn't been heat- or alkali-treated. If it isn't in the budget, stick to the best pure cocoa powder you can find.

The Real Muffin

Most muffins would be more correctly labeled as cupcakes because they are little more than sugar and white flour. Add the fact they are four times an appropriate serving size and you have a recipe for, well . . .anti-inflammatory disaster. Love muffins? Make them yourself from whole ingredients.

Makes 12 muffins

1 cup whole spelt or whole wheat flour, sprouted if available
¾ cup oat flour—*see tip*
½ cup hemp seeds
½ cup chopped dried apple or other dried fruit
½ cup chopped walnuts or other nuts
1 teaspoon baking powder
1 teaspoon baking soda
⅛ teaspoon salt
1½ teaspoons cinnamon
1-14 oz. (398 ml) can pumpkin or sweet potato puree
2 eggs or 2 chia/flax eggs—*see tip*
6 tablespoons olive oil
¼ cup maple syrup
1½ teaspoons vanilla
1 teaspoon grated fresh gingerroot

Preheat oven to 350°F.

In a large bowl, whisk together flours, hemp seeds, dried apple, walnuts, baking powder and soda, salt, and cinnamon. In a medium bowl, whisk together pumpkin, eggs, oil, maple syrup, vanilla, and gingerroot. Add wet to dry ingredients and stir until just combined, about 18–20 stirs. Don't over-mix! Batter will be thick.

Divide batter into a greased muffin tin or a baking sheet lined with silicone muffin cups. Bake for 18–22 minutes or until a toothpick inserted in the center of a muffin comes out clean.

Tip: These muffins freeze well; keep your freezer stocked for emergency breakfasts or healthy snacks!

Tip: If you can't find oat flour, you can make it yourself by pulsing oats in a food processor until they are fine as flour. A few small pieces of oats in the flour are still ok.

Tip: To replace one egg, place 1 tablespoon ground flax or ground chia seeds in a cup. Add 3 tablespoons of warm water, stir and let sit for 5 minutes.

It's Easy Being Green Smoothie

Eating your daily greens will make a world of difference in how you look and feel. The easiest way to boost your greens score? Drink them! Spinach is a great place to start because it is easy to blend and inexpensive; when you are feeling adventurous, switch up the greens! A little green tea makes this a great morning drink with just a hint of caffeine to give you even more of a boost. Have fun with flavored teas too . . . passion fruit green tea makes for a delicious drink.

Makes one breakfast or two snack smoothies

½ banana, fresh or frozen
1 small apple (3-inch diameter), cored and cut into large chunks
½ lemon, peeled with most of white pith removed
4-inch piece cucumber, cut into chunks
2–3 cups packed baby spinach
1 cup cooled green tea

Place everything in a blender and blend until smooth. Two cups of spinach will yield a green smoothie that is lighter in flavor.

Tip: Freeze your bananas for a creamier smoothie! Let bananas get very ripe and then freeze peeled halves in a freezer-proof storage container or zipper bag. This smoothie also tastes good with a bit of fresh mint added.

South of the Border Tofu Scramble

Eggs aren't the only food you can scramble! Tofu scrambles up beautifully with a hearty dose of spice and flavorful extras that are sure to satisfy, thanks to a winning combination of protein and fiber. The black bean and corn combo makes it a hit with kids. Great for brunch or make it once and enjoy it all week long!

Makes 4–6 servings

1 tablespoon extra virgin olive oil
1 onion, diced
1 package organic or non-GMO extra-firm tofu
1 cup frozen corn, thawed
1-14 oz. (398 ml) can black beans, rinsed and drained or 1½ cups cooked
1 teaspoon Mexican chili powder
½ teaspoon cumin
salt to taste
1 cup cherry tomatoes, halved
1 cup fresh cilantro leaves
1 lime, cut into wedges
Salsa

In a medium frying pan, heat oil and sauté onions until soft and lightly golden, about 5–7 minutes.

Using fingers, crumble tofu into small crumbles and add to the pan. Sprinkle with chili powder and cumin. If you prefer a spicier dish, add an additional ¼–½ teaspoon of chili powder.

Cook, stirring often, until tofu loses its moisture and mixture looks dry, about 5 minutes. Add corn and black beans and stir through; cook for 5–7 minutes to allow flavors to blend. Season with salt.

Serve with tomato, cilantro, salsa, and a lime wedge. Goes well with a green salad and warmed corn tortillas.

Brilliant Breakfast Bars

No time for breakfast? No excuses! You can make these nutritious breakfast bars on the weekend and then just grab and go during the week. These bars feature real whole grains (and can be gluten-free if need be), protein, and omega-3 rich hemp seeds and almost no added sugars. A far cry from your standard café fare—these are baked goods that make you feel good!

Makes twelve cookies or bars

¾ cup oat flour—*see tip*
¾ cup large flake oats
¾ cup unsweetened shredded coconut
1 tablespoon ground flaxseed
½ cup hemp seeds
½ teaspoon cinnamon
½ teaspoon salt
¼ cup chopped walnuts
½ cup dried apricots, chopped
3 very ripe bananas, mashed
¼ cup extra virgin olive oil
1 tablespoon honey
1 teaspoon vanilla extract

Preheat oven to 350°F.

In a large bowl, whisk together oat flour, oats, coconut, flax, hemp, cinnamon, and salt. Stir in walnuts and dried apricots.

In another bowl, mash bananas with a fork and stir in olive oil, honey, and vanilla. Add banana mixture to flour mixture and fold until combined. The dough for these bars is pretty easy to handle so don't be afraid to get in there with your hands for a more thorough mix!

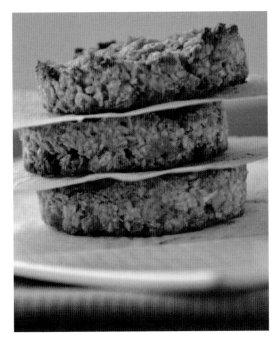

Line a 9 × 13 inch baking dish or 8 × 12 inch small rimmed baking sheet with parchment paper. Press cookie mixture into the pan evenly. Bake for 25 minutes or until edges are golden brown. Allow to cool 5 minutes. Score into 12 bars and then transfer to a cooling rack to cool completely. Alternately, you can form 12 bars or cookies by hand and bake on a parchment paper lined baking sheet for 25 minutes or until edges are golden brown.

Tip: If you can't find oat flour, you can make it yourself by pulsing oats in a food processor until they are fine as flour. A few small pieces of oats in the flour are still ok.

Tip: The bars will keep for one to two months in the freezer. Make a huge batch to save time and simply remove from the freezer the night before to grab'n go for a quick breakfast in the morning.

Feel Good Pancakes

I am late to the pancake party; I have never cared for sweet breakfasts so it wasn't until I started experimenting with my own recipes that I learned to love them. These pancakes are hearty and satisfying and offer a good dose of protein. Great for a family . . . and grown-ups too!

Makes twelve pancakes

1 cup oat flour—*see tip*
½ cup almond flour—*see tip*
1 teaspoon baking powder
2 eggs, beaten or 2 chia/flax eggs—*see tip*
¾ cup milk
1 cup cottage cheese
1 teaspoon vanilla
Coconut oil or butter for frying

Blend flours and baking powder in a medium-sized bowl. In a separate bowl, use a fork to whisk together eggs, milk, cottage cheese, and vanilla. Add the wet ingredients to the flour mixture and whisk lightly with a fork to mix well.

Preheat a large skillet or frying pan over medium heat and add a dollop of coconut oil or butter. Drop pancakes onto pan in ¼ cup increments. Wait until bubbles form and then flip over. Keep warm in a 200°F oven until all the pancakes are ready.

Serve sprinkled with cinnamon and your favorite fresh fruit, maple syrup, or honey.

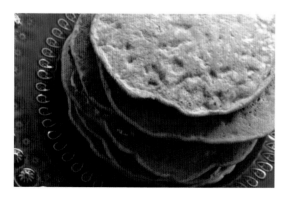

Tip: If you can't find oat flour, you can make it yourself by pulsing oats in a food

processor until they are fine as flour. A few small pieces of oats in the flour are still ok.

Tip: If you can't find almond flour, you can also use ground almonds or almond meal and pulse 2–3 times in a food processor to make it finer like flour.

Tip: To replace one egg, place 1 tablespoon ground flax or ground chia seeds in a cup. Add 3 tablespoons of warm water, stir and let sit for 5 minutes.

Tip: Since butter tends to brown, carefully wipe it out of the pan after cooking a batch of pancakes and add fresh butter so it doesn't overbrown the next batch or smoke.

Say "Yes" to Salad for Breakfast

Salad for breakfast? Of course! A bed of greens is the perfect foil for a runny egg yolk and tempeh bacon. Start your day with an energizing protein and produce combination instead of stupefying sweets.

Makes 4 servings

3 tablespoons plain yogurt
1 tablespoons grainy mustard
2 teaspoons Dijon mustard
1 tablespoon lemon juice
Drizzle of honey
4 cups packed baby arugula
1 package tempeh bacon or ½ package turkey bacon, chopped
1 tablespoon olive oil
1 cup sliced crimini mushrooms
4 eggs

Whisk together plain yogurt, mustards, lemon juice, and honey. Toss dressing with the arugula. Arrange on four plates.

Meanwhile, sauté bacon in a medium frying pan according to package directions and set aside. In the same pan, add olive oil if needed and sauté mushrooms until they release their juices and the juices start to evaporate. Remove from the pan and set aside.

Next, cook eggs to your preference—fried or poached. Arrange arugula on plates with bacon, mushrooms, and top with an egg.

Tip: If you like them, a rich, runny yolk really adds something to the overall salad. Poach eggs soft or fry eggs sunny side up.

Sprouted Buckwheat Granola

Store bought granolas can be absolutely loaded with sugar and the wrong kinds of fat but at their hearts, they are a healthy food. Making granola yourself is surprisingly simple. Here, we have replaced raw oats with sprouted grains for a delicious change. Sprinkle this over yogurt, fruit, or enjoy with your favorite veggie milk.

Makes about four cups

3 cups sprouted buckwheat or oat groats from 1 cup raw grains—*see tip*
¼ cup honey
2 tablespoons extra virgin olive oil
¼ teaspoon cinnamon
1 teaspoon grated fresh gingerroot
½ cup chopped dried fruit
¼ cup chopped walnuts or your favorite nuts
¼ cup hemp seeds
¼ cup pumpkin seeds

Preheat oven to 300°F. Line a rimmed baking sheet with parchment paper or a silpat.

Combine all ingredients in a mixing bowl and stir to combine. Spread on prepared baking sheet.

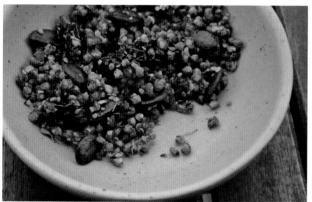

Bake for 45 minutes, stirring every 15 minutes. If the granola is not crispy enough, bake for an extra 5 minutes. Let cool completely before transferring to a sealed container for up to 2 weeks.

Tip: Sprouting grains is simple. Add grains to a large clean mason jar and fill with water. Cover the jar with cheesecloth and an elastic band and let the grains soak for 8–12 hours. Rinse grains very well: add water, stir with a chopstick to agitate grains, and rinse well and drain. Repeat this step 2–3 times and then replace cheesecloth. Let the jar rest on its side for half a day and then repeat rinsing step, always resting jar on its side afterwards. We find that setting a reminder on your smart phone helps you remember! Repeat this rinsing step twice a day until the grains sprout tails at least as long as the grain itself, about 2–3 days from initial soak. Rinse and refrigerate until ready to use.

Note: Sprouts are not recommended for pregnant women or immunocompromised individuals.

Snappy Lunches

Grown-Up Lunch Box
Remember those "make your own" lunch kits you used to eat as a kid? Not so healthy. But a grown up, anti-inflammatory version is perfect for a busy workday. Munch as you have time and have fun customizing your favorite fixins! Snacky lunches never get boring.

Makes one healthy lunch

½ cup hummus
Handful of whole grain crackers—*see resources for suggestions*
1 cup chopped or sliced veggies: peppers, cucumbers and kohlrabi are favorites
¼ cup good quality black olives
3 sesame tofu sticks (recipe on page 243)
¼ cup almonds
4 dried apricots

Pack everything into reusable lunch containers the night before and enjoy a tasty, snacky lunch!

Almost Instant Spinach Salad!
Makes one hearty salad

4 handfuls of baby spinach
½ cup halved cherry tomatoes

¼ cup raw sunflower seeds
½ cup cooked or canned chickpeas, drained and rinsed
¼ cup chopped dried apples
¼ cup feta cheese or goat cheese, optional
1½ tablespoons extra virgin olive oil
1½ tablespoons freshly squeezed lemon juice
Drizzle of honey if the lemon juice is too tart
¼ teaspoons dried thyme or 1 teaspoon fresh thyme leaves
½ small shallot, minced
Salt and pepper to taste

Place all the salad ingredients including baby spinach, tomatoes, sunflower seeds, chickpeas, dried apples, and cheese into a large resealable bowl. Place the remaining dressing ingredients into a small cup with tight-fitting lid or a small jam jar. Pack both for lunch and give the dressing a good shaking before tossing with the salad.

Spicy Korean Tempeh "Reuben"

Sandwiches are incredibly underrated; they are quick to prepare and super delicious, when you go beyond the basics. Calling this a Reuben is kind of a stretch because I have changed every component of the classic dish, but at its heart, it is a fermented pickle with a richly flavored protein. This sandwich is filling, protein packed and full of zip from the chili sauce and kimchi. Serve with sliced veggies or baked fries.

Makes one sandwich

1 teaspoon avocado or olive oil
4 slices tempeh bacon or 1 slice sesame tofu (recipe on page 243, prepared in large slices not sticks)
1 tablespoon real mayo or Vegenaise
½ teaspoon Korean chili sauce or sriracha (rooster) sauce
2 slices sprouted grain bread, toasted
¼ cup grated carrot
¼ cup kimchi (recipe on page 243)

If making sandwich with tempeh bacon, heat oil in a frying pan over medium heat. Add tempeh bacon and fry for 2–3 minutes a side.

Meanwhile, mix mayo/Vegenaise and chili sauce and spread on toasted bread. Layer with grated carrot, kimchi, and fried tempeh bacon or sesame tofu.

Salmon and Sprout Salad

This salad may be light and refreshing but it is not lightweight in the flavor department! The bean sprouts add an earthy crunch to the sweetness of the red pepper and the richness of the salmon. Protein and produce make for a full and satisfied belly!

Makes 4–6 servings

½ cup uncooked quinoa or 3 cups leftover cooked quinoa
1 cup mixed bean and lentil sprouts
½ cup chopped green onions
1 celery stalk, finely chopped
¼ of a red bell pepper, chopped
⅓ cup chopped cilantro
Grated zest and juice from 1 lemon
1 tablespoon extra virgin olive oil
Salt to taste
2 (213 g) cans wild salmon or 2 cups cooked salmon, broken up into pieces

Cook quinoa according to package directions. Alternately, combine quinoa and ¾ cup water in a saucepan and bring to a boil. Cover, reduce heat and simmer for 10 minutes. Turn off heat and allow to sit covered for 5 minutes. Fluff and cool to room temperature or chill in the refrigerator.

In a medium-sized serving bowl, toss the cooked and cooled quinoa, sprouts, vegetables, and cilantro together. Sprinkle with lemon zest and drizzle with lemon juice and olive oil.

Gently toss with salmon and season with salt to taste. If you prefer, you can also substitute salmon with 2 cups cooked or canned chickpeas.

Sister Act Quesadilla

Squash, beans, and corn are known as the three sisters; the moniker comes from their unique ability to assist each other's growth when planted together. The trio is pretty delicious and nutritious too. The filling will keep well through the week; make it on a Sunday night and have quesadillas all week!

Makes 6 servings

3 cups cubed butternut squash
¾ teaspoon ground coriander
¾ teaspoon ground cumin

1-14 oz. (398 ml) can pinto beans, drained and rinsed or 1½ cups cooked
2 tablespoons fresh lemon or lime juice
½ cup canned or frozen corn
1 tomato, diced
1 cup grated white cheddar or vegan cheese
6 brown rice, corn or sprouted grain tortillas
Salsa

Preheat oven to 375°F. Grease a baking pan.

Roast cubed butternut squash for 30 minutes, turning occasionally, until tender and golden brown. Leftover cooked squash can easily be used in place of roasting squash.

In a large skillet over medium heat, toast cumin and coriander until fragrant, about 30 to 45 seconds. This helps to bring out their flavor.

In a large bowl, mash pinto beans with a potato masher or fork. Add toasted spices and lemon or lime juice and mix well. Add corn, squash, tomato, and cheese and fold to mix. Divide bean and vegetable mixture between 3 tortillas and spread mixture evenly over tortillas.

In the same large skillet over medium heat, grill tortillas for 6 to 8 minutes, top with second tortilla and turn over. Grill other side for 4 to 6 minutes until golden brown. Using a knife or pizza wheel cut into 6 pieces and serve with salsa.

Tip: To speed things along, look for frozen cubed butternut squash or sweet potatoes . . . they cook up quickly, and no chopping required!

Something Light

Broccoli Crunch Salad

Broccoli salad is such a familiar, crowd-pleasing dish that you almost forget it's healthy. This is a perfect way to get more broccoli into the less-inclined as the sweetness of the grapes and honey masks any hint of bitterness that might be detected in the broccoli. This recipe is great for potlucks, picnics, and lunches—anytime really!

Makes 4–6 servings

5 cups bite-size broccoli florets
1 red delicious apple, unpeeled and diced

1 cup purple grapes, sliced in half
⅓ cup real mayo or Vegenaise
1 tablespoon white wine or apple cider vinegar
1 tablespoon honey
¼ cup toasted sesame seeds
¼ cup toasted shelled pumpkin seeds

Prepare all vegetables and fruit and toss together in a large serving bowl.

In a small bowl, whisk together mayo/Vegenaise and vinegar. Add honey to taste. Drizzle dressing over salad and gently toss to coat well.

Just before serving, sprinkle with sesame and pumpkin seeds and fold to spread throughout the salad.

Tip: This salad will keep in the refrigerator for five days.

Roasted Vegetable and Barley Salad

Salads don't have to be all leaves and crunch, this grainy salad is a hearty addition to any meal . . . or a perfect meal on its own! Barley is a phenomenal grain for keeping blood sugars balanced and lowering cholesterol, due to its high content of beta-glucan, a soluble fiber. This filling and delicious salad is sure to make you a barley fan.

Makes 3–4 meal-sized servings

⅔ cup pearl barley
1½ cups water
½ medium eggplant, cut into 1 inch chunks
1½ cups grape or cherry tomatoes, halved
1 orange, yellow or red bell peppers, chopped
1 small red onion, chopped
2 tablespoons extra virgin olive oil
1 garlic clove, minced
1 tablespoon freshly squeezed lemon juice
1 teaspoon honey
¼ cup fresh basil, chiffonade or chopped
¼ cup crumbled feta cheese, optional
1½ cups baby spinach or arugula

Preheat oven to 425°F.

Bring barley and water to a boil in a medium pot. Reduce heat and simmer, covered until all of the liquid is absorbed and barley is tender, about 30–40 minutes. Remove from heat and transfer to a baking sheet with roasted vegetables to cool.

Meanwhile, toss eggplant, tomatoes, bell pepper, onion, and garlic with 1½ tablespoons olive oil and spread on a large rimmed baking sheet. Season with salt and pepper. Roast vegetables until golden brown and tender, stirring halfway through, about 25 minutes.

Whisk together lemon juice, remaining ½ tablespoon olive oil, and honey. Pour over barley and veggies along with the basil, feta cheese, and spinach or arugula. Mix gently. Season with salt and pepper.

Cauliflower Tabbouleh

Oh this is a delightful new spin on a classic salad. Filled with colorful veggies, fresh herbs, and lemon zest and juice, this salad is bursting with fresh flavor. And the star of the salad—the bold cauliflower—is a super healthy cruciferous vegetable loaded with cancer fighting power including phytonutrients and antioxidants.

Makes 4–6 servings

½ head of cauliflower
3 cups curly parsley, chopped finely—about one large bunch
½ cucumber, chopped
1 cup of cherry tomatoes, quartered
½ cup packed fresh mint, finely sliced
¼ cup fresh lemon juice
¼ cup olive oil
½ clove garlic crushed or grated on a microplane
¼ teaspoon cumin
1 teaspoon allspice
salt and pepper

Wash and trim the cauliflower. Grate the cauliflower using a stand-up grater or a food processor. Transfer to a large serving bowl and add the parsley, mint, cucumber and tomatoes.

In a small bowl, whisk together the lemon juice, oil, and cumin. Add garlic and allspice. Season with salt and pepper. Drizzle over cauliflower salad and toss to coat well.

Tofu Sesame Sticks

Tofu is the ultimate blank canvas; knowing how to impart flavor is the trick to making tofu lovers out of anyone. This protein and calcium rich dish makes a great protein at dinnertime, a great snack, or sandwich meat.

Makes 4 servings

1 package organic or non-GMO extra-firm tofu
3 tablespoons soy sauce
3 tablespoons toasted sesame oil
3 tablespoons sesame seeds
1 teaspoon ground cumin
½ teaspoon pepper

Preheat oven to 350°F.

Slice tofu into sticks. Whisk together soy sauce, oil, seeds, cumin, and pepper. Toss tofu sticks with sauce and marinate for at least 30 minutes or overnight.

Place tofu on a baking sheet and bake for 15–20 minutes or until golden brown.

Homegrown Kimchi

Kimchi is a traditional Korean condiment; it is eaten at each meal and every family has their own variation. It is an easy way to get started with fermented foods at home; it is hard to get it wrong! This is a pungent, spicy, and delicious side dish to meals and is so easy to prepare at home . . . and homemade is always more delicious than store-bought!

2 lb. suey choy (napa cabbage) or 2 lb. brussels sprouts
3 green onions
1 small lo boc radish or purple top turnip
1 carrot
2 or more garlic cloves, minced
1 inch or more of fresh gingerroot, minced
2 tablespoons salt
2½ tablespoons Korean red pepper (gojuchang)
½–1 teaspoon cayenne pepper

Chop the napa cabbage into bite-sized pieces. If using brussels sprouts, shred them using a food processor or practice your knife skills and chop by hand. Fill a large bowl with 1.5 liters water (~50.8 ounces) and 3 tablespoons salt. Add napa cabbage or brussels sprouts and soak for 1–2 hours. Drain and rinse.

Prepare the green onions by cutting the green tops into ½ inch pieces and cutting the white part in half lengthwise and then into ½ inch pieces. Peel and julienne the radish or turnip and carrot.

In a small bowl, stir the garlic, ginger, and salt and peppers together. Put all ingredients into a large bowl. Using gloves, massage the spices into the cabbage or brussels sprout mixture.

Pack mixture into a large, very clean jar. Add one cup of water if using brussels sprouts. Pack down the mixture and add a weight to keep the veggies in the brine. A small glass container usually works well as a weight. Leave the jar at room temperature with the lid loose to let it ferment for 2–4 days. Taste and when you like the tangy flavor, move to the refrigerator and enjoy within 1 month.

Tip: If you cannot find Korean red pepper, try this variation: 2 tablespoons red chili flakes with ½ teaspoon hot smoked paprika and ½ teaspoon regular paprika instead of the cayenne pepper.

Kale and Avocado Salad

Kale literally blows lesser salad greens out of the water when it comes to nutrition. Packed with vitamins and anti-inflammatory phytochemicals, kale deserves to be a part of the regular greens rotation. The key to a sweeter and more tender salad is massaging a healthy oil, in this case avocado, into the leaves to help soften them. This salad will make believers out of kale skeptics.

Makes 2–4 servings

7 cups bite-sized kale pieces (about one bunch of kale, washed and torn)
1 avocado, chopped
1 bell pepper (red, yellow or orange), diced
½ cup chopped fresh parsley
1 tablespoon extra virgin olive oil
2 tablespoons fresh lemon juice or orange juice
Pinch cayenne pepper or dried chili flakes
Salt and pepper to taste

Toss kale and avocado together in a large bowl. Here's your opportunity to get your hands dirty by massaging the avocado into kale leaves until they soften. Feel free to lick your fingers afterwards—we always do! Add peppers and parsley to kale.

In a small bowl, whisk together oil and lemon juice with salt, pepper, and cayenne pepper. Drizzle over salad and enjoy!

Spiced Tomato Soup

This soup is a far cry from the version you grew up with! Peanut butter adds a satisfying richness without cream and the white beans add body, filling fiber, and protein that makes this soup a meal on its own.

Makes 8 servings

1½ tablespoons olive oil
1 yellow onion, chopped
2 garlic cloves, minced
1 teaspoon chili powder or ancho chili powder
½ teaspoon cumin
½ teaspoon cinnamon
2 cups low sodium veggie or chicken stock
2 cups water
1-28 oz. (798 ml) can plum tomatoes
1 medium sweet potato, peeled and chopped into ½ inch pieces
⅓ cup natural peanut butter
1-14 oz. (398 ml) can white beans, drained and rinsed or 1½ cups cooked
1–2 tablespoons harissa—*see tip*

Heat oil in a large soup pot over medium heat. Add onions and sauté until translucent and lightly caramelized, about 5–7 minutes. Stir in garlic, chili powder, cumin and cinnamon and sauté until fragrant, about 1 minute.

Deglaze the pot with a little bit of stock. Add remaining stock, water, and tomatoes. If diced or whole, break up the tomatoes with the back of your spoon. Add sweet potato and stir. Bring to a boil and simmer for 20 minutes or until sweet potato is tender.

Use an immersion blender to puree soup. Or puree soup in a food processor in batches. Once soup is smooth to your liking, stir in peanut butter and white beans. Simmer for 5 minutes.

Serve drizzled with harissa.

Tip: Harissa is a spicy and aromatic paste made from chili, spices, and herbs. It's often used to flavor stews, soups and couscous. If you cannot find it at your local store, you can substitute sriracha (rooster) sauce—it will have a different taste but still delicious!

Edible Medicine Soup

Food really is medicine and this warming soup has it in spades! Garlic, ginger, greens, and mushrooms are all potent medicinal foods in their own right. Consider your chicken soup recipe a thing of the past.

Makes 6 hearty servings

2 tablespoons olive oil
1 large yellow onion, chopped
1 tablespoon cumin seeds
1 lb. mixed mushrooms, sliced (use crimini as a base and add shiitakes and other exotic varieties as availability and budget allows)
4 garlic cloves, minced
1 liter low sodium veggie stock
2 cups water
1 tablespoon finely grated fresh gingerroot
1 bunch lacinato (black or dinosaur) kale, sliced into ½ inch pieces
1-19 oz. (540 ml) can white beans, or 2 cups cooked
1 teaspoon red chili flakes
Salt to taste

Heat oil in a large soup pot over medium heat; add onion and cumin seeds and sauté until onion is glossy and transparent, about 5 minutes. Add mushrooms and continue to sauté until mushrooms release their liquid, about 3 minutes. Stir in garlic and continue to stir until most of the liquid has evaporated.

Deglaze the pot with a little bit of veggie stock. Add remaining stock and 2 cups of fresh water. Bring to a boil. Stir in fresh gingerroot and kale. Return soup to a boil; reduce heat and simmer for 10 minutes. Add white beans and red chili flakes and simmer for another 10 minutes. Season with salt. If desired, skip the salt and serve soup sprinkled with a little grated parmesan cheese. This soup tastes even better the next day.

Arugula Blackberry Salad

This unique salad pairs a variety of tastes together including bitter arugula, sweet blackberries and vanilla, and tart lemon juice with a little hint of spice from chili flakes.

Makes 2 meal-sized servings

8 cups baby arugula
2 cups fresh blackberries or other berries in season
2 cups cucumber, chopped
½ cup hazelnuts, toasted if desired
½ cup feta cheese or goat cheese
4 tablespoons extra virgin olive oil
2 tablespoons freshly squeezed lemon juice
⅛ teaspoon vanilla extract
⅛ teaspoon chili flakes
Salt and pepper to taste

In a medium-sized serving bowl, combine salad ingredients including arugula, blackberries, cucumber, hazelnuts, and cheese.

In a small bowl, whisk together olive oil, lemon juice, vanilla, and chili flakes. Season with salt and pepper. Drizzle over salad and toss gently.

Colorful Winter Slaw

You know that point in the winter when the harvest season is long gone and spring plantings are still a ways off? That is when you need this amazingly satisfying, crunchy slaw. It turns winter staples into a fresh and flavorful salad that is wonderful in lunches or as a side dish. Fennel is a fantastic veggie to help soothe tummy troubles and aid with digestion.

Makes 5 servings

¾ cup plain yogurt
2 teaspoons Dijon mustard
1 tablespoon freshly squeezed lemon juice
2 teaspoons honey
¼ cup packed and chopped fresh dill
Salt and pepper to taste
1 small fennel bulb

1 broccoli stalk, peeled
1 carrot, peeled
¼ head red cabbage

In a small bowl, whisk together yogurt, mustard, lemon juice, honey, and fresh dill. Cover and store in the refrigerator to allow flavors to blend.

Use a mandolin or food processor with slicer attachment to slice vegetables into thin julienne or matchstick pieces. Start with the lightest colored vegetables: fennel, broccoli stalk, carrot, and finally red cabbage. Once sliced, place fennel, broccoli, and carrot in a colander under cold running water, tossing occasionally. This will crisp up vegetables so they are nice and crunchy. When ready to serve, drain, and toss with red cabbage.

Season yogurt dill dressing with salt and pepper to taste and add to vegetables; tossing to combine well.

One Dish Wonders

Eat Your Greens Frittata

Frittata is on heavy dinner rotation in our houses; there is nothing simpler and more accommodating to whatever you might have lying around your fridge. It is also a great way to serve greens to those who aren't greens fans yet. Perfect served cold for lunches the next day.

Makes 4–6 servings

1 tablespoon olive oil
1 small yellow onion, coarsely chopped
2 garlic cloves, minced
1 bunch kale, washed, de-stemmed and torn into bite sized pieces

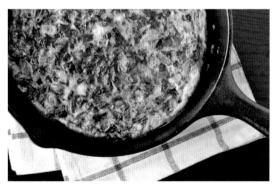

1 yellow pepper, diced
8 eggs
¼ cup of good quality pesto (vegan or regular)

In a large heavy skillet or cast iron frying pan, sauté onion in oil over medium-high heat until soft and golden, about 5–7 minutes. Add garlic, stir through for one minute and add kale. Cover with a lid for 3 minutes to steam. Remove lid and continue to sauté until totally wilted, about 3 more minutes.

Add yellow pepper and sauté for 1 minute. Season vegetable mixture with a pinch of salt and freshly ground pepper. Preheat broiler.

Beat eggs in a large mixing bowl with pesto. Add vegetable mix to the eggs, mix through and return to the skillet. Cook, undisturbed, on medium heat until the top is almost set, about 10 minutes. Finish under the broiler until the top is golden. Serve with a side salad or roasted yams.

Sweet Potato and Chickpea Curry

This is a hearty and flavorful meal to warm you up when it is cold out. It is both sweet and savory and everything you could want in a filling, nutritious, and delicious meal. Eat it as a stew with your favorite whole grain; to make it more kid friendly, use just half a jalapeño.

Makes 8 servings

2 teaspoons olive oil
1 onion, chopped
1–2 jalapeño, seeded and minced
4 garlic cloves, minced
1 tablespoon grated fresh gingerroot
1 red bell pepper, chopped
1-19 oz. (540 ml) can whole tomatoes
2 cups peeled and cubed sweet potatoes
1 teaspoon ground cumin
½ teaspoon ground coriander
1 teaspoon ground garam masala
½ teaspoon salt
1-19 oz. (540 ml) can chickpeas, rinsed and drained or 2 cups cooked—*see tip page 264*
1 fresh mango (or 1 cup frozen), chopped finely or pureed
1 cup coconut milk
Fresh cilantro, chopped

Heat oil in heavy soup pot over medium heat. Add onion, jalapeño, ginger, and garlic cloves and sauté for 2–3 minutes. Add red bell pepper and sauté for another 5 minutes until onions are translucent. Add tomatoes and sweet potatoes; cook for 5 minutes. Add spices and chickpeas.

Bring to a boil and simmer for 10 minutes, stirring occasionally. Add mango and coconut milk; stir to combine. Bring back to a boil and simmer until thickened. Adjust seasoning with salt and pepper. Serve over brown basmati rice and sprinkled with fresh cilantro.

Portuguese Baked Beans

This recipe is my childhood in a bowl. My grandmother would simmer these beans until the oil glistened on top (and added big hunks of Portuguese sausage). Now, she makes these beans for me without the meat and it is astounding how something so simple can be so delicious. Try them, you won't be disappointed—it's all about the onions for flavor. Serve with a nice salad.

Makes 4–6 servings

¼ cup olive oil
1 cup diced yellow onion
1 garlic clove, minced
2 19 oz. (540 ml) cans kidney beans, drained and rinsed or 4 cups cooked beans
1 teaspoon cumin
½–1 teaspoon salt—*see tip*
½ cup passata (strained) tomato sauce

Preheat oven to 350°F.

Heat oil in a large skillet over medium-high heat. Add onions and sauté until they are soft and just starting to caramelize, about 5–7 minutes. Stir in garlic, cumin and salt and cook for 1 minute or until fragrant. Add beans and tomato sauce. Give it a good stir and remove from heat.

Transfer beans to a 9 × 9 inch square casserole dish, cover with aluminum foil and bake for one hour.

Tip: The amount of salt to add will vary depending on the beans you choose to use. If you are using salted canned beans, add ½ teaspoon of salt. For home cooked beans or unsalted canned beans, you can add up to 1 teaspoon of salt.

Tip: For a quick weekday-friendly recipe, simply simmer the beans for 20 minutes on the stovetop, with the lid on. Add water in ¼ cup increments if the beans look dry.

Chipotle Maple Baked Beans

Beans are foundational in an anti-inflammatory eating plan, so you will need few good recipes to help you make them a dinnertime staple! This sweet and spicy casserole is Heather's favourite take on a classic dish.

Makes 8 servings

2-14 oz. (398 ml) cans white kidney beans or navy beans, drained and rinsed—*see tip*
½–1 chipotle pepper in adobo sauce
1 cup tomatoes, peeled, seeded and diced (or canned tomatoes, seeded and diced)
1 tablespoon olive oil
1 large onion, minced
2 garlic cloves, minced
½ cup maple syrup
2 tablespoons brown sugar
2 teaspoons apple cider vinegar
1½ cups low sodium veggie or chicken stock
Salt and pepper to taste

Preheat oven to 300°F. Place beans in a medium sized casserole dish.

In a blender or food processor, puree chipotle pepper with tomato. If you like spice, use a whole chipotle pepper. If you prefer a mild flavor, use only half a chipotle pepper.

Heat oil in a sauté pan over medium heat. Add onions and cook for 5–7 minutes until onions are soft. Add pureed chipotle tomato mixture and remaining ingredients. Bring to a simmer. Remove from heat and pour over beans in casserole dish. Stir to combine.

Cover and bake for 2 hours. Uncover and bake for another 45 minutes to 1 hour until most of the liquid is absorbed and beans are brown in color. Season with salt and pepper and serve.

Tip: To cook your own beans for this recipe, soak 1 cup of navy beans in lots of cold water overnight. Drain soaked beans and rinse well under cold water. Discard any shriveled beans or those that did not swell. Place navy beans in a saucepot and cover with a large amount of fresh water, about 3 inches above beans. Bring to a boil; simmer until tender, about 40 minutes. Drain and place in a casserole dish.

Main Events

Rockin' Tempeh Tacos

This is such a quick and easy way to enjoy healthy tacos at home you won't ever look back. Tempeh is a wonderful fermented soybean cake that is common in Indonesia and incredibly nutritious. If you have been scared off by tempeh in the past, this recipe will change your mind. The spices pair perfectly with the earthiness of the tempeh.

Makes 4 servings

1½ tablespoons oregano
1½ tablespoons ground cumin
2 teaspoons ground coriander
½ –1 teaspoon cayenne pepper
salt and pepper to taste
1 tablespoon lime juice
1 tablespoon unsalted tomato paste
½ cup water
1 tablespoon olive oil
1 onion, diced
2 garlic cloves, minced
1 red bell pepper, diced
1 package tempeh, crumbled

Fixings: Corn tortillas or collard leaves, salsa, shredded lettuce or cabbage, grated cheese or vegan cheese, and lime wedges.

In a small bowl, combine spices. In another small bowl, combine lime juice, tomato paste, and water. Set the bowls aside. Preparing your fixings so they are ready to go!

Heat oil in a frying pan over medium heat. Add onion and sauté for 3 minutes; add garlic and bell pepper and sauté for 3 more minutes. Add crumbled tempeh and the spice mixture and cook for 2–3 minutes.

Stir in lime and tomato water. Cook until most of the moisture has absorbed, about 5 minutes. Season with salt and pepper. Serve in corn tortillas or collard leaves with salsa, shredded lettuce, and grated cheese.

Tip: Tired of corn tortillas breaking and spilling their contents? Give them a collard wrap! Use trimmed collard greens as the bottom layer, add corn tortilla and fixings. The collards are more flexible than corn tortillas and give you an extra serving of good-for-you greens.

Comfort, Better Known as Stuffed Sweet Potatoes

I love baked potatoes but they don't always scream healthy. This recipe takes a more nutrient dense option, the sweet potato, and loads it full of anti-inflammatory goodness. These spuds are a meal in themselves but would be delicious with the kale and avocado salad. Eat these when you want to feel full and satisfied!

Makes 4 servings

4 small to medium sized sweet potatoes
2 cups cooked lentils—*see tip*
1 tablespoon olive oil
1 yellow onion, diced
2 cups diced crimini or shitake mushrooms
Splash of red wine
½ teaspoon cinnamon
¼ teaspoon cardamom
½ teaspoon cumin
salt and pepper to taste
2 tablespoons maple syrup

Preheat oven to 400°F. Bake sweet potatoes for 30–45 minutes or until tender. Set aside.
Meanwhile, prepare lentils if you are cooking them from dry.

Heat oil in a saucepan over medium heat. Add onions and sauté until translucent and lightly caramelized, about 5–7 minutes. Add mushrooms and sauté until they release their juices and the liquid reduces. Deglaze the pan with a splash of red wine. Stir in cooked lentils, spices, and season with salt and pepper. Turn off the heat. Divide the lentil mixture in half, placing half in a bowl.

Gently cut the top portion of skin off the sweet potatoes. Scoop out the sweet potato, taking care to leave the skin intact and add to the bowl with half the lentil mixture. Add maple syrup and gently stir to combine. Stuff potato skins with the sweet potato mixture and top with remaining lentil mixture. Serve with a colorful green salad.

Tip: Lentils are super easy to cook as they don't require soaking. We recommend using French lentils if you can find them. They hold their shape well after cooking. To make 2 cups cooked lentils, bring ¾ cup dried French green lentils and 2¼ cups water in a saucepan and bring to a boil. Reduce heat and simmer for 30–40 minutes or until tender. Drain away any excess water.

Colorful Spiced Chicken Lettuce Cups

Trying to break the starchy meal cycle? Lettuce wrap it! This is a protein and produce feast that is fun food for a crowd. The richly spiced flavors are a perfect complement to the crunch of crisp lettuce.

Makes 4 servings

1 lb. lean ground chicken or turkey
1 tablespoon grated fresh gingerroot
2 teaspoons olive or coconut oil
½ red onion, diced
1 red bell pepper, diced
1 yellow bell pepper, diced
1-8 oz. (227 ml) can sliced water chestnuts, chopped
¼ cup hoisin sauce
¼ cup water
¾ teaspoon Chinese five spice
¼–½ teaspoon sambal oelek or dried chilies
1 carrot, grated
1 head iceberg or butter lettuce, leaves left whole, washed and dried

In a skillet over medium heat, cook ground chicken and ginger for 5 to 6 minutes or until cooked through. Set aside.

In the same skillet, heat oil over medium heat. Add onion and sauté for 2 minutes. Add bell peppers and sauté for 3 more minutes. Add cooked chicken and water chestnuts and stir to mix. Add hoisin sauce, water, Chinese five spice and desired amount of sambal oelek or dried chilies. Stir to combine. Cook until heated through.

Place the grated carrots and lettuce leaves on a large platter with the chicken and vegetable mixture in a bowl. The lettuce wraps are best assembled individually at the table. Top each leaf with chicken and vegetable mixture and grated carrot, wrap, and enjoy.

Lettuce wraps can be served hot or cold, as a meal or an appetizer.

Gloriously Green Herb-Crusted Tof-alibut

This is flexitarian, anti-inflammatory food at its finest! Healthy can be beautiful, flavorful, and impress your dinner guests. Serve tofu for vegetarian friends, halibut for the omnivores. Both are delicious and the herb crust is packed with antioxidant rich herbs.

Makes 4 servings

⅓ cup raw pumpkin seeds
1 cup packed mint leaves
1 cup packed cilantro leaves
4 tablespoons extra virgin olive oil
1 tablespoon freshly squeezed lime juice
¼ teaspoon salt
1 package organic or non-GMO extra-firm tofu or 4 halibut fillets (about 4–5 oz. each)

In a food processor or high speed blender, pulse pumpkin seeds first until they are coarsely ground then add herbs. Pulse as you drizzle in olive oil and lime juice until a thick paste forms. Season with salt.

Preheat oven to 400°F.

To make herb-crusted tofu, place brick of tofu on a cutting board. Cut in half so you have two square pieces. Then take each square piece and slice on the horizontal so you end up with four, one inch thick tofu steaks. Season each side of the steaks with salt and pepper. Preheat oven-proof frying pan or cast iron pan until hot. Fry tofu steaks for 5 minutes on each side. Spread a thick layer of herb paste on the top of each steak. Transfer to preheated oven and bake for 15 minutes.

To make herb-crusted halibut, preheat oven-proof frying pan or cast iron pan until hot. Place halibut fillets, skin side up and sear for 2–4 minutes or until nicely browned. Flip over and spread a thick layer of herb paste on top of each seared fillet. Transfer to preheated oven and bake for 15 minutes for 1½ inch thick halibut fillets.

Tip: This recipe makes a good amount of herb pesto. If you're only making one or two servings of herb-crusted tofu or fish, extra pesto is delicious as a sauce for pasta or spreading on sandwiches.

Miso Ginger Salmon Collard Packets

This recipe is ridiculously good. The wrapping takes a few extra minutes but it is worth it. Some weird sort of alchemy happens when the salmon steams in the miso ginger sauce packaged perfectly in the collard wrap. This recipe is sure to please and is such a nutritious foundation to a meal.

Makes 2 servings

2 large collard green leaves
2 12-inch long green onions (or 4 smaller ones), optional
¼ cup white miso paste
¼ cup rice vinegar
1 tablespoon grated fresh gingerroot
1 tablespoon maple syrup
1 teaspoon sesame oil
1 cup thinly sliced shiitake or crimini mushrooms
2 salmon fillets, cut into a rectangle shape (about 4–5 oz. each)

Preheat oven to 400°F. Line a rimmed baking sheet with parchment paper.

Place the collard green on a cutting board, smooth side down. With a sharp knife, carefully slice off the protruding portion of the collard stem as this will make the leaves more flexible for wrapping. Remove the white portions of the green onions and save for another use. Prepare a large bowl of cold water.

Bring a large pot of water to a boil. Add collard greens and blanch for 90 seconds. Remove immediately and place in the cold water bath to stop the cooking process. Blanch green onions for 60 seconds and immediately place in the cold water bath.

In a small bowl, mix together miso paste, rice vinegar, gingerroot, maple syrup, and sesame oil. Set aside.

To assemble the salmon packets, place a blanched collard leave lengthwise in front of you. Place a few slices of mushrooms along the stem and add salmon fillet on top of the mushrooms. The salmon should hide the mushrooms so tuck them in if they stick out. Layer a few more mushrooms slices on top of the salmon and drizzle 1 tablespoon of sauce over top. Fold the collard wrap, short sides first and then long sides so that you have a tidy wrapped package.

You can use two toothpicks to secure the packages. If you want to get fancy, tie the packages with the blanched green onions. If you have short green onions, tie the ends of 2 green onions together to make a long one.

Bake salmon packets for 20 minutes. Drizzle with another tablespoon of miso sauce and enjoy.

Tip: The sauce is enough to make four portions if company is coming. If not, use the remainder to dress an Asian-inspired salad or soba noodles . . . which would be delicious served with the salmon packets!

Turmeric Chicken Skillet

Turmeric is not just an anti-inflammatory superstar, it is pretty too! Turmeric gives this curry a lovely color with just the right amount of heat. Don't let the long list of ingredients deter you; most of them are spices you probably already have in your pantry and the recipe comes together in less than 30 minutes! Healthy curry in a hurry . . .

Makes 4 servings

2 tablespoons avocado or coconut oil
1 lb. boneless, skinless chicken thighs or breasts, cut into strips or cubes
1 large onion, thinly sliced
1 apple, unpeeled and grated
3 garlic cloves, minced
1 tablespoon grated fresh gingerroot
1 tablespoon turmeric
1 teaspoon ground coriander
½ teaspoon cumin
¼ teaspoon cinnamon
¼ teaspoon ground ginger
¼ teaspoon ground cardamom
⅛ teaspoon cayenne pepper
⅛ teaspoon ground cloves
⅛ teaspoon ground pepper
2 tablespoons all-purpose flour
2 cups low sodium chicken stock
4 cups spinach or other greens
Fresh cilantro leaves

Heat 1 tablespoon of oil in a large skillet or Dutch oven over medium-high heat. Add chicken and sear until lightly golden brown, about 1–2 minutes. Set aside.

Reduce heat to medium and heat remaining 1 tablespoon of oil in the same skillet or Dutch oven. Add onions and sauté until they soften, about 3 minutes. Add apple, garlic, gingerroot, and spices and stir to combine until fragrant, about 1 minute. Stir in flour and cook for 2 minutes to remove the floury taste. Slowly add chicken stock, stirring constantly to combine. Bring to a boil and simmer for 2 minutes or until the sauce has thickened.

Return the chicken and any accumulated juices to the skillet, stir and cook for 10 minutes or until the chicken is cooked through. Stir in the spinach or greens and cook for 1 more minute or until greens are wilted. Serve with barley or brown rice and garnish with cilantro leaves.

Greens and Beans Casserole

I first encountered greens and beans in university and have been making some haphazard variation of it ever since; I thought it was high time to standardize what has become a Nielsen family staple. Hearty, comforting, and utterly nutritious—with a bit of cheese on top.

Makes 8 servings

1 tablespoon olive oil
1 yellow onion, diced
1 celery stalk, diced
1 carrot, diced
8 cups packed baby kale
2 garlic cloves, minced
4 cups cooked lentils—*see tip on page 254*
2 cups low sodium veggie stock
1 teaspoon cumin
1 bay leaf
4 cups cooked brown rice
2 cups shredded extra aged white cheddar or Monterey Jack vegan cheese

Preheat oven to 375°F.

Cook brown rice and lentils according to package directions if you need to. Heat olive oil in a large frying pan over medium heat. Add onion, carrot, and celery and sauté until soft, about 5–7 minutes. Add half the kale and sauté until it wilts; add the other half and sauté until it wilts.

Stir in garlic and sauté for 1 minute. Add lentils, stock and spices. Bring to a gentle boil, reduce heat and simmer for 15 minutes. Adjust seasoning to taste with salt and pepper and remove bay leaf.

Press rice into the bottom of a 9 × 13 baking dish. Pour lentil and kale mixture over the rice and spread evenly. Bake for 30 minutes. Sprinkle with cheese and bake another 15 minutes or until the moisture is absorbed and cheese is melted.

Tip: This recipe is really flexible. Feel free to use any combination of beans, greens and grains you wish. Sage goes really well with white beans or you could go Tex-Mex with kidney beans!

Super Snacks

Spiced White Bean Dip

Who doesn't love a dip? And who decided that they have to be loaded with fat? White beans are the perfect dip base as they are creamy, comforting, and rich without adding gobs of unhealthy fats. Get your fiber the fun way!

Makes two cups

2 cups cooked white beans or 1-19 oz. (540 ml) can white kidney beans—*see tip on page 251*
2 tablespoons extra virgin olive oil
Grated zest of ½ a lemon
2 tablespoons freshly squeezed lemon juice
1 garlic clove, crushed—really good if roasted
1 tablespoon chopped fresh thyme
¼ teaspoon red pepper flakes
¼ teaspoon cumin
¼ – ½ teaspoon salt
¼ cup pumpkin seeds, whole or chopped

In a food processor, combine all ingredients except pumpkin seeds and pulse a few times. If needed, add water, 1 tablespoon at a time, pulsing until the mixture is the consistency desired. Taste and adjust the lemon juice and salt. If using salted canned beans, add ¼ teaspoon salt. If using unsalted canned or cooked beans, add ½ teaspoon salt. Place in serving dish and top with pumpkin seeds for crunch and add a drizzle of olive oil. Serve with fresh chopped veggies.

Tip: If you don't have a food processor, an immersion blender will also work well. Tip the bowl so you create a pool of liquid ingredients, start your blending there and eventually work the rest of the beans into the puree.

Energy to Spare Trail Mix

Is trail mix a recipe? Maybe we just need a reminder that we don't have to pay $6.99 for a tiny bag of mixed goodies when you can customize your own to your tastes. I have included golden berries, one of my favorite superfood treats. If they aren't available or too expensive at your local store, substitute an unsweetened dried fruit like golden sultanas or apricots.

Makes two cups

½ cup almonds
½ cup pumpkin seeds
¼ cup shaved coconut
½ cup golden berries (or golden sultana raisins)
¼ cup cacao nibs

Mix all the fixings into a resealable container and keep on hand (or in your desk drawer) for snack fixes.

Tip: Trail mix is the easiest thing going—the key is not to overload it with sweets so that it resembles candy. Keep the ratio of non-sweet to sweet fixings at 3:1. Making your own trail mix saves you money, lets you to customize to your favorites, and avoids nasty ingredients like soy oil and high fructose corn syrup.

Baked Mexican Dip

I love me some seven layer dip but not the junk that normally goes into them. This is my anti-inflammatory take on that creamy goodness that tastes just as good as the original. Snacking can be nutritious!

Makes 4–6 servings

1 cup cashews
1-14 oz. (398 ml) can black refried beans—the spicy version is a great pick
1 tablespoon olive oil
1 bunch of collard greens, finely chopped or your favorite greens
1 teaspoon chili powder
¼ teaspoon salt
½ teaspoon garlic powder
¼ teaspoon ground cumin
¼ teaspoon paprika

1 cup queso fresco, feta cheese, or Monterey Jack vegan cheese
1 avocado
juice of ½ lime
1 cup chopped tomatoes
3 green onions, sliced
salsa, optional

Soak cashews in a bowl with water to cover for 30–60 minutes.
Preheat oven to 375°F. Spread black beans in a 9 × 9 inch baking dish.
Heat oil in a skillet or sauté pan over medium. Add chopped collards and sauté until they are wilted. Season with salt and pepper and layer over beans.

Drain cashews but reserve the soaking liquid. Place soaked cashews in a blender or food processor and add just enough of the soaking liquid to barely cover the cashews. Blend until thick and smooth and add spices. Layer over greens. Sprinkle with cheese. Bake until cheese bubbles, about 20–30 minutes.

Meanwhile, mash avocado with the lime juice. When dip is ready, allow to cool for 5 minutes before layering with mashed avocado, chopped tomatoes, and green onions. Top with salsa if desired.

Serve with organic tortilla chips, rye crackers, or chopped veggies. Endive leaves make great dippers too!

Banana Sushi

My son loves sushi: I have seen him eat three rolls at one sitting! (He is four.) So this idea takes the shape of sushi to transform a fairly traditional lunchtime staple—a PB & B. Hemp seeds add a boost of omega-3 in a kid-friendly package. This is great for kids and adults alike.

Makes one serving

1 small banana
2 tablespoons natural and unsweetened nut, seed, or pea butter
1 teaspoon runny honey
1 tablespoon hemp seeds
1 8-inch sprouted grain or whole wheat tortilla

If the tortillas are too stiff to roll, give them a quick steam over some boiling water or in a hot moist towel. Spread tortilla with nut butter, drizzle with honey, and sprinkle with hemp seeds. Place banana along one edge of the tortilla and roll the tortilla around the banana. Slice into 8 pieces and arrange in a lunch container. Serve with chopsticks for fun!

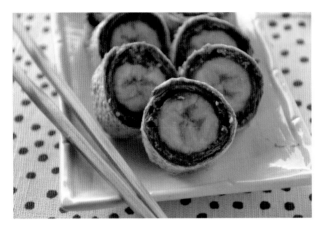

Allergy Friendly Tip: There are butters made from almost anything you can think of nowadays. For a totally nut free option, try Sunbutter (from sunflower seeds), pumpkin seed butter (a stronger flavor) or NoNuts (golden peas).

Salted Chocolate Almond Gems

Craving chocolate? How about chocolate with a side of healthy? These are so simple to make and keep well for whenever a chocolate craving strikes. Dates are a mineral rich alternative to refined sugars and the sea salt makes these raw truffles extra delectable.

Makes ten to twelve bites

10 pitted medjool dates
3 tablespoons natural almond butter
2 tablespoons raw cacao or cocoa powder
½ teaspoon vanilla or scraped vanilla bean
¼ teaspoon sea salt
Extra raw cacao, cocoa powder, or chopped almonds for rolling

Place the pitted dates in a food processor and pulse until the dates are about the size of peas. Add almond butter, cacao or cocoa powder, vanilla, and salt. Pulse until combined. Mixture will be crumbly.

Roll mixture into ½-inch balls and then roll in raw cacao, cocoa powder, or chopped almonds. Store in the refrigerator for up to 2 weeks or freeze to enjoy later on.

Shockingly Good Pink Walnut Dip

This is one time that a shocking pink color is not the work of food dyes! This is an unexpected and delicious way to eat your beets; classic Mediterranean ingredients combine for a newfangled take on snack time. High in anti-inflammatory nutrition and super fun to eat.

Makes three cups

2 cups chopped raw beets, about one large (4-inch diameter)
½ cup walnuts
1-14 oz. (398 ml) can white cannellini or navy beans, drained and rinsed—*see tip on page 251*
1 tablespoon extra virgin olive oil
1 tablespoon freshly squeezed lemon juice
3 tablespoons maple syrup
½–1 garlic clove, minced
salt and pepper to taste

Place all ingredients in a blender or food processor and blend until smooth or nearly smooth. Serve with veggies or crackers or use as a sandwich spread.

The Amazing Roasted Chickpea

Sometimes you just want to snack on something amazing. So many snack foods are completely devoid of nutrition but who says a snack can't be tasty and healthy? Chickpeas are full of protein, minerals, and fiber and are so versatile; whatever flavors you crave, chickpeas can pair well with them.

Makes three cups

2-14 oz. (398 ml) cans chickpeas, drained and rinsed or 3 cups cooked chickpeas—*see tip*
2 tablespoons extra virgin olive oil
salt and pepper to taste or your favorite seasonings

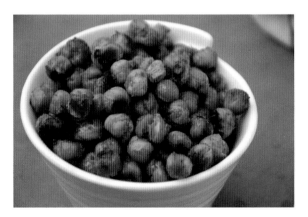

Preheat oven to 375°F. Line a baking sheet with parchment paper or a Silpat mat.

In a large bowl, combine chickpeas with flavorful ingredients and toss to coat well.

Spread chickpeas on prepared baking sheet and bake for 35–45 minutes, stirring half way through.

Cool slightly before eating. Store in an airtight container and enjoy within 2 weeks.

Tip: These make a fantastic, protein rich snack! Try different flavorings such as 1 tablespoon chopped fresh rosemary and 1 teaspoon crushed garlic, 1 teaspoon each cinnamon and honey, or 1 tablespoon curry powder.

Tip: To cook your own chickpeas, soak one cup dried chickpeas in lots of cold water overnight. Drain soaked chickpeas and rinse well under cold water. Discard any shriveled chickpeas or those that did not swell. Place soaked chickpeas in a saucepot and cover with a large amount of fresh water, about three inches above chickpeas. Bring to a boil; simmer until tender, about eighty minutes. Drain and they are ready to use. One cup of dried chickpeas equals about three cups cooked chickpeas.

Sweet Nothings

Black Bean Brownies

I wanted to create sweets that you could feel good about eating and this is it! Totally grain free, low in sugar, and packed with chocolate. The beans provide a fudgy texture and plenty of protein and fiber to keep blood sugars stable. Go ahead, eat a brownie a day . . . dietitian's orders!

Makes twelve brownies

1-14 oz. (398 ml) can black beans, drained and rinsed or 1½ cups cooked black beans
1 cup chopped medjool dates
⅓ cup extra virgin olive oil
1 teaspoon vanilla
100 g bar 85 percent cocoa dark chocolate, broken into small pieces
2 tablespoons unsweetened chocolate almond milk
⅓ cup almond flour—*see tip on page 235*
¼ teaspoon salt
½ teaspoon cinnamon
1 egg, beaten or 1 chia/flax egg—*see tip on page 235*
½ cup chopped raw pecans or walnuts, optional

Preheat oven to 350°F. Grease an 8 × 8 inch square baking pan with olive oil or coconut oil.

Place beans, dates, oil, and vanilla in a food processor and puree. Alternatively, you could puree the mixture in a narrow bowl with an immersion blender. It will be a bit slow going, but it works well. You should have a smooth, thick paste without any pieces of bean or date left.

In a double boiler or bowl set over a small amount of simmering water, melt dark chocolate with almond milk, stirring frequently. Add to the bean mixture and stir well. Stir in almond flour, salt, cinnamon, and egg. If desired you can mix in the nuts or sprinkle them on top of brownie. Pour the brownie in the prepared baking pan. Bake for 20–25 minutes. The brownie top should be totally set but the brownies will have a fudgy texture.

Frozen Blueberry Yogurt

Strangely, most frozen yogurts on store shelves have very little to do with actual yogurt. Instead of fillers and food cosmetics, why not make your own using real ingredients? This is one of the easiest treats to make: no ice cream maker required!

Makes 2 cups or 4 small servings

2 cups frozen blueberries
1 cup plain yogurt, preferably 2–3.5 percent milk fat—the little bit of fat makes this treat creamier than if you use fat-free yogurt.

Place the blueberries in a food processor and pulse several times to break up the blueberries. Add the plain yogurt. Blend until mixture is smooth and looks like delicious blueberry ice cream. Serve immediately.

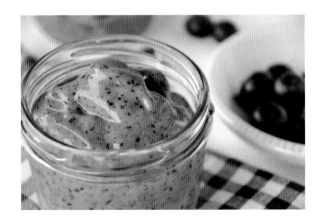

Tip: This is a simple and easy recipe that has lots of room to be creative. Blueberry is Heather's favorite but this recipe is also delicious using frozen peaches, strawberries, blackberries, cherries, or other local fruit. Raspberries are also fun for a tart frozen treat.

Baked Apple Oat Pudding

This pudding has all the flavors of an apple pie, with a fraction of the sugar and plenty of soluble fiber from the oats. This is a warm, comforting dessert you can feel good about.

Makes 4–6 hearty breakfast servings or 6–9 dessert servings

1 cup large flake oats
1 teaspoon baking powder
¼ teaspoon salt
1 teaspoon cinnamon
2 medium (or 3 small) apples, coarsely grated
¼ cup chopped walnuts
1 egg, beaten
3 cups vanilla almond milk or regular milk with 1 teaspoon vanilla
¼–⅓ cup maple syrup

Preheat oven to 375°F.

In a medium bowl, combine oats, baking powder, salt, cinnamon, apples, and walnuts. In another bowl, whisk together egg, milk, and maple syrup until well combined. Pour wet ingredients into dry and stir to combine.

Pour into a greased 9 × 9 inch baking dish. Bake for 35–45 minutes until set in the center.

Tip: This dessert is excellent served with honeyed greek yogurt or cashew cream.

Coconut Black Rice Pudding

Makes 6 servings

1½ cups Thai black sweet rice
1-14 oz. (398 ml) can coconut milk
⅓ cup maple syrup
½ cup unsweetened shredded coconut
¼ teaspoon salt
fresh mango, sliced or chopped dried mango
pistachios

Rinse rice in a colander and place in a medium saucepan with 3 cups of cold water. Soak overnight or for 6–8 hours during the day. Remove 1½ cups of water.

Stir in coconut milk, maple syrup, coconut, and salt. Bring to a boil. Reduce heat, cover, and simmer for one hour. Rice will be tender but chewy. Serve with fresh sliced mango or chopped dried mango and pistachios.

Crunchy Nut Candy Bars

Makes twelve small bars

1 cup sliced natural almonds
½ cup walnut pieces
½ cup pumpkin seeds
1 tablespoon natural almond butter
2 tablespoons honey
1 tablespoon coconut oil
100g bar 85 percent cocoa dark chocolate, broken into small pieces

Grease a loaf pan or a 9 × 9 inch baking pan with coconut oil.

In a medium-sized bowl, combine almonds, walnuts, and pumpkin seeds. Combine almond butter, honey, and coconut oil in a small saucepan and melt over low heat to mix well. Add to nut and seed mixture and stir to coat well. Spread into prepared pan. If using a 9 × 9 inch baking pan, spread mixture into half of the pan. Place in the freezer for 30 minutes to set.

In a double boiler or bowl set over a small amount of simmering water, melt dark chocolate, stirring frequently. Pour over nut and seed mixture. Return to the freezer for 30 minutes or until set. Cut into 12 small bars. Store in the freezer. Best enjoyed chilled.

Paperback Edition Bonus Recipes

Mediterranean Stuffed Dates

Nothing wrong with a little healthy indulgence . . . this Mediterranean-inspired appetizer is perfect whenever you're craving something rich and creamy. If you don't want to stuff the dates, stir ½ cup chopped dates into the cashew cheese and serve as a dip or spread with crackers and veggies.

Makes approximately 2/3 cup of cashew cheese

½ cup raw unsalted cashews

2 tablespoons water

1 teaspoon nutritional yeast

2 tablespoons freshly squeezed lemon juice

1 teaspoon apple cider vinegar

½ teaspoon salt

1 teaspoon tahini (sesame butter)

¼ cup finely chopped walnuts

chili flakes to taste *(I like ½ teaspoon)*

18 large fresh dates such as Medjool or Deglet Noor

Soak the cashews: place cashews in a small bowl and add enough water to cover. Soak for at least 4 hours. If soaking for more than 4 hours, place bowl in refrigerator while soaking.

Drain and rinse cashews and place in a food processor or high speed blender. Add the rest of the ingredients and purée until really smooth. Chill for 30 minutes so the cashew cheese can set.

Carefully slice dates lengthwise to the center and remove pit. Don't cut all the way through—you are making a slit to add the cheese to, not cutting the dates in half. Add 1 teaspoon of cashew cheese mixture in the center of each date and serve.

Tip: The cashews will continue to hydrate the longer you soak them. After a long soak, start with 1 tablespoon of water so you don't end up with runny cashew cheese. If after pureeing for a couple of minutes, the cheese mixture seems too dry, add water in 1 tablespoon increments.

Note: After stuffing 18 dates, you'll probably have some cashew cheese left over . . . use as a spread or dip within 3 days!

Energizing Cauliflower Salad

Salad doesn't fill you up? Meet your match. Crunchy, hearty veggies combined with protein- and fibre-packed beans means that this salad will satisfy. I like whipping up a batch of this on Sunday night so I can have it for lunch all week.

Makes 4–6 servings

1 medium head of cauliflower, riced

1 small bulb (3–4 inch) kohlrabi, peeled and cubed
1 - 14 oz. (398ml) can of navy beans or other soft white bean, drained and rinsed
½ large English cucumber, chopped
1 cup parsley leaves
1 cup feta (optional)

½ cup of your favorite hummus
juice of 1 lemon

Make the cauliflower rice: wash and trim the cauliflower. Chop into florets and place in food processor. Pulse until cauliflower looks close to the size and texture of rice. You can also grate the cauliflower using a box grater.

In a large salad bowl, add cauliflower, kohlrabi, beans, cucumber, parsley, and feta (if using).

In a small bowl, combine hummus and lemon juice. If starting with a firmer hummus, thin mixture with a bit of water until it has the consistency of a creamy and slightly thick salad dressing. Season with salt and pepper to taste.

Toss dressing with salad and serve.

Tip: No kohlrabi? Substitute peeled broccoli stalks.

Cucumber "Noodles" with Almond Miso

In the middle of the summer, there is nothing more refreshing than cucumber! And be warned: you will want to use this sauce on everything. Drizzle it over roasted sweet potatoes, use it to roast tofu, or as a dipping sauce for salad rolls. Serve with fish or tofu for a complete meal.

Makes 4 main-dish servings

2 large English cucumbers
¼ cup almond butter
¼ cup white (shiro) miso
¼ cup water
1 teaspoon rice vinegar
1 teaspoon maple syrup
2 teaspoons freshly squeezed lime juice

1 teaspoon minced garlic
chili flakes, to taste
1 cup cilantro leaves
½ cup chopped almonds

Trim cucumbers and run them through a spiralizer to create long "noodles." Place in a large salad bowl.

In a small bowl, add dressing ingredients and blend with a whisk or hand-held blender. Toss cucumbers with half of the dressing. Add more dressing if desired or reserve remainder for another use.

Serve sprinkled with chopped almonds and some cilantro.

Tip: No spiralizer? Thinly slice cucumbers instead . . . not quite as fun as slurping noodles but just as tasty! Zucchini works well instead of cucumber, too.

Lemon Cardamom Muffins

Almond meal makes these muffins protein and fiber packed! These gluten-free treats are lightly sweetened and have the texture of cornbread. These citrusy snacks help keep energy levels stable when you're on the go.

Makes 9 muffins

2½ cups almond meal
2 teaspoons baking powder
¼ teaspoon salt
¾ teaspoon cardamom
1/3 cup ground flax seed
1/3 cup freshly squeezed lemon juice
¼ cup milk, soymilk, or coconut-based milk alternative
zest of one lemon
¼ cup refined avocado oil or extra virgin olive oil
1/3 cup maple syrup

Preheat oven to 350 degrees. Use a nonstick muffin pan or line pan with silicone baking cups.

Blend dry ingredients together in a medium-sized mixing bowl. Mix wet ingredients together in a small bowl. Add wet ingredients to dry and stir until well blended.

Fill muffin pan using a ¼ cup measure. Bake for 25 minutes. Muffins should be starting to get golden on the edges.

Remove from heat and let rest in pan for 5 minutes. Carefully loosen around the edges with a knife and remove muffins to a cooling rack. Let cool completely so they can firm up.

Harissa-Roasted Eggplant and Chickpeas

Harissa is a fire-y North African spice paste that adds a nice bite to eggplant. It comes in a variety of strengths so be sure to taste it before you set your recipe on fire! You could eat this as a hearty side dish, stuff it into wraps, or try my pasta suggestion.

Makes 4 main-dish servings

1 large eggplant, chopped into 1 inch pieces
2 - 14 oz. (398ml) cans of chickpeas, drained and rinsed
1 tablespoon harissa paste
2 tablespoons freshly squeezed lemon juice
2 tablespoons extra virgin olive oil
2 large cloves garlic, crushed or finely grated
¼–½ teaspoon salt (see note)
2 tablespoons tomato paste
¼ teaspoon cumin
dash chili flakes . . . if the harissa isn't already too hot!

For pasta:
4 cups of your favorite cooked pasta
1½ cups canned diced tomatoes
1 cup feta cheese (optional)

If you want to improve the flavor and texture of eggplant, don't skip the salting step. Place cubed eggplant into a bowl and sprinkle on ½ tablespoon of salt. Toss to coat and let rest 1 hour.

Place eggplant in a colander and rinse off excess salt. Preheat oven to 400 degrees.

In a large mixing bowl, combine harissa, lemon, oil, garlic, salt, tomato paste, cumin, and chili flakes. Mix to combine.

Add chickpeas and eggplant to the spice paste and mix until well coated with spice mixture.

Place in a roasting pan and roast for 20 minutes, stir, and continue to cook for 10 to 20 minutes. You want to get to the point where the chickpeas are starting to crisp up . . . but before the mixture dries out.

If serving as a pasta, combine diced tomatoes with hot pasta and divide among serving plates. Add on a generous amount of chickpeas and eggplant and top with a bit of feta, if using.

Note: I use unsalted beans, so I add ½ teaspoon of salt. If using salted canned beans, stick to ¼ teaspoon.

Matcha Mango Chia Pudding

This is the ultimate on the go breakfast: caffeine and a meal, rolled into one! Matcha powder is ground whole green tea leaves, making it even more anti-oxidant-packed than brewed green tea.

Makes 1 (generous) serving

1 cup light coconut milk (from a can)
½ cup frozen or fresh mango
1 teaspoon maple syrup or honey (and more, to taste)
1 teaspoon matcha powder
1 tablespoon shredded coconut
3 tablespoons chia seed

In a mason jar or re-sealable container, use a handheld blender to blend the coconut milk, mango, and maple syrup until smooth. Add matcha and give another quick whir.

Next, stir in chia seed and coconut and whisk vigorously for about 1 minute. Wait a few minutes and repeat stirring session.

Go ahead and repeat this cycle once more for chia pudding perfection. (You do this to ensure that the chia doesn't clump together as it hydrates.)

Place in the fridge and you've got breakfast the next morning.

Tip: If you tasted the matcha mix before you added the chia, you'll note it tastes sweet. This sweetness dissipates by the next morning . . . it will taste like an unsweetened matcha latte. Which is awesome, if that's how you like it. Need a bit more sweetness? Stir in some more maple syrup in the AM.

Glorious Greens Soup

This simple soup is the perfect warm up when you don't have a lot of time to cook. White beans give it a creamy texture . . . without the addition of cream! This recipe is super flexible. Try baby kale, arugula, green chickpeas . . . whatever you have lying around. If using bitter greens, a tiny drizzle of maple syrup before serving will balance it out.

Makes 4–6 servings

¼ cup extra virgin olive oil
1 medium onion, chopped
¼ teaspoon salt
2 cloves garlic, chopped
2 cups broccoli florets and stalk
1–5 oz. clamshell baby spinach
1 - 14 oz. (398ml) can soft white beans (like navy or cannellini), drained and
   rinsed
1 cup frozen peas
32 oz. (946ml) container of low sodium vegetable broth
¼–3/4 teaspoon ground cumin
¼–½ teaspoon ground nutmeg
chili flakes, to taste

Heat oil in a soup pot and sauté onion until glossy and translucent, about 5 to 7 minutes. Season with ¼ teaspoon salt.

Add garlic and broccoli and sauté for about 3 minutes. Next, add spinach and stir until wilted, about 5 minutes. Add beans and peas and stir until heated through.

Add spices and broth, turn off the heat once it's heated through. Purée with an immersion blender to desired consistency. I like the soup about 3/4 purée, so there is still some texture.

Taste and adjust both spice and salt, if necessary.

Turmeric Tonic

Ginger and turmeric are mainstays in an anti-inflammatory regime. You can take this tonic as a wellness shot . . . but brace yourself, it's super strong. You might also try adding a shot of this to a big mug of hot water or sparkling water to take it as a tonic. However you enjoy it, get this into your belly and feel the burn.

Makes approximately 3/4 cup

1 3-inch piece of ginger, peeled (scant ¼ cup when finely grated)
1 tablespoon ground turmeric
¼ cup honey
¼ cup lemon juice
¼ cup water

Use a fine microplane grater to grate ginger into a large jam jar. Mix in remaining ingredients.

Alternatively, purée all ingredients together in a blender or small food processor.

Pour into an airtight container and store in the fridge for up to 1 week. Stir well before using.

Tip: Use as is, or, to make a more syrup-like texture, strain the mixture through an extra fine sieve, squeezing as much liquid out of the pulp as you can.

Creamy Triple Seed Risotto with Roasted Asparagus

Arborio rice, the usual ingredient in a risotto, isn't exactly the most nutritious food on the planet. Swapping in seeds boosts healthy fats, fiber, and minerals. Sure, it's not exactly authentic, but it's super tasty. Asparagus not in season? Roast your favorite seasonal veggies—it's all good!

Makes 4 servings

1 cup raw pumpkin seeds
1 cup raw sunflower seeds
1 large bunch of asparagus (about 20 stalks)
2 tablespoons extra virgin olive oil + more for roasting
1 medium yellow onion, diced
2 cloves of garlic, minced
2 cups low sodium vegetable stock
½ cup raw tahini (sesame butter)

2 tablespoons freshly squeezed lemon juice
dash sesame oil

Soak the seeds: Boil a kettle of water and let it cool for five minutes. In a bowl, soak the pumpkin and sunflower seeds in enough water to fully cover by at least 1 inch, for at least 4 hours or all day (do this in the morning so you are ready for dinner at night!). If soaking more than 4 hours, place in refrigerator.

When you're ready to cook, start by prepping the asparagus: preheat oven to 400 degrees.

Wash asparagus and trim ends. Place on a rimmed cookie sheet and toss with extra virgin olive oil, salt, and pepper. Roast for 15 to 30 minutes, watching for desired doneness. You want them to soften, get a bit roasted, but remain vibrant and not look too wilted. How long it takes depends on how large the asparagus are. When done, slice into 2 inch pieces and set aside.

For the risotto, heat 2 tablespoons olive oil in a large sauté pan or a medium sauce pan over medium heat. Sauté the onion and garlic until translucent and glossy, about 5 to 7 minutes.

Drain and rinse seeds in a colander and add to onions, along with stock. Turn heat to medium-low, stir, cover the pot, and simmer the seeds for 20 minutes.

Remove cover, stir, and simmer for another 10 minutes. Remove from heat. Most of the liquid will have been absorbed, but not all . . . don't worry, it will come together with the tahini sauce!

In a jar or small bowl, mix together the tahini with lemon juice and sesame oil, and season to taste with salt and pepper.

Stir tahini sauce into risotto, adjust seasoning with salt, pepper, and lemon juice (I like a lot of lemon!) and serve with asparagus.

Tip: if you want a more uniformly textured "risotto", you can use all sunflower seeds but I like the extra texture—and omega 3s! —the pumpkin seeds offer.

Ka-Pow Energy Smoothie

Sometimes, you just need a nutritional kick in the pants. This will give you that kick.

Makes 1 serving

½ cup water
2 tablespoons freshly grated ginger
½ red grapefruit, peeled and pith removed

½ cup fresh or frozen cranberries

½ apple, seeded and chopped with skin on

1 scoop of your favorite protein if eating as a meal

Combine all ingredients in your blender and blend until liquefied. It's that easy.

APPENDIX

HEALTHY EATING AND HEALTHY FOOD RESOURCES

Information about Food Systems, Sustainability, and Food Safety

Environmental Working Group
Dirty Dozen, Meat Eater's Guide, Eating on a Budget Guide: www.ewg.org

Food Politics
Blog on food and nutrition policy and politics from Marion Nestle, MPH, PhD: *www.foodpolitics.com*

Monterey Bay Aquarium (USA)
Sustainable seafood guide and app: www.montereybayaquarium.org

Non-GMO Project
Information about genetically engineered foods and how to avoid them: www.nongmoproject.org

Ocean Wise (Canada)
Sustainable seafood guide and app: www.oceanwise.ca

Products for Your Healthy Kitchen

Attune Foods
Super Grains cereals with simple ingredients: www.attunefoods.com

Blue Diamond
Unsweetened Chocolate Almond Breeze is my favorite almond milk*:* www.almondbreeze.com

Bragg's
Excellent unpasteurized apple cider vinegar: www.bragg.com

Bob's Red Mill
Good quality gluten-free and regular grain flours: www.bobsredmill.com

Cookin' Greens
Frozen super greens, no chopping required! www.cookingreens.com

Daiya Foods
My favorite vegan cheese alternative. No soy, no gluten: www.daiyafoods.com

Eden Foods
Good organic products, including whole soy foods, grains and canned beans. Uses BPA-free cans: www.edenfoods.com

Enjoy Life
High fiber, gluten-free cereal and allergen free products: www.enjoylifefoods.com

Food for Life
Sprouted grain and gluten-free breads and wraps: www.foodforlife.com

Guayaki
Ethically sourced organic yerba mate teas: www.guayaki.com

Izze Soda
A great, fruit-based option for weaning yourself off of conventional sodas: www.izze.com

Jovial Foods
Ancient grain and gluten-free pastas: www.jovialfoods.com

Larabar
Whole food snack bars with simple ingredients: www.larabar.com

Light Life
Organic Tempeh Bacon: www.lightlife.com

Macrobar
Vegan, macrobiotic snack and protein bars: www.gomacro.com

Manna Breads
Unleavened sprouted grain breads: www.mannaorganicbakery.com

Manitoba Harvest Hemp
Good quality hemp seeds, hemp protein and hemp milk: www.manitobaharvest.com

Mary's Organic Crackers
Whole grain, vegan, gluten-free crackers: www.marysgonecrackers.com

Melt
Excellent non-GMO spread with an inventive blend of oils: www.meltorganic.com

Nature's Path
Superseed cereal without added oils or sugars, high fiber cereals, organic oats and flax seeds: www.naturespath.com

Numi Organic Tea
Ethically sourced teas . . . I love the chocolate pu-erh: www.numitea.com

Nutiva
Good quality hemp and coconut products. Try the coconut manna, trust me! www.nutiva.com

Prana
High quality vegan nut and seed products: www.pranana.com/en/

Ryvita
Whole grain crackers: www.ryvita.com

Silver Hills
Canadian sprouted grain breads, bagels and buns. Gluten-free options. www.silverhillsbakery.ca

Spectrum Naturals
High quality cooking oils, expeller pressed and organic: www.spectrumorganics.com

Traditional Medicinals
Ethically sourced medicinal grade herbal teas and tea remedies: www.traditionalmedicinals.com

Turtle Island
Crazy good tempeh bacon: www.tofurky.com

Wasa
Whole grain crackers without added flavorings: www.wasa.com

Super Supplements

Ascenta Omega-3 Oils
I like the NutraSea + D oil and the NutraVege oil: www.ascentahealth.com

Bio K Plus Probiotics
Bio-K+ is my preferred brand and the probiotics company I work with regularly; high potency (50 billion CFU) fresh fermented probiotic, manufactured in Canada: www.biokplus.com

New Chapter
Organic multivitamins, anti-inflammatory herbs and an environmentally conscious omega-3 oil: www.newchapter.com

Vega
Excellent line of clean vegan proteins for smoothies and delicious maca chocolate: www.myvega.com

Fermented Foods

Some of my favorite kombucha choices . . .
RISE Kombucha: www.risekombucha.com
GT's Kombucha www.synergydrinks.com

Karthein's Sauerkraut
Excellent brand of fermented sauerkraut in Canada
www.belandorganicfoods.com/en/organic-products/kartheins/overview

Liberte
Organic Kefir, Greek and Probiotic yogurt: www.liberteyogurt.com

Nancy's Yogurt
Organic Yogurt: www.nancysyogurt.com

PHOTO CREDITS

Heather McColl:

All photos in the recipes section, except for page 237.

Learn more about Heather's work on her blog: *www.freshsheetnutrition.com*

Melissa Quantz:

All photos in chapter 6

Learn more about Melissa's work on her website: www.thebountyhunter.ca

REFERENCES

Chapter One

1. Survey of Household Spending, 2010. *The Daily (April 25, 2012)*. Accessed on January 8, 2013 at www.statcan.gc.ca/daily-quotidien/120425/dq120425a-eng.htm

2. *2011 Restaurant Industry Pocket Factbook*. National Restaurant Association. Accessed on January 8, 2013 at http://restaurant.org/pdfs/research/2011forecast_pfb.pdf

3. Special K Protein Plus Cereal Ingredients List obtained on January 8, 2013 from www.specialk.com

4. Keebler Cinnamon Roll Cookies Ingredients List obtained on January 8, 2013 from www.keebler.com

5. Nabisco Honey Butter Ritz Crackers Ingredients List obtained on January 8, 2013 from www.nabiscoworld.com/ritz/

6. Quaker Cinnamon Granola Bites Ingredients List obtained on January 8, 2013 from www.quakeroats.com

7. Dunkin Donuts Cinnamon Cake Donut Ingredients List obtained on January 8, 2013 from www.dunkindonuts.com

8. Top Agricultural Commodity Production Statistics. USA 2010. *Food and Agricultural Production Statistics from UN FAO* Accessed on January 8, 2013 from http://faostat.fao.org/site/339/default.aspx

9. *Food Inc* (Movie) Corn-derived ingredients handout. Accessed at www.pbs.org/pov/pdf/foodinc/foodinc_corn_derived_handout.pdf

10. *Obesity in Canada Report.* Public Health Agency of Canada/Canadian Institute for Health Information 2011.

11. Ogden C, Carroll M, Kit B, Flegal K. "Prevalence of Obesity in the United States, 2009–2010." Centers for Disease Control and Prevention. NCHS 82; January 2012. Accessed at www.cdc.gov/nchs/data/databriefs/db82.pdf

12. Lim, Stephen S., *et al.* "A comparative risk assessment of burden of disease and injury attributable to 67 risk factors and risk factor clusters in 21 regions, 1990–2010: a systematic analysis for the Global Burden of Disease Study 2010." *The Lancet* 380.9859 (2013): 2224–2260.

13. "Declining Medicine Use and Costs: For Better or For Worse?" Report by the IMS Institute for Health Informatics May 2013.

14. Kessler, David A. *The end of overeating: Taking control of the insatiable American appetite*. Rodale, 2009.

15. Coca Cola Company, 2012, 10K Report.

16. PepsiCo, 2012, 10K Report.

17. General Mills, 2012, 10K Report.

18. Kraft Foods, 2012, 10K Report.

Chapter Two

1. Esfahani A. "Glycemic Index: Physiological significance." Journal of the American College of Nutrition 2009; 28(4):439S–445S.

2. "About the Glycemic Index." University of Sydney. Accessed on January 29, 2013 at www.glycemicindex.com/about.php

3. Lustig R. "The Bitter Truth" (recorded lecture). Accessed on January 29, 2013 at http://youtu.be/dBnniua6-oM

4. Caton, Paul W., *et al.* "Fructose induces gluconeogenesis and lipogenesis through a SIRT1-dependent mechanism." *Journal of Endocrinology* 208.3 (2011): 273–283.

5. Tappy, Luc, and Kim-Anne Lê. "Metabolic effects of fructose and the worldwide increase in obesity." *Physiological Reviews* 90.1 (2010): 23–46.

6. Tappy L. Q&A: "Toxic" Effects of Sugar: Should We be Afraid of Fructose? *BMC Biology* 2012; 10:42.

7. 2008 Clinical Practice Guidelines. Canadian Diabetes Association.

8. Celiac Disease (Webpage). National Digestive Diseases Information Clearinghouse (Website). Accessed at http://digestive.niddk.nih.gov/ddiseases/pubs/celiac/#other

9. Rubio-Tapia A, *et al.* "Increased prevalence and mortality in undiagnosed celiac disease." *Gastroenterology* 2009; 137(1):88-93.

10. Sapone A, *et al.* "Spectrum of gluten-related disorders: consensus on new nomenclature and classification." *BMC Medicine* 2012;10(1): 13.

11. Atchison J, Head L, Gates A. "Wheat as food, wheat as industrial substance; comparative geographies of transformation and mobility." *Geoforum*. 2010; 41: 236–246.

12. van den Broeck, H, *et al.* "Presence of celiac disease epitopes in modern and old hexaploid wheat varieties: wheat breeding may have contributed

to increased prevalence of celiac disease." *Theoretical and Applied Genetics* 2010; 121(8): 1527–1539.

13. Kasarda D. "Can an increase in celiac disease be attributed to an increase in the gluten content of wheat as a consequence of wheat breeding? A perspective." *Journal of Agriculture and Food Chemistry* 2013; 61(6): 1155–1159.

14. Nanda R, Shu L, and Thomas J. A "FODMAP Diet Update: Craze or Credible?" *Practical Gastroenterology* 2012; 37.

15. Elango R, Humayun M A, Ball R, Pencharz P. "Evidence that protein requirements have been significantly underestimated." *Current Opinion in Clinical Nutrition* 2010;13(1):52-7.

16. Hamerschlag K. *Meat Eater's Guide to Climate Change and Health*. Environmental Working Group Report. July 2011.

17. Henry, Amanda G., Alison S. Brooks, and Dolores R. Piperno. "Microfossils in calculus demonstrate consumption of plants and cooked foods in Neanderthal diets (Shanidar III, Iraq; Spy I and II, Belgium)." *Proceedings of the National Academy of Sciences* 108.2 (2011): 486–491.

18. Nutrient Profile: Soybeans, green (edamame), boiled, drained (Food code 2209). Canadian Nutrient Datafile.

19. Kang J, Badger T, Ronis M, and Wu X. "Non-isoflavone Phytochemicals in Soy and Their Health Effects." *Journal of Agriculture and Food Chemistry* 2010; 58: 8119–8133.

20. Souza, M. A., Carvalho, F. C., Ruas, L. P., Ricci-Azevedo, R., and Roque-Barreira, M. C. "The immunomodulatory effect of plant lectins: a review with emphasis on ArtinM properties." *Glycoconjugate Journal 2013;* 1–17.

21. Patisaul, Heather B., and Wendy Jefferson. "The pros and cons of phytoestrogens." *Frontiers in Neuroendocrinology* 31.4 (2010): 400–419.

22. Patterson, E., *et al.* "Health implications of high dietary omega-6 polyunsaturated fatty acids." *Journal of Nutrition and Metabolism* 2012 (2012).

23. Manore, M.M, Barr, S.I., Butterfield, G.E. (2009) "Position of the American Dietetic Association, Dietitians of Canada, and the American College of Sports Medicine: Nutrition and Athletic Performance." *Journal of the American Dietetics Association.* P. 509–527.

24. Remig V. *et al.* "Trans Fats in America: A Review of Their Use, Consumption, Health Implications, and Regulation." *Journal of the American Dietetics Association* 2010;110:585–592.

25. Myers J, Allen J. "Nutrition and Inflammation: Insights on Dietary Pattern, Obesity, and Asthma." *American Journal of Lifestyle Medicine.* 2012;6(14).

26. Siri-Tarino PW, Sun Q, Hu FB, Krauss RM: "Meta-analysis of prospective cohort studies evaluating the association of saturated fat with cardiovascular disease." *American Journal of Clinical Nutrition,* 2010; 91:535–546.

27. Feranil AB, Duazo PL, Kuzawa CW, Adair LS. "Coconut oil is associated with a beneficial lipid profile in pre-menopausal women in the Philippines." *Asia Pacific Journal of Clinical Nutrition.* 2011;20(2):190–5.

28. Assunção ML, Ferreira HS, dos Santos AF, Cabral CR Jr, Florêncio TM. "Effects of dietary coconut oil on the biochemical and anthropometric profiles of women presenting abdominal obesity." *Lipids.* 2009 Jul;44(7):593–601.

29. Willett W. "Dietary fats and coronary artery disease (Review)". Journal of Internal Medicine, 2012; 27213–24.

30. Mozaffarian D, Tao Hao P, Rimm E, Willett W, Hu F. "Changes in Diet and Lifestyle and Long- Term Weight Gain in Women and Men." *New England Journal of Medicine,* 2011; 364: 2392–404.

Chapter Three

1. Forchielli M, Walker W. "The role of gut-associated lymphoid tissues and mucosal defense" *British Journal of Nutrition* 2005; 93(1): S41–S48.

2. Kokkinos A *et al.* "Eating Slowly Increases the Postprandial Response of the Anorexigenic Gut Hormones, Peptide YY and Glucagon-Like Peptide-1." *Journal of Clinical Endocrinology and Metabolism* 2010;95(1) 333–337.

3. Li, J *et al.* "Improvement in chewing activity reduces energy intake in one meal and modulates plasma gut hormone concentrations in obese and lean young Chinese men." *American Journal of Clinical Nutrition* 2011;94(3): 709–716.

4. Yang Q. "Gain weight by 'going diet?' Artificial sweeteners and the neurobiology of sugar cravings." *Yale Journal of Biology and Medicine* 2010; 83(2): 101–108.

5. Aagaard K, Riehle K, Ma J, Segata N, Mistretta T-A, *et al.* (2012) "A Metagenomic Approach to Characterization of the Vaginal Microbiome Signature in Pregnancy." PLoS ONE 7(6): e36466. doi:10.1371/journal.pone.0036466.

6. Dominguez-Bello, M. "Delivery mode shapes the acquisition and structure of the initial microbiota across multiple body habitats in newborns." *Proceedings of the National Academy of Sciences U S A*. 2010; 107(26): 11971–11975.

7. Penders, John, *et al*. "Quantification of Bifidobacterium spp., Escherichia coli and Clostridium difficile in faecal samples of breast-fed and formula-fed infants by real-time PCR." *FEMS Microbiology Letters* 243.1 (2005): 141–147.

8. Penders, John, *et al*. "Factors influencing the composition of the intestinal microbiota in early infancy." *Pediatrics* 118.2 (2006): 511–521.

9. Savino F. "*Lactobacillus reuteri* DSM 17938 in Infantile Colic: A Randomized, Double-Blind, Placebo-Controlled Trial." *Pediatrics,* 2010;126(3):e526–e533.

10. Clemente, J, Ursell, L, Wegener Parfrey. L, Knight, R. "The Impact of the Gut Microbiota on Human Health: An Integrative View." *Cell,* 2012; 148(6):1258–70.

11. Brown, K, DeCoffe, D, Molcan, E, Gibson, D. "Diet-Induced Dysbiosis of the Intestinal Microbiota and the Effects on Immunity and Disease." *Nutrients* 2012;4: 1095–1119.

12. Mayer, E. A. "The neurobiology of stress and gastrointestinal disease." *Gut* 47.6 (2000): 861–869.

13. Dallman, Mary F. "Stress-induced obesity and the emotional nervous system." *Trends in Endocrinology & Metabolism* 21.3 (2010): 159–165.

14. Brunner, Eric J., Tarani Chandola, and Michael G. Marmot. "Prospective effect of job strain on general and central obesity in the Whitehall II Study." *American Journal of Epidemiology* 1657 (2007): 828–837.

15. Ness-Jensen, E, Lindam, A, Lagergren, J, *et al*. "Changes in prevalence, incidence and spontaneous loss of gastro-esophageal reflux symptoms: a prospective population-based cohort study, the HUNT study." *Gut* 2011.

16. Rubio-Tapia A. "Increased prevalence and mortality in undiagnosed celiac disease." *Gastroenterology*. 2009;137(1):88–93.

17. *Gluten Free Food and Beverages in the US, 4th ed.* Packaged Facts Report (abstract). Accessed on March 5, 2013 at http://www.packagedfacts.com/Gluten-Free-Foods-7144767/

18. Sapone, A, *et al*. "Spectrum of gluten-related disorders: consensus on nomenclature and classification." *BMC Medicine*. 2012; 10(13).

19. Kasarda, D. "Can an Increase in Celiac Disease Be Attributed to an Increase in the Gluten Content of Wheat as a Consequence of Wheat Breeding?" *J Agriculture and Food Chemistry* 2013; 61(6): 1155–1159.

20. Sapone, *et al.* "Spectrum of gluten-related disorders: consensus on new nomenclature and classification." *BMC Medicine* 2012; 10(13).

21. Lactose Intolerance (Web Page). *Genetics Home Reference.* US National Library of Medicine. Accessed on March 12, 2013 at http://ghr.nlm.nih.gov/condition/lactose-intolerance

22. Thompson, WG, Irvine, EJ, Pare, P, Ferrazzi, S, Rance, L. "Functional gastrointestinal disorders in Canada." *Digestive Diseases and Sciences.* 2002;47(1):225–35.

23. Grundmann O, Yoon SL. "Irritable bowel syndrome: epidemiology, diagnosis, and treatment: an update for health-care practitioners." *Journal of Gastroenterology and Hepatology.* 2010;25: 691–699.

24. Nanda, Rakesh, Lin H. Shu, and J. Reggie Thomas. "A FODMAP Diet Update: Craze or Credible?." *Practical Gastroenterology* (2012): 37.

25. Hou, Jason K., Bincy Abraham, and Hashem El-Serag. "Dietary intake and risk of developing inflammatory bowel disease: a systematic review of the literature." *The American Journal of Gastroenterology* 106.4 (2011): 563–573.

26. Hansen, Tanja Stenbaek, *et al.* "Environmental factors in inflammatory bowel disease: a case-control study based on a Danish inception cohort." *Journal of Crohn's and Colitis* 5.6 (2011): 577–584.

27. Ng, Siew C., *et al.* "Geographical variability and environmental risk factors in inflammatory bowel disease." *Gut* 62.4 (2013): 630–649.

Chapter Four

1. Campos, S, Doxey, J, Hammond, D. "Nutrition Labels on Pre-packaged foods: a systematic review." *Public Health Nutrition* 2011;14(8): 1496–1506.

2. Brownawell, Amy M., *et al.* "Prebiotics and the health benefits of fiber: current regulatory status, future research, and goals." *The Journal of Nutrition* 142.5 (2012): 962–974.

Chapter Five

1. Shoelson S, Herrero L, Naaz A. "Obesity, inflammation, and insulin resistance." *Gastroenterology* 2007;132: 2169–2180.

2. Van Gaal, Luc F., Ilse L. Mertens, and E. Christophe. "Mechanisms linking obesity with cardiovascular disease." *Nature* 444.7121 (2006): 875–880.

3. Calder, Philip C., *et al.* "Inflammatory disease processes and interactions with nutrition." *British Journal of Nutrition* 101.S1 (2009): 1–45.

4. Cancello, R., and K. Clement. "Review article: Is obesity an inflammatory illness? Role of low-grade inflammation and macrophage infiltration in human white adipose tissue." *BJOG: An International Journal of Obstetrics & Gynaecology* 113.10 (2006): 1141–1147.

5. Hooper, Lora V., Dan R. Littman, and Andrew J. Macpherson. "Interactions between the microbiota and the immune system." *Science* 336.6086 (2012): 1268–1273.

6. Cerf-Bensussan, Nadine, and Valérie Gaboriau-Routhiau. "The immune system and the gut microbiota: friends or foes?." *nATuRE REvIEws | Immunology* 10 (2010): 735.

7. Round, June L., and Sarkis K. Mazmanian. "The gut microbiota shapes intestinal immune responses during health and disease." *Nature Reviews Immunology* 9.5 (2009): 313–323.

8. Neish, Andrew S. "Microbes in gastrointestinal health and disease." *Gastroenterology* 136.1 (2009): 65–80.

9. Lupp, Claudia, *et al.* "Host-mediated inflammation disrupts the intestinal microbiota and promotes the overgrowth of Enterobacteriaceae." *Cell Host & Microbe* 2.2 (2007): 119–129.

10. Brown, Kirsty, *et al.* "Diet-induced dysbiosis of the intestinal microbiota and the effects on immunity and disease." *Nutrients* 4.8 (2012): 1095–1119.

11. Zhang, Chenhong, *et al.* "Interactions between gut microbiota, host genetics and diet relevant to development of metabolic syndromes in mice." *The ISME Journal* 4.2 (2009): 232–241.

12. Cani, Patrice D., and Nathalie M. Delzenne. "The gut microbiome as therapeutic target." *Pharmacology & Therapeutics* 130.2 (2011): 202–12.

13. Capaldo, Christopher T., and Asma Nusrat. "Cytokine regulation of tight junctions." *Biochimica et Biophysica Acta (BBA)-Biomembranes* 1788.4 (2009): 864–871.

14. Fasano, Alessio. "Zonulin and its regulation of intestinal barrier function: the biological door to inflammation, autoimmunity, and cancer." *Physiological Reviews* 91.1 (2011): 151–175.

15. Food Allergies and Intolerances. *Health Canada (web page)*. www.hc-sc. gc.ca/fn-an/securit/allerg/index-eng.php

16. Dickinson, Scott, *et al.* "High–glycemic index carbohydrate increases nuclear factor-κB activation in mononuclear cells of young, lean healthy subjects." *The American Journal of Clinical Nutrition* 87.5 (2008): 1188–1193.

17. Vijay-Kumar, Matam, *et al.* "Fish oil rich diet in comparison to saturated fat rich diet offered protection against lipopolysaccharide-induced inflammation and insulin resistance in mice." *Nutrition & Metabolism* 8.1 (2011): 16.

18. Erridge, Clett, *et al.* "A high-fat meal induces low-grade endotoxemia: evidence of a novel mechanism of postprandial inflammation." *The American Journal of Clinical Nutrition* 86.5 (2007): 1286–1292.

19. Erridge, Clett, and Nilesh J. Samani. "Saturated fatty acids do not directly stimulate toll-like receptor signaling." *Arteriosclerosis, Thrombosis, and Vascular Biology* 29.11 (2009): 1944–1949.

20. Siri-Tarino PW, Sun Q, Hu FB, Krauss, RM: "Meta-analysis of prospective cohort studies evaluating the association of saturated fat with cardiovascular disease." *American Journal of Clinical Nutrition* 2010; 91:535–546.

21. Willett W. "Dietary fats and coronary artery disease (Review)." *Journal of Internal Medicine* 2012; 27213–24.

22. Enos, Reilly T., *et al.* "Influence of dietary saturated fat content on adiposity, macrophage behavior, inflammation, and metabolism: composition matters." *Journal of Lipid Research* 54.1 (2013): 152–163.

23. Shrestha, Chandan, *et al.* "Saturated fatty acid palmitate induces extracellular release of histone H3: A possible mechanistic basis for high-fat diet-induced inflammation and thrombosis." *Biochemical and Biophysical Research Communications* (2013).

24. Egger, Garry, and J. Dixon. "Non-nutrient causes of low-grade, systemic inflammation: support for a 'canary in the mineshaft' view of obesity in chronic disease." *Obesity Reviews* 12.5 (2011): 339–345.

25. Hopkins, Myfanwy H., *et al.* "Antioxidant micronutrients and biomarkers of oxidative stress and inflammation in colorectal adenoma patients: results from a randomized, controlled clinical trial." *Cancer Epidemiology Biomarkers & Prevention* 19.3 (2010): 850–858.

26. Pashkow, Fredric J. "Oxidative stress and inflammation in heart disease: do antioxidants have a role in treatment and/or prevention?." *International Journal of Inflammation* 2011 (2011).

27. Davis, Donald R., Melvin D. Epp, and Hugh D. Riordan. "Changes in USDA food composition data for 43 garden crops, 1950 to 1999." *Journal of the American College of Nutrition* 23.6 (2004): 669–682.

28. Davis, Donald R. "Declining fruit and vegetable nutrient composition: What is the evidence?." *Horticultural Science* 44.1 (2009): 15–19.

29. Pottala, James V., *et al*. "Blood EPA and DHA Independently Predict All-Cause Mortality in Patients with Stable Coronary Heart Disease. The Heart and Soul Study." *Circulation, Cardiovascular Quality and Outcomes* 3.4 (2010): 406.

30. Mas, Emilie, *et al*. "The omega-3 fatty acids EPA and DHA decrease plasma F2-isoprostanes: Results from two placebo-controlled interventions." *Free Radical Research* 44.9 (2010): 983–990.

31. Serhan, Charles N., Nan Chiang, and Thomas E. Van Dyke. "Resolving inflammation: dual anti-inflammatory and pro-resolution lipid mediators." *Nature Reviews Immunology* 8.5 (2008): 349–361.

32. Mullen, Anne, Christine E. Loscher, and Helen M. Roche. "Anti-inflammatory effects of EPA and DHA are dependent upon time and dose-response elements associated with LPS stimulation in THP-1-derived macrophages." *The Journal of Nutritional Biochemistry* 21.5 (2010): 444–450.

33. Kiecolt-Glaser, Janice K., *et al*. "Omega-3 supplementation lowers inflammation and anxiety in medical students: a randomized controlled trial." *Brain, Behavior, and Immunity* 25.8 (2011): 1725–1734.

34. Guillot, Xavier, *et al*. "Vitamin D and inflammation." *Joint Bone Spine* 77.6 (2010): 552–557.

35. Health Canada. "Updated Recommendations for Calcium and Vitamin D" (web page) www.hc-sc.gc.ca/fn-an/nutrition/vitamin/vita-d-eng.php

Additional Resources for Chapter Five.

Kau, Andrew L., *et al*. "Human nutrition, the gut microbiome and the immune system." *Nature* 474.

Konturek, P. C., T. Brzozowski, and S. J. Konturek. "Stress and the gut: pathophysiology, clinical consequences, diagnostic approach and treatment options." *Journal of Physiology and Pharmacology* 62.6 (2011): 591–599.

Chapter Six

1. González-Gallego, Javier, *et al*. "Fruit polyphenols, immunity and inflammation." *British Journal of Nutrition* 104.supplement 3 (2010): S15–S27.

2. Hidalgo, Maria, *et al.* "Potential anti-inflammatory, anti-adhesive, anti/estrogenic, and angiotensin-converting enzyme inhibitory activities of anthocyanins and their gut metabolites." *Genes & Nutrition* 7.2 (2012): 295–306.

3. Liu, Yixiang, *et al.* "Blueberry anthocyanins: protection against ageing and light-induced damage in retinal pigment epithelial cells." *British Journal of Nutrition* 108.1 (2012): 16.

4. Poulose, Shibu M., Amanda N. Carey, and Barbara Shukitt-Hale. "Improving brain signaling in aging: could berries be the answer?." *Expert Review of Neurotherapeutics* 12.8 (2012): 887–889.

5. Basu, Arpita, Michael Rhone, and Timothy J. Lyons. "Berries: emerging impact on cardiovascular health." *Nutrition Reviews* 68.3 (2010): 168–177.

6. Stoner, Gary D., and Li-Shu Wang. "Chemoprevention of Esophageal Squamous Cell Carcinoma with Berries." *Natural Products in Cancer Prevention and Therapy.* Springer Berlin Heidelberg, 2013. 1–20.

7. Sikora, Ewa, Giovanni Scapagnini, and Mario Barbagallo. "Curcumin, inflammation, ageing and age-related diseases." *Immunity & Ageing* 7.1 (2010): 1.

8. Julie, S., and M. T. Jurenka. "Anti-inflammatory Properties of Curcumin, a Major Constituent." *Alternative Medicine Review* 14.2 (2009).

9. Basnet, Purusotam, and Natasa Skalko-Basnet. "Curcumin: an anti-inflammatory molecule from a curry spice on the path to cancer treatment." *Molecules* 16.6 (2011): 4567–4598.

10. Kelkel, Mareike, *et al.* "Antioxidant and anti-proliferative properties of lycopene." *Free Radical Research* 45.8 (2011): 925–940.

11. Shokri Mashhadi, Nafiseh, *et al.* "Influence of Ginger and Cinnamon Intake on Inflammation and Muscle Soreness Endued by Exercise in Iranian Female Athletes." *International Journal of Preventive Medicine* 1.1 (2013): S18–S22.

12. Weng, Chia-Jui, *et al.* "Anti-invasion effects of 6-shogaol and 6-gingerol, two active components in ginger, on human hepatocarcinoma cells." *Molecular Nutrition & Food Research* 54.11 (2010): 1618–1627.

13. Zick, Suzanna M., *et al.* "Phase II study of the effects of ginger root extract on eicosanoids in colon mucosa in people at normal risk for colorectal cancer." *Cancer Prevention Research* 4.11 (2011): 1929–1937.

14. Gerber, Mariette. "Omega-3 fatty acids and cancers: a systematic update

review of epidemiological studies." *British Journal of Nutrition* 107.Suppl 2 (2012): S228–S239.

15. Zheng, Ju-Sheng, *et al.* "Intake of fish and marine n-3 polyunsaturated fatty acids and risk of breast cancer: meta-analysis of data from 21 independent prospective cohort studies." *British Medical Journal* 346 (2013).

16. Engell, Rebecca E., *et al.* "Seafood omega-3 intake and risk of coronary heart disease death: an updated meta-analysis with implications for attributable burden." *The Lancet* 381 (2013): S45.

17. Bradbury, Joanne. "Docosahexaenoic acid (DHA): an ancient nutrient for the modern human brain." *Nutrients* 3.5 (2011): 529–554.

18. Sublette, M. Elizabeth, *et al.* "Meta-analysis: Effects of Eicosapentaenoic Acid in Clinical Trials in Depression." *The Journal of Clinical Psychiatry* 72.12 (2011): 1577.

19. Hurst, S., *et al.* "Dietary fatty acids and arthritis." *Prostaglandins, Leukotrienes and Essential Fatty Acids* 82.4 (2010): 315–318.

20. Miles, Elizabeth A., and Philip C. Calder. "Influence of marine n-3 polyunsaturated fatty acids on immune function and a systematic review of their effects on clinical outcomes in rheumatoid arthritis." *British Journal of Nutrition* 107.S2 (2012): S171–S184.

21. Rop, Otakar, Jiri Mlcek, and Tunde Jurikova. "Beta-glucans in higher fungi and their health effects." *Nutrition Reviews* 67.11 (2009): 624–631.

22. Wang, Ji-Lian, *et al.* "Combination therapy with lentinan improves outcomes in patients with esophageal carcinoma." *Molecular Medicine Reports* 5.3 (2012): 745–748.

23. Oba, Koji, *et al.* "Individual patient based meta-analysis of lentinan for unresectable/recurrent gastric cancer." *Anticancer Research* 29.7 (2009): 2739–2745.

24. CFR Ferreira, Isabel, *et al.* "Compounds from wild mushrooms with antitumor potential." *Anti-Cancer Agents in Medicinal Chemistry (Formerly Current Medicinal Chemistry-Anti-Cancer Agents)* 10.5 (2010): 424–436.

25. Harvey, Kevin A., *et al.* "Oleic acid inhibits stearic acid-induced inhibition of cell growth and pro-inflammatory responses in human aortic endothelial cells." *Journal of Lipid Research* 51.12 (2010): 3470–3480.

26. Cintra, Dennys E., *et al.* "Unsaturated fatty acids revert diet-induced hypothalamic inflammation in obesity." *PloS One* 7.1 (2012): e30571.

27. Fahey, Jed W., *et al.* "Protection of humans by plant glucosinolates: ef-

ficiency of conversion of glucosinolates to isothiocyanates by the gastro-intestinal microflora." *Cancer Prevention Research* 5.4 (2012): 603–611.

28. Tsai, Jo-Ting, Hui-Ching Liu, and Yue-Hwa Chen. "Suppression of inflammatory mediators by cruciferous vegetable-derived indole-3-carbinol and phenylethyl isothiocyanate in lipopolysaccharide-activated macrophages." *Mediators of Inflammation* (2010).

29. Chakole, Rita, Shubhangi Zade, and Manoj Charde. "Antioxidant and anti-inflammatory activity of ethanolic extract of beta vulgaris linn roots" *International Journal of Biomedical and Advance Research* 2.4 (2011): 124–130.

30. Detopoulou, Paraskevi, *et al.* "Dietary choline and betaine intakes in relation to concentrations of inflammatory markers in healthy adults: the ATTICA study." *The American Journal of Clinical Nutrition* 87.2 (2008): 424–430.

31. Yi, Eui-Yeun, and Yung-Jin Kim. "Betaine inhibits in vitro and in vivo angiogenesis through suppression of the NF-κB and Akt signaling pathways." *International Journal of Oncology* 41.5 (2012): 1879–1885.

32. Subramoniam, Appian, et al. "Chlorophyll Revisited: Anti-inflammatory Activities of Chlorophyll a and Inhibition of Expression of TNF-α Gene by the Same." *Inflammation* 35.3 (2012): 959-966.

33. Cho, Jae Youl. "Radical Scavenging Activity-Based and AP-1-Targeted Anti-Inflammatory Effects of Lutein in Macrophage-Like and Skin Keratinocytic Cells." *Mediators of Inflammation* 2013 (2013).

34. Brandenburg, Lars-Ove, *et al.* "Sulforaphane suppresses LPS-induced inflammation in primary rat microglia." *Inflammation Research* 59.6 (2010): 443–450.

35. Vazquez-Prieto, Marcela Alejandra, *et al.* "Garlic and onion attenuates vascular inflammation and oxidative stress in fructose-fed rats." *Journal of Nutrition and Metabolism* 2011 (2011).

36. Keophiphath, Mayoura, *et al.* "1, 2-vinyldithiin from garlic inhibits differentiation and inflammation of human preadipocytes." *The Journal of Nutrition* 139.11 (2009): 2055–2060.

37. Ng, Kevin TP, *et al.* "A garlic derivative, S-allylcysteine (SAC), suppresses proliferation and metastasis of hepatocellular carcinoma." *PloS One* 7.2 (2012): e31655.

38. Casas-Agustench, Patricia, Mònica Bulló, and Jordi Salas-Salvadó. "Nuts,

inflammation and insulin resistance." *Asia Pacific Journal of Clinical Nutrition* 19.1 (2010): 124.

39. Esmaillzadeh, Ahmad, and Leila Azadbakht. "Legume consumption is inversely associated with serum concentrations of adhesion molecules and inflammatory biomarkers among Iranian women." *The Journal of Nutrition* 142.2 (2012): 334–339.

40. Hermsdorff, Helen Hermana M., *et al.* "A legume-based hypocaloric diet reduces proinflammatory status and improves metabolic features in overweight/obese subjects." *European Journal of Nutrition* 50.1 (2011): 61–69.

41. Stote, K. S., *et al.* "Effect of cocoa and green tea on biomarkers of glucose regulation, oxidative stress, inflammation and hemostasis in obese adults at risk for insulin resistance." *European Journal of Clinical Nutrition* 66.10 (2012): 1153–1159.

42. Vázquez-Agell, M., *et al.* "Cocoa consumption reduces NF-κB activation in peripheral blood mononuclear cells in humans." *Nutrition, Metabolism and Cardiovascular Diseases* (2011).

43. Pérez-Cano, Francisco J., *et al.* "The effects of cocoa on the immune system." *Frontiers in Pharmacology* 4 (2013).

44. Hyson, Dianne A. "A comprehensive review of apples and apple components and their relationship to human health." *Advances in Nutrition: An International Review Journal* 2.5 (2011): 408–420.

45. Sim, Jang Seop, *et al.* "Inhibitory effect of the phenolic compounds from apples against oxidative damage and inflammation." *Korean Journal of Plant Research* 23.6 (2010): 487–497.

46. El Khoury, D., *et al.* "Beta glucan: health benefits in obesity and metabolic syndrome." *Journal of Nutrition and Metabolism* 2012 (2011).

47. Shen, Y., *et al.* "Beneficial Effects of Cinnamon on the Metabolic Syndrome, Inflammation, and Pain, and Mechanisms Underlying These Effects—A Review." *Journal of Traditional and Complementary Medicine* 2.1 (2012): 27.

48. Ho, Su-Chen, and Pei-Wen Chang. "Inhibitory Effects of Several Spices on Inflammation Caused by Advanced Glycation End Products." *American Journal of Plant Sciences* 3 (2012): 995–1002.

Chapter Seven

1. Burke, Lora E., Jing Wang, and Mary Ann Sevick. "Self-monitoring in weight loss: a systematic review of the literature." *Journal of the American Dietetic Association* 111.1 (2011): 92–102.

2. Dulloo A. "Explaining the failures of obesity therapy: willpower attenuation, target miscalculation or metabolic compensation?" *International Journal of Obesity* 36 (2012): 1418–1420.

Chapter Twelve

1. Institute of Medicine of the National Academies. Dietary Reference Intakes: The essential guide to nutrient requirements. The National Academies Press, Washington DC, 2006.

2. Whelton, Paul K., *et al.* "Sodium, Blood Pressure, and Cardiovascular Disease Further Evidence Supporting the American Heart Association Sodium Reduction Recommendations." *Circulation* 126.24 (2012): 2880–2889.

3. Dietary Guidelines for Americans, 2010. U.S. Department of Health and Human Services.

4. Siri-Tarino PW, Sun Q, Hu FB, Krauss RM: "Meta-analysis of prospective cohort studies evaluating the association of saturated fat with cardiovascular disease." *Am J Clin Nutr* 2010; 91:535–546.

5. Shrestha, Chandan, *et al.* "Saturated fatty acid palmitate induces extracellular release of histone H3: A possible mechanistic basis for high-fat diet-induced inflammation and thrombosis." *Biochemical and Biophysical Research Communications* (2013).

6. Enos, Reilly T., *et al.* "Influence of dietary saturated fat content on adiposity, macrophage behavior, inflammation, and metabolism: composition matters." *Journal of Lipid Research* 54.1 (2013): 152–163.

7. Johnson, Rachel K., *et al.* "Dietary sugars intake and cardiovascular health a scientific statement from the American Heart Association." *Circulation* 120.11 (2009): 1011–1020.

8. Health Canada. Dietary Reference Intakes: Fiber.

IN GRATITUDE

To my incredible husband Jim and our son, Elliott—without whom there would be no point in trying to achieve anything extraordinary in this life. You are the center of my world and all the joy it contains.

To my mother, for believing I could do anything and not skipping a beat when my passions changed from astronaut/lawyer/first Canadian Miss America/genetic engineer/model to dietitian and author. To my father, for being a bigger part of my life and who I am as a person than he might realize.

To my wonderful parents-in-law, Svein and Wendy Nielsen, for all the extra babysitting, the hours spent reading my work and testing my recipes (and actually laughing at my jokes) and eating my rabbit food. I couldn't be happier to be a part of your family.

To Heather McColl, my longtime mentor, colleague, and dear friend for inspiring me beyond the usual path and teaching me how to build recipes that other people could actually figure out (and correcting them when they can't). You are a cherished friend, and I am so thrilled that the universe brought us together!

To Melissa Quantz, for being such a treasured friend that shares as intense a love of food as I do. Thank you for bringing so much inspiration to my life and to the beautiful photos in these pages.

To Lori Petryk MSc RD, Veronica Kacinik MSc RD, Matthieu Millette PhD, and Jason Tetro BSc for taking the time to provide invaluable feedback and guidance that made this work better and for being such valued friends and colleagues. To Francois-Pierre Chevalier, Isabele Chevalier, David Christie and Lisa Chisholm-Neal, for your gracious support and advice to help me get this book out into the world. Thank you to Jason Lau and Esther Huang, my student volunteers, for helping support this newbie entrepreneur; staying connected to the next generation of dietitians keeps us "old" folks on our toes!

To the friends and family who helped test my recipes to make sure they work outside of my taste buds and kitchen—thanks for being my guinea pigs!

To my editor at Skyhorse, Nicole Frail, and the rest of the Skyhorse team for finding me in the digital universe and making my literary dreams a reality.

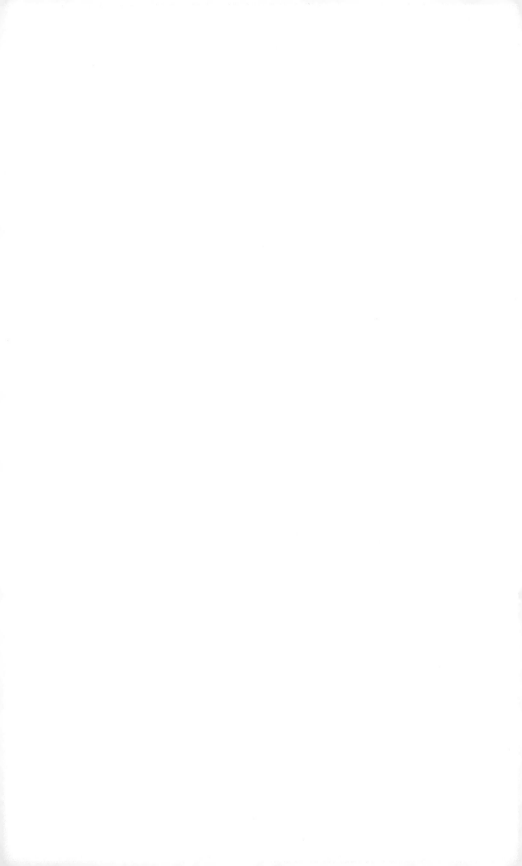

INDEX

Recipes are in **bold**. Photos are in *italics*. Boxes are marked b. Titles are marked t.

Numbers

1,2-vinyldithiin, 124
14-day kick-start, 184–193, 190t
28-day meal plan, 194–200
80/20 plan, 175–183, 215–225

A

acid reflux, 65–66
addiction, 23
adipocytes, 87–88
advertising, 24b
air pollution, 103
ALA (alpha-linoleic acid), 47–48, 109
alcohol, 50b–51b, 51, 104b, 179t, 188
All Bran Buds, 159
allergies, 94, 95b
alliin, 124
allspice, **242**
almond butter. *see* butter, almond
almond milk. *see* milk, almond
almond oil. *see* oil, almond
almonds, 169
  Candy Bars, Crunchy Nut, **267**
  Lunch Box, Grown-Up, **237**
  Trail Mix, Energy to Spare, **260**
Almost Instant Spinach Salad, **237–38**
alpha-linoleic acid (ALA), 47–48, 109
amaranth, 180t
Amazing Roasted Chick-pea, **263–64**, *263*
amino acids, 37, 37b, 39
animal protein. *see* protein, animal-based

anthocyanins, 15, 114, 126, 130
anti-inflammitory foods, 114–133. *see also* inflammation
  apples, 130, *131*
  avocados, 126, *127*
  beans, 126
  beets, 124, *125*
  berries, 114, *115*
  broccoli, 122–24
  cherries, 114
  cinnamon, 132, *133*
  cocoa, 128
  fermented foods, 118–19
  fish, 116–18
  garlic, 124
  ginger, 116
  grains, 128–130
  greens, 120–21, *123*
  green tea, 119
  herbs, 128, *129*
  mushrooms, 120, *121*
  nuts, 124–26
  olive oil, 119
  seeds, 122
  spinach, 122
  sweet potatoes, 130
  tomatoes, 116, *117*
  turmeric, 114
apigenin, 106–7
appetite, 59
apples, 130, *131*, 164
  Chicken Skillet, Turmeric, **257–58**
  Muffin, Real, **230–31**
  Pudding, Baked Apple Oat, **266**
  Salad, Almost Instant Spinach, **237–38**
  Salad, Broccoli Crunch, **240–41**
  Smoothie, It's Easy Being Green, **231**

apricots
  Breakfast Bars, Brilliant, **232–34**
  Lunch Box, Grown-Up, **237**
artificial sweeteners, 31, 58–59
arugula, 122
  Salad, Arugula Black-berry, **247**
  Salad, Roasted Vegetable and Barley, **241–42**
  Salad for Breakfast, **235–36**
Ascenta Omega-3 Oils, 280
astaxanthin, 118
athletes, 45
Attune Foods, 268
avocado oil. *see* oil, avocado
avocados, 126, *127*, 166, 181t
  Dip, Baked Mexican, **260–61**
  Reuben, Spicy Korean Tempeh, **238**
  Salad, Kale and Avocado, **244–45**

B

bacteria, 60–63, 90–91
  diet and, 92
  dysbiosis and, 72, 91
  fermented foods and, 118–19
  immunity and, 89
  probiotics, 110–11, 168, 271
bagels, 159
Baked Apple Oat Pudding, **266**
Baked Beans
  Chipotle Maple, **251**
  Portuguese, **250**

bananas
Banana Sushi, **261–62**
Breakfast Bars, Brilliant,
232–34
Smoothie, Cocoaberry,
229–230
Smoothie, It's Easy Being
Green, **231**
barley, 128, 180t
Salad, Roasted Vegetable
and Barley, **241–42**
barramundi, 116, 163
basil, 128
Salad, Roasted Vegetable
and Barley, **241–42**
beans, 126, 179t, 211
beans, black, 126
Brownies, Black Bean,
264–65
Scramble, Tofu, **232**
beans, kidney
Baked Beans, Chipotle
Maple, **251**
Baked Beans, Portu-
guese, **250**
Dip, White Bean, **259**
beans, navy
Baked Beans, Chipotle
Maple, **251**
Dip, Pink Walnut, **262–63**
beans, pinto
Quesadilla, Sister Act,
239–240
beans, refried
Dip, Baked Mexican,
260–61
beans, white
Dip, Pink Walnut, **262–63**
Dip, White Bean, **259**
Soup, Edible Medicine,
246
Soup, Spiced Tomato,
245–46
beef, 162
beer. *see* alcohol
beet greens, 120
beets, 124, *125*

Dip, Pink Walnut, **262–63**
Smoothie, Liquid Gold,
229
berries, 114, *115*, 164
Salad, Arugula Black-
berry, **247**
Smoothie, Cocoaberry,
229–230
Trail Mix, Energy to
Spare, **260**
Yogurt, Frozen, **265**
beta-carotene, 106–7
beta-glucans, 128
betaine, 124
betalains, 124
Bio K Plus Probiotics, 280
black beans. *see* beans,
black
blackberries. *see* berries
black cod, 116, 163
black tea. *see* tea
blame, 147–48
bliss point, 23
blood sugar, 28–29, 96–97
blueberries. *see* berries,
164
Blue Diamond, 277
BMI (Body Mass Index),
17, 18t, 19
Bob's Red Mill, 278
Body Mass Index (BMI),
17, 18t, 19
Bombeck, Erma, 201
boswellia, 112
Bragg's, 277
bread, 159, 181t, 209–10
Reuben, Spicy Korean
Tempeh, **238**
breakfast
Breakfast Bars, Brilliant,
232–34, *233*
Granola, Sprouted Buck-
wheat, **236–37**, *236*
Muffin, Real, **230–31**
Pancakes, Feel Good,
234–35, *234*
Salad for Breakfast,

235–36
Scramble, Tofu, **232**
Smoothie, Cocoaberry,
229–230
Smoothie, It's Easy Being
Green, **231**
Smoothie, Liquid Gold, **229**
Brilliant Breakfast Bars,
232–34, *233*
broccoli, 122–24
Salad, Broccoli Crunch,
240–41
Slaw, Colorful Winter,
247–48
bromelain, 112
Brownies, Black Bean,
264–65
brown sugar. *see* sugar,
brown
brussels sprouts
Kimchi, Homegrown,
243–44
buckwheat, 180t
Granola, Sprouted Buck-
wheat, **236–37**
bulk foods, 207–8
butter, 166, 172, 179t, 209
butter, almond
Almond Gems, Salted
Chocolate, **262**
Candy Bars, Crunchy
Nut, **267**
butter, coconut, 166
butter, nut, 166
Banana Sushi, **261–62**
butter, peanut, 172
Soup, Spiced Tomato,
245–46
butternut squash
Quesadilla, Sister Act,
239–240

C
cabbage
Slaw, Colorful Winter,
247–48
cacao, 170–71. *see also*

chocolate; cocoa
Almond Gems, Salted
    Chocolate, **262**
Smoothie, Cocoaberry,
    229–230
Trail Mix, Energy to
    Spare, **260**
caesarean section, 61
caffeine, 104b, 161–62,
    188
cakes, 179t
calcium, 79b
Canadian Digestive
    Health Foundation, 72
cancer, 44–45
Candy Bars, Crunchy Nut,
    267
canned food, 211
carbohydrates, 27–36
  blood sugar, 28–29
  "chew test," 34b
  complex, 27–28
  gluten, 35–36
  low-carb diets, 32b–33b
  simple, 27–28, 30–31,
    205t
  unprocessed, 29–30
  whole grains, 33–34
cardamom
  Chicken Skillet, Turmeric,
    257–58
  Sweet Potatoes, Stuffed,
    253–54
cardiovascular disease, 88
carotenoids, 106–7, 122,
    126
Carr, Kris, 20
carrots
  Casserole, Greens and
    Beans, **258–59**
  Chicken Lettuce Cups,
    254–55
  Kimchi, Homegrown,
    243–44
  Reuben, Spicy Korean
    Tempeh, **238**
  Slaw, Colorful Winter,

247–48
Smoothie, Liquid Gold,
    229
cashews
  Dip, Baked Mexican,
    260–61
  Casserole, Greens and
    Beans, **258–59**
catechins, 106–7, 126, 130
cauliflower, **242**
cayenne pepper
  Chicken Skillet, Turmeric,
    257–58
  Salad, Kale and Avocado,
    244–45
  Tacos, Tempeh, **252–53**
CDC (Centers for Disease
    Control and Preven-
    tion), 16
celery
  Casserole, Greens and
    Beans, **258–59**
celiac disease, 35, 66–68,
    94
Center for Celiac Re-
    search, 67
Centers for Disease Con-
    trol and Prevention
    (CDC), 16
cereal, 160, 181t, 209–10
chard, 120, 124, 165
cheese, 167, 179t, 209
  Casserole, Greens and
    Beans, **258–59**
  Dip, Baked Mexican,
    260–61
  Quesadilla, Sister Act,
    239–240
  Salad, Almost Instant
    Spinach, **237–38**
  Salad, Arugula Black-
    berry, **247**
  Salad, Roasted Vegetable
    and Barley, **241–42**
cherries, 114. see also
    berries
Smoothie, Cocoaberry,

229–230
chia seeds. see seeds,
    chia
chicken
  Chicken Lettuce Cups,
    254–55
  Turmeric Chicken Skillet,
    257–58
chicken stock. see stock,
    chicken
chickpeas, 126
  Curry, Sweet Potato and
    Chickpea, **249–250**
  Roasted, **263–64**, *263*
  Salad, Almost Instant
    Spinach, **237–38**
Child, Julia, 53
children
  cooking with, 150
  diabetes in, 21
  healthy eating, 222–23,
    224b–25b
  obesity, 16
chilies
  Chicken Lettuce Cups,
    254–55
chili flakes
  Salad, Kale and Avocado,
    244–45
  Soup, Edible Medicine,
    246
chili powder
  Dip, Baked Mexican,
    260–61
  Soup, Spiced Tomato,
    245–46
Chinese five spice
  Chicken Lettuce Cups,
    254–55
chipotle
  Baked Beans, Chipotle
    Maple, **251**
chips, 171, 210
chlorogenic acid, 130
chlorophyll, 122
chocolate, 128, 170–71,
    181t, 210. see also

cacao, cocoa
cholesterol, 42, 46, 48, 49, 79b
chronic disease, 99–100,
　104–5
　BMI and, 19
　medication and, 22
　obesity and, 16
　weight and, 21
cilantro
　Chicken Skillet, Turmeric,
　　257–58
　Curry, Sweet Potato and
　　Chickpea, **249–250**
　Salad, Salmon and
　　Sprout, **239**
　Tof-alibut, Herb-Crusted,
　　255
cinnamon, 132, *133*
　Breakfast Bars, Brilliant,
　　232–34
　Brownies, Black Bean,
　　264–65
　Chicken Skillet, Turmeric,
　　257–58
　Granola, Sprouted Buck-
　　wheat, **236–37**
　Muffin, Real, **230–31**
　Pudding, Baked Apple
　　Oat, **266**
　Soup, Spiced Tomato,
　　245–46
　Sweet Potatoes, Stuffed,
　　253–54
Clostridium difficile, 61
cloves
　Chicken Skillet, Turmeric,
　　257–58
Coca Cola Company, 24b
cocoa, 128, 182t. *see also*
　cacao, chocolate
　Almond Gems, Salted
　　Chocolate, **262**
　Brownies, Black Bean,
　　264–65
　Candy Bars, Crunchy
　　Nut, **267**
　Cocoaberry Smoothie,

229–230
coconut
　Breakfast Bars, Brilliant,
　　232–34
　Pudding, Coconut Black
　　Rice, **266–67**
　Trail Mix, Energy to
　　Spare, **260**
coconut butter. *see* butter,
　coconut
coconut milk. *see* milk,
　coconut
coconut oil. *see* oil, coconut
cod, black, 116, 163
coffee, 161–62, 182t,
　188
colic, 62
collards, 120
　Dip, Baked Mexican,
　　260–61
　Salmon Collard Packets,
　　256–57
　Tacos, Tempeh, **252–53**
　Colorful Spiced Chicken
　　Lettuce Cups, **254–55**
　Colorful Winter Slaw,
　　247–48
Comfort, Better Known as
　Stuffed Sweet Pota-
　toes, **253–54**
complex carbohydrates.
　see carbohydrates,
　complex
condiments, 211
cookies, 170, 179t
cooking, 11, 149, 150b
Cookin' Greens, 278
coriander
　Chicken Skillet, Turmeric,
　　257–58
　Curry, Sweet Potato and
　　Chickpea, **249–250**
　Quesadilla, Sister Act,
　　239–240
　Tacos, Tempeh, **252–53**
corn, 14–15, 211
　Quesadilla, Sister Act,

239–240
　Scramble, Tofu, **232**
cottage cheese, 163
　Pancakes, Feel Good,
　　234–35
crackers, 160, 181t, 210
　Lunch Box, Grown-Up, **237**
Creamy Triple Seed
　Risotto with Roasted
　Asparagus, **274**
Crohn's disease, 72–73
Crunchy Nut Candy Bars,
　267
cucumbers
　Cucumber "Noodles" with
　　Almond Miso, **269**
　Lunch Box, Grown-Up, **237**
　Salad, Arugula Black-
　　berry, **247**
　Smoothie, It's Easy Being
　　Green, **231**
　Tabbouleh, Cauliflower, **242**
cumin
　Baked Beans, Portu-
　　guese, **250**
　Casserole, Greens and
　　Beans, **258–59**
　Chicken Skillet, Turmeric,
　　257–58
　Curry, Sweet Potato and
　　Chickpea, **249–250**
　Dip, Baked Mexican,
　　260–61
　Dip, White Bean, **259**
　Quesadilla, Sister Act,
　　239–240
　Scramble, Tofu, **232**
　Soup, Edible Medicine, **246**
　Soup, Spiced Tomato,
　　245–46
　Sweet Potatoes, Stuffed,
　　253–54
　Tabbouleh, Cauliflower, **242**
　Tacos, Tempeh, **252–53**
curcumin, 114
　Curry, Sweet Potato and
　　Chickpea, **249–250**

D

daidzein, 43
dairy swaps, 166–67
Daiya Foods, 278
dandelion, 122
dates, medjool
  Almond Gems, Salted
    Chocolate, **262**
  Brownies, Black Bean,
    264–65
desserts
  Brownies, Black Bean,
    264–65
  Candy Bars, Crunchy
    Nut, **267**
  Pudding, Baked Apple
    Oat, **266**
  Pudding, Coconut Black
    Rice, **266–67**
  Yogurt, Frozen Blueberry,
    265, *265*
DHA (docosahexae-
  noic acid), 48, 109–10,
  116–18, 168
diabetes, 21, 27, 31, 32b,
  88
diallylsulfide, 124
diets, 83–84, 144, 214
  FODMAPS, 36, 72
  low-carb, 32b–33b
  paleo, 39–41
digestive system, 53–73
  acid reflux, 65–66
  bacteria and, 60–63, 72, 89
  celiac disease, 66–68
  excretion, 59–60
  gluten intolerance, 66–68
  IBD, 72–73
  IBS, 71–72, 71b
  immunity and, 54, 61–62
  inflammation, 88–89
  lactose intolerance,
    68–69, 70b
  nervous system and,
    54–55
  senses and, 57
  stages, 55–56
  stress and, 57, 63–64

dill, 128, *129*
Slaw, Colorful Winter,
  247–48
dinner. *see* main dishes;
  side dishes
dips
  Baked Mexican Dip,
    260–61
  Pink Walnut Dip, **262–63**
  White Bean Dip, **259**
diversity, nutritional. *see*
  variety, nutritional
docosahexaenoic acid
  (DHA), 48, 109–10,
  116–18, 168
drink swaps, 160–62
dysbiosis, 72, 91. *see also*
  bacteria

E

eating, mindful, 152b–53b
eating out. *see* restau-
  rants
eating personality quiz,
  138–140
eating plans, 144–45
  14-day kick-start,
    184–193
  28-day meal plan,
    194–200
  80/20 plan, 175–183,
    215–225
  menu plans, 190t, 196t–
    99t
  swaps, 156–174
Eat Your Greens Frittata,
  248–49
edamame, 181t
Eden Foods, 278
Edible Medicine Soup, **246**
EGCG (epigallocatechin-
  3-gallate), 119, 162
eggplant
  Salad, Roasted Vegetable
    and Barley, **241–42**
eggs, 164, 180t, 209
  Frittata, Eat Your
    Greens, **248–49**

eicosapentaenoic acid
  (EPA), 48, 109–10,
  116–18
eighty/twenty plan,
  175–183, 215–225
einkorn, 180t, 211
enablers, 150
Energizing Cauliflower
  Salad, **268**
energy, **21**
energy drinks, 161
Energy to Spare Trail Mix,
  260
Enjoy Life, 159, 278
enteric nervous system,
  54–55
environmental factors, 103
Environmental Working
  Group, 277
EPA (eicosapentae-
  noic acid), 48, 109–10,
  116–18
epigallocatechin-3-gallate
  (EGCG), 119, 162
epithelium, 93–94
esophagus, 55
excretion, 59–60
exercise, 102, 103, 187
extremes, diet, 148–49

F

fast food, 11, 181t
fat cells, 87–88
fats, 46–50
  inflammation and,
    97–100, 107
  monounsaturated, 49
  omega-3. *see* omega-3
    fats
  omega-6, 47, 98,
    98b–99b, 107, 122
  saturated, 48, 99, 204t
  SCFA (short chain fatty
    acids), 62, 90
  trans, 46–47, 79b
Feel Good Pancakes,
  234–35, *234*
fennel

Slaw, Colorful Winter,
247–48
fermented foods, 108,
118–19, 167, 182t, 271
feta cheese
Dip, Baked Mexican,
260–61
Salad, Almost Instant
Spinach, 237–38
Salad, Arugula Black-
berry, 247
Salad, Roasted Vegetable
and Barley, 241–42
fiber
daily amount, 205t
excretion and, 60
sources, 15, 122, 126, 130
swaps for, 159
fish
anti-inflammitory, 107,
116–18
canned, 211
eating plans, 180t, 182t
Salmon Collard Packets,
256–57
swaps, 163
Tof-alibut, Herb-Crusted,
255
flavonoids, 106–7, 122, 128
flavor. see taste
flavor scientists, 12
flax seeds. see seeds, flax
flour, 14, 211
Breakfast Bars, Brilliant,
232–34
Muffin, Real, 230–31
Pancakes, Feel Good,
234–35
FODMAPS, 36, 72
folate, 124
Food for Life, 278
food journal, 135–37, 177
food philosophy quiz,
140–43
Food Politics, 277
food safety, 277
food swaps, 156–174
food systems, 277

fourteen-day kick-start,
184–193, 190t
fries, 165
frittata
Eat Your Greens Frittata,
248–49, 248
Frozen Blueberry Yogurt,
265
fructans, 36
fructose, 31
fruits
anti-inflammitory, 106–7
eating plans, 179t
shopping for, 206–7
swaps, 164–65, 167, 169
fruit snacks, 210

G
gallbladder, 56
GALT (gut-associated
lymphoid tissue), 89
garam masala
Curry, Sweet Potato and
Chickpea, 249–250
garbanzo beans. see
chickpeas, 126
garlic, 124, 182t
Baked Beans, Chipotle
Maple, 251
Baked Beans, Portu-
guese, 250
Casserole, Greens and
Beans, 258–59
Curry, Sweet Potato and
Chickpea, 249–250
Dip, Baked Mexican,
260–61
Dip, Pink Walnut, 262–63
Dip, White Bean, 259
Kimchi, Homegrown,
243–44
Salad, Roasted Vegetable
and Barley, 241–42
Soup, Edible Medicine, 246
Soup, Spiced Tomato,
245–46
Tabbouleh, Cauliflower, 242
Tacos, Tempeh, 252–53

gatroesophageal reflux
disease (GERD), 65–66
General Mills, 24b
genetically modified
organisms (GMO), 171,
268
genistein, 43
GERD (gatroesophageal
reflux disease),
65–66
GI (glycemic index),
28–29, 97
Gibson, Peter, 72
ginger, 116, 182t
Chicken Skillet, Turmeric,
257–58
Granola, Sprouted Buck-
wheat, 236–37
Kimchi, Homegrown,
243–44
Muffin, Real, 230–31
Salmon Collard Packets,
256–57
Soup, Edible Medicine,
246
Gleason, Jackie, 156
Glorious Greens Soup, 273
glucagon, 32b
glucose, 31
glucosinolates, 120
gluten, 35–36, 66–68
glycemic index (GI),
28–29, 97
GMO (genetically modified
organisms), 171, 268
goat cheese
Salad, Almost Instant
Spinach, 237–38
Salad, Arugula Black-
berry, 247
gojuchang
Kimchi, Homegrown,
243–44
golden berries. see berries
grains, 128–130, 159–160,
181t, 207
grains, whole, 33–34, 107,
159, 180t

Granola, Sprouted Buck-
wheat, **236–37**, *236*
granola bar, 169, 210
grapes
Salad, Broccoli Crunch,
240–41
Greek yogurt. *see* yogurt,
Greek
greens, 120–21, *123*
Greens and Beans Cas-
serole, **258–59**
green tea. *see* tea
Grown Up Lunch Box,
237
GT's Kombucha, 280
Guayaki, 278
gut-associated lymphoid
tissue (GALT), 54, 89

H
habits, forming, 146b–47b
harissa
Harissa-Roasted Egg-
plant and Chickpeas,
271
Soup, Spiced Tomato,
245–46
halibut
Tof-alibut, Herb-Crusted,
255
hazelnuts
Salad, Arugula Black-
berry, **247**
HDL cholesterol. *see* cholesterol
hemp seeds. *see* seeds,
hemp
herbs, *129*, 182t
herring, 116, 163
high fructose corn syrup
(HFCS), 31
Hippocrates, 113
hoisin sauce
Chicken Lettuce Cups,
254–55
holidays, 216–17, 217b–18b
Homegrown Kimchi,
243–44

honey, 172, 211
Banana Sushi, **261–62**
Candy Bars, Crunchy
Nut, **267**
Granola, Sprouted Buck-
wheat, **236–37**
Salad, Broccoli Crunch,
240–41
Salad, Roasted Vegetable
and Barley, **241–42**
Salad for Breakfast,
235–36
Slaw, Colorful Winter,
247–48
hummus, 165, 166
Lunch Box, Grown-Up,
237
Hyman, Mark, 30

I
IBD (inflammatory bowel
disease), 72–73, 94
IBS (irritable bowel syn-
drome), 36, 39, 71–72,
71b
ice cream, 170, 179t
IL-6, 126, 132
IL-10, 119
immune system, 54, 61–62
inactivity, 103. *see also*
exercise
indole-3-carbinol, 120, 122
inflammation, 85–112. *see
also* anti-inflammtory
foods
bacteria and, 90–91, 92
blood sugar and, 96–97
causes, 90b
chronic, 86–87, 88, 91,
93, 104–5
diet and, 96, 105–8
digestive tract and,
88–89
environmental factors, 103
fats and, 97–100, 107–8
inactivity and, 103
leaky gut, 93–94
medicines, natural,

111–12
sensitivities and, 96–97
sleep and, 103
stress and, 100
supplements and,
108–11
weight and, 87–88
inflammatory bowel dis-
ease (IBD), 72–73, 94
information overload, 26
ingredients
list. *see* labeling, food
quiz, 12b–15b
Institute of Medicine, 110
insulin, 28–29, 31, 32b
intestines, 56
intolerance, 94, 95b. *see
also* gluten; lactose
intolerance
IP-6 (supplement), 43
irritable bowel syndrome
(IBS), 36, 39, 71–72, 71b
isothiocyanates, 120
It's Easy Being Green
Smoothie, **231**
Izze Soda, 278
J
jalapeños
Curry, Sweet Potato and
Chickpea, **249–250**
jam, 172
Jenkins, David, 28
journal, food, 135–37, 177
Jovial Foods, 278
juice
Smoothie, Liquid Gold, **229**
swaps, 161

K
kaempferol, 120, 126
kale, 120, *123*, 165
Casserole, Greens and
Beans, **258–59**
Frittata, Eat Your
Greens, **248–49**
Salad, Kale and Avocado,
244–45
Soup, Edible Medicine, **246**

Ka-Pow Energy Smoothie, **275**
Karthein's Sauerkraut, 280
kefir, 118, 167, 182t
ketosis, 33b
kidney beans. *see* beans, kidney
kids. *see* children
kimchi, 118, 167, 182t
  Homegrown, **243–44**
  Reuben, Spicy Korean Tempeh, **238**
kohlrabi
  Lunch Box, Grown-Up, **237**
kombucha, 118, 167, 182t, 271
Kraft Foods, 24b

L
labeling, food, 79b, 80–82, 81b, 202–6
Lactobacillus johnsonii, 61
lactose intolerance, 68–69, 70b
Larabar, 278
large intestine, 56
LDL cholesterol. *see* cholesterol
leaky gut, 93–94
Lebowitz, Fran, 26
lectins, 42
legumes, 107
lemon
  Lemon Cardamom Muffins, **270**
  Smoothie, It's Easy Being Green, **231**
  Smoothie, Liquid Gold, **229**
lentils, 163, 179t
  Casserole, Greens and Beans, **258–59**
  Sweet Potatoes, Stuffed, **253–54**
lentinan, 120
lettuce
  Chicken Lettuce Cups, **254–55**
L-glutamine, 112
Liberte, 280
Light Life, 278
lignans, 43–44
lipopolysaccharides (LPS), 92, 98, 99, 124, 130
Liquid Gold Smoothie, **229**
liquor. *see* alcohol
liver, 55
low-carb diets, 32b–33b
LPS (lipopolysaccharides), 92, 98, 99, 124, 130
L-theanine, 119
lunch
  Lunch Box, Grown-Up, **237**
  Quesadilla, Sister Act, **239–240**
  Reuben, Spicy Korean Tempeh, **238**
  Salad, Almost Instant Spinach, **237–38**
  Salad, Salmon and Sprout, **239**
Lustig, Robert, 30
lutein, 106–7, 116, 120, 122, 126
lycopene, 106–7, 116
lysine, 39

M
mackerel, 116, 163
Macrobar, 278
magnesium, 124
main dishes
  Baked Beans, Chipotle Maple, **251**
  Baked Beans, Portuguese, **250**
  Casserole, Greens and Beans, **258–59**
  Chicken Lettuce Cups, **254–55**
  Chicken Skillet, Turmeric, **257–58**
  Curry, Sweet Potato and Chickpea, **249–250**
Frittata, Eat Your Greens, **248–49**, *248*
  Salmon Collard Packets, **256–57**
  Sweet Potatoes, Stuffed, **253–54**
  Tacos, Tempeh, **252–53**
  Tof-alibut, Herb-Crusted, **255**
malnutrition, 20
manganese, 124
mango
  Curry, Sweet Potato and Chickpea, **249–250**
  Pudding, Coconut Black Rice, **266–67**
Manitoba Harvest Hemp, 279
Manna Breads, 278
manufactured food. *see* processed food
maple syrup, 172, 211
  Baked Beans, Chipotle Maple, **251**
  Dip, Pink Walnut, **262–63**
  Muffin, Real, **230–31**
  Pudding, Baked Apple Oat, **266**
  Salmon Collard Packets, **256–57**
  Sweet Potatoes, Stuffed, **253–54**
margarine, 166
marketing, 24b
Mary's Organic Crackers, 160, 279
Matcha Mango Chia Pudding, **272**
mayo, 166
  Reuben, Spicy Korean Tempeh, **238**
  Salad, Broccoli Crunch, **240–41**
McColl, Heather, 228
Mead, Margaret, 134
meat, 40–41, 162–63, 180t, 208. *see also* protein
medication

natural, 111–12
prescriptions, 22
meditation, 102
Mediterranean Stuffed Dates, **267**
medjool dates
Almond Gems, Salted Chocolate, **262**
Brownies, Black Bean, **264–65**
Melt, 279
menu plans, 190t, 196t–99t. *see also* eating plans
methionine, 39
microbes. *see* bacteria
milk, 166, 179t, 182t, 208
Pancakes, Feel Good, **234–35**
Pudding, Baked Apple Oat, **266**
milk, almond
Brownies, Black Bean, **264–65**
Smoothie, Cocoaberry, **229–230**
milk, coconut
Curry, Sweet Potato and Chickpea, **249–250**
Pudding, Coconut Black Rice, **266–67**
mindful eating, 152b–53b
mint, 128
Tabbouleh, Cauliflower, **242**
Tof-alibut, Herb-Crusted, **255**
misinformation, 26
miso, 167, 181t
Salmon Collard Packets, **256–57**
moderation, 148–49
monounsaturated fats. *see* fats, monounsaturated
Monterey Bay Aquarium, 277
mouth, 55

muesli, 209
muffins, 160, 171, 179t
Real Muffin, **230–31**
multivitamins, 109
mushrooms, 120, *121*
Salad for Breakfast, **235–36**
Salmon Collard Packets, **256–57**
Soup, Edible Medicine, **246**
Sweet Potatoes, Stuffed, **253–54**
mustard
Salad for Breakfast, **235–36**
Slaw, Colorful Winter, **247–48**

N
Nancy's Yogurt, 280
napa cabbage
Kimchi, Homegrown, **243–44**
naringenin, 116
National Restaurant Association, 11
natural medication, 111–12
Nature's Path, 159, 279
navy beans. *see* beans, navy
nervous system, 54–55
Nestle, Marion, 268
New Chapter, 280
New Year's resolutions, 134–35
Non-GMO Project, 171, 277
Numi Organic Tea, 279
nut butter. *see* butter, nut
Nutiva, 279
nutrients, 20
Nutrition Action Health Letter, 12b
nutritional label. *see* labeling, food
nutritionism, 76–78
nuts, 124–26, 179t, 181t,

207
Granola, Sprouted Buckwheat, **236–37**

O
oats, 128–130, 160, 209–10
Breakfast Bars, Brilliant, **232–34**
Pudding, Baked Apple Oat, **266**
obesity, 16–17. *see also* weight
Ocean Wise, 107, 277
oil, almond, 172, 181t
oil, avocado, 172, 181t
oil, coconut, 172
oil, olive, 119, 172, 181t
oil, soy, 44
oleic acid, 119, 126
olive oil. *see* oil, olive
olives, 181t
Lunch Box, Grown-Up, **237**
omega-3 fats, 47–48, 98, 107. *see also* fats
sources, 98b–99b, 116–18, 122, 126
supplements, 109–10, 168, 271
omega-6 fats, 47, 98, 98b–99b, 107, 122. *see also* fats
orange juice
Smoothie, Liquid Gold, **229**
oregano
Tacos, Tempeh, **252–53**
organic food, 207
overweight. *see* weight

P
paleo diet, 39–41
palmitic acid, 99
Pancakes, Feel Good, **234–35**, *234*
pancreas, 56
paprika
Dip, Baked Mexican, **260–61**

parsley, 120–22
Salad, Kale and Avocado, **244–45**
Tabbouleh, Cauliflower, **242**
pasta, 159, 181t
pastries, 179t
peanut butter. *see* butter, peanut
pears, 164
pecans
Brownies, Black Bean, **264–65**
pepper flakes
Dip, White Bean, **259**
peppers
Chicken Lettuce Cups, **254–55**
Curry, Sweet Potato and Chickpea, **249–250**
Frittata, Eat Your Greens, **248–49**
Lunch Box, Grown-Up, **237**
Salad, Kale and Avocado, **244–45**
Salad, Roasted Vegetable and Barley, **241–42**
Salad, Salmon and Sprout, **239**
Tacos, Tempeh, **252–53**
PepsiCo, 24b
Perricone, Nicholas, 96
personality, eating, 138–140
pesto
Frittata, Eat Your Greens, **248–49**
Peyer's patches, 89
philosophy, food, 140–43
phytates, 42–43
phytochemicals, 120
phytoestrogens, 43–44
Pink Walnut Dip, **262–63**
pinto beans. *see* beans, pinto
pistachios
Pudding, Coconut Black

Rice, **266–67**
plans, eating. *see* eating plans
plant-based proteins, 37–39, 38b–39b, 41, 41t
Pollan, Michael, 74
polyphenols, 128
poop, 59–60
popcorn, 171, 210
Portuguese Baked Beans, **250**
potatoes, 130
Prana, 279
prescriptions, 22
probiotics, 110–11, 168, 271. *see also* bacteria
processed food, 12, 14–15, 23, 23–25, 24b, 181t
protein, 36–45
amino acids, 37, 37b, 39
animal-based, 41, 41t, 180t, 208
athletes and, 45
daily amount, 38
inflammation and, 107
paleo diet, 39–41
plant-based, 37–39, 38b–39b, 41, 41t
soy, 42–45
superfoods, 39
swaps, 162–64
pudding
Baked Apple Oat, **266**
Coconut Black Rice, **266–67**
pumpkin puree
Muffin, Real, **230–31**
pumpkin seeds. *see* seeds, pumpkin
purslane, 122
Pycnogenol, 112

Q
quercetin, 106–7, 120, 126, 130

Quesadilla, Sister Act, **239–240**
queso fresco
Dip, Baked Mexican, **260–61**
quinoa, 180t
Salad, Salmon and Sprout, **239**
quiz
eating personality, 138–140
food philosophy, 140–43
ingredients, 12b–15b

R
radishes
Kimchi, Homegrown, **243–44**
raspberries, 114
Real Muffin, **230–31**
Recovery (medicine), 112
rectum, 56
refried beans. *see* beans, refried
relaxation. *see* stress
research, nutritional, 74–76
resolutions, 134–35
responsibility, 147–48
restaurants, 11, 215, 216b
Reuben, Spicy Korean Tempeh, **238**
rhubarb, 124
rice, 180t
Casserole, Greens and Beans, **258–59**
Pudding, Coconut Black Rice, **266–67**
RISE Kombucha, 280
road trips, 219–220, 220b
Roasted Vegetable and Barley Salad, **241–42**
Roberts, Wayne, 10
Rockin' Tempeh Tacos, **252–53**
romaine, 165
rosemary, 128
rye, 180t
Ryvita, 160, 279

S
sablefish, 116, 163
SAD (standard American diet), 14, 92
safety, food, 268
salad dressing, 211
salads, 120–22, 165
  Arugala Blackberry, **247**
  Barley and Roasted Vegetable, **241–42**
  Breakfast Salad, **235–36**
  Broccoli Crunch, **240–41**
  Cauliflower Tabbouleh, **242**
  Kale and Avocado, **244–45**
  Salmon and Sprout, **239**
  Spinach, Almost Instant, **237–38**
salmon, 116, 163
  Salad, Salmon and Sprout, **239**
  Salmon Collard Packets, **256–57**
Salted Chocolate Almond Gems, **262**
sambal oelek
  Chicken Lettuce Cups, **254–55**
sandwich
  Reuben, Spicy Korean Tempeh, **238**
saponins, 42
sardines, 116, 163
saturated fats. see fats, saturated
sauerkraut, 108, 118–19, 167, 182t, 271
Say "Yes" to Salad for Breakfast, **235–36**
SCFA (short chain fatty acids), 62, 90. see also fats
SCOBY, 118
scones, 159, 179t
scramble
  South of the Border Tofu Scramble, **232**

seafood. see fish
Seafood Watch, 107
seeds, 122, 179t, 207
seeds, chia, 122
seeds, flax, 122
  Breakfast Bars, Brilliant, **232–34**
seeds, hemp, 122, 167
  Banana Sushi, **261–62**
  Breakfast Bars, Brilliant, **232–34**
  Granola, Sprouted Buckwheat, **236–37**
  Muffin, Real, **230–31**
seeds, pumpkin
  Candy Bars, Crunchy Nut, **267**
  Dip, White Bean, **259**
  Granola, Sprouted Buckwheat, **236–37**
  Salad, Broccoli Crunch, **240–41**
  Tof-alibut, Herb-Crusted, **255**
  Trail Mix, Energy to Spare, **260**
seeds, sesame
  Salad, Broccoli Crunch, **240–41**
  Tofu Sesame Sticks, **243**
seeds, sunflower
  Salad, Almost Instant Spinach, **237–38**
selenium, 120
self-blame, 147–48
self-responsibilty, 147–48
sensitivity, 95b, 96–97
sesame seeds. see seeds, sesame
shallot
  Salad, Almost Instant Spinach, **237–38**
Shepherd, Sue, 72
Shockingly Good Pink Walnut Dip, **262–63**
shopping, 168–69, 201–13
  bread, 209–10

  bulk foods, 207–8
  canned food, 211
  cereal, 209–10
  labels, reading, 202–6
  lists, 191t–93t, 212, 213t
  meat, 208
  produce, 206–7
  refridgerated section, 208–9
  snacks, 210–11
  tips, 202b
short chain fatty acids (SCFA), 62, 90. see also fats
side dishes
  Kimchi, Homegrown, **243–44**
  Salad, Arugula Blackberry, **247**
  Salad, Broccoli Crunch, **240–41**
  Salad, Kale and Avocado, **244–45**
  Salad, Roasted Vegetable and Barley, **241–42**
  Slaw, Colorful Winter, **247–48**
  Soup, Edible Medicine, **246**
  Soup, Spiced Tomato, **245–46**
  Tabbouleh, Cauliflower, **242**
  Tofu Sesame Sticks, **243**
Silver Hills, 279
simple carbohydrates. see carbohydrates, simple
Sister Act Quesadilla, **239–240**
Slaw, Colorful Winter, **247–48**
sleep, 102, 103, 104b, 168, 187
small intestine, 56
smoking, 103
smoothies, 165, 168
  Cocoaberry, **229–230**
  It's Easy Being Green, **231**

Liquid Gold, **229**
snacks, 169–171, 191, 220b
  Almond Gems, Salted
    Chocolate, **262**
  Banana Sushi, **261–62**, *262*
  Chickpeas, Roasted,
    263–64, *263*
  Dip, Baked Mexican,
    260–61
  Dip, Pink Walnut, **262–63**
  Dip, White Bean, **259**
  Trail Mix, Energy to
    Spare, **260**
social eating, 215, 216b
soda, 160–61
sodium, 204t
soluble fiber. *see* fiber
soups, 211
  Edible Medicine, **246**
  Tomato, Spiced, **245–46**
South of the Border Tofu
    Scramble, **232**
soy, 42–45, 181t
  antinutrients, 42–43
  phytoestrogens, 43–44
  whole soy, 44–45
soy oil. *see* oil, soy
soy sauce
  Tofu Sesame Sticks, **243**
Spectrum Naturals, 279
spelt, 180t, 211
Spiced Tomato Soup,
    245–46
Spiced White Bean Dip, **259**
spices, 182t, 211–12
Spicy Korean Tempeh
    Reuben, **238**
spinach, 122, 164, 165
  Chicken Skillet, Turmeric,
    257–58
  Salad, Almost Instant
    Spinach, **237–38**
  Salad, Roasted Vegetable
    and Barley, **241–42**
  Smoothie, It's Easy Being
    Green, **231**
Sprouted Buckwheat Gra-
    nola, **236–37**, *236*

sprouts
  Salad, Salmon and
    Sprout, **239**
squash
  Quesadilla, Sister Act,
    239–240
sriracha
  Reuben, Spicy Korean
    Tempeh, **238**
standard American diet
    (SAD), 14, 92
Staphylococcus, 61
starches. *see* carbohy-
    drates, complex
stevia, 58–59
Stiles, Tara, 101–2
stock, chicken
  Baked Beans, Chipotle
    Maple, **251**
  Chicken Skillet, Turmeric,
    257–58
  Soup, Spiced Tomato,
    245–46
stock, veggie
  Baked Beans, Chipotle
    Maple, **251**
  Casserole, Greens and
    Beans, **258–59**
  Soup, Edible Medicine, **246**
  Soup, Spiced Tomato,
    245–46
stomach, 55
strawberries. *see* berries
stress
  digestion and, 57, 63–64
  excretion and, 60
  inflammation and, 100
  management, 101–2
Stuffed Sweet Potatoes,
    253–54
suey choy
  Kimchi, Homegrown,
    243–44
sugar, 30–31, 172, 206b.
    see also carbohy-
    drates, simple
sugar, brown
  Baked Beans, Chipotle

Maple, **251**
sulforaphane, 124
sunflower seeds. *see*
    seeds, sunflower
superfoods, 39
supplements, 52–53,
    108–11, 167–68, 271
sustainability, 268
swaps, food, 156–174
sweeteners, artificial, 31,
    58–59
sweet potatoes, 130
  Curry, Sweet Potato and
    Chickpea, **249–250**
  Muffin, Real, **230–31**
  Soup, Spiced Tomato,
    245–46
  Stuffed, **253–54**
sweets. *see* desserts
syrup, maple. *see* maple
    syrup
systems, food, 268

T
Tabbouleh, Cauliflower,
    242
Tacos, Rockin' Tempeh,
    252–53
taste, 11–12, 23, 31, 58
tea, 119, 162, 182t, 270
  Smoothie, It's Easy Being
    Green, **231**
tempeh, 107, 181t, 209
  Reuben, Spicy Korean
    Tempeh, **238**
  Salad for Breakfast,
    235–36
  Tacos, Tempeh, **252–53**
thiacremonone, 124
thyme, 128
  Dip, White Bean, **259**
  Salad, Almost Instant
    Spinach, **237–38**
tight junction, 94
time management, 11, 22,
    149
TLRs (toll-like receptors),
    91, 97–98, 99

tofu, 107, 163, 165, 181t, 209
  Lunch Box, Grown-Up,
    237
  Reuben, Spicy Korean
    Tempeh, **238**
  Scramble, Tofu, **232**
  Tof-alibut, Herb-Crusted,
    255
  Tofu Sesame Sticks, **243**
toll-like receptors (TLRs),
  91, 97–98, 99
tomatoes, 116, *117*, 211
  Baked Beans, Chipotle
    Maple, **251**
  Curry, Sweet Potato and
    Chickpea, **249–250**
  Dip, Baked Mexican,
    260–61
  Quesadilla, Sister Act,
    239–240
  Salad, Almost Instant
    Spinach, **237–38**
  Salad, Roasted Vegetable
    and Barley, **241–42**
  Scramble, Tofu, **232**
  Soup, Spiced Tomato,
    245–46
  Tabbouleh, Cauliflower,
    242
tomato sauce
  Baked Beans, Portu-
    guese, **250**
tortillas, 181t
  Banana Sushi, **261–62**
  Quesadilla, Sister Act,
    239–240
  Tacos, Tempeh, **252–53**
Traditional Medicinals, 279
trail mixes, 169, 210
  Trail Mix, Energy to
    Spare, **260**
trans fats. *see* fats, trans
traveling, 218–222, 220b,
  221b–22b
turkey, 162
  Lettuce Cups, **254–55**
  Salad for Breakfast,
    235–36

turmeric, 114, 182t
  Chicken Skillet, Turmeric,
    257–58
  Smoothie, Liquid Gold, **229**
  Turmeric Tonic, **273**
turnips
  Kimchi, Homegrown,
    243–44
Turtle Island, 280
twenty-eight day meal
  plan, 194–200

V
variety, nutritional, 14, 15
Vega, 280
Vegenaise
  Reuben, Spicy Korean
    Tempeh, **238**
  Salad, Broccoli Crunch,
    240–41
vegetables
  anti-inflammatory, 106–7
  eating plans, 179t
  Lunch Box, Grown-Up, **237**
  shopping for, 206–7
  swaps, 164–65, 167, 169
vegetarian diets, 92, 164
veggie stock. *see* stock,
  veggie
vitamin A, 120, 122
vitamin B12, 15
vitamin C, 78, 122
vitamin D, 110
vitamin D1, 120
vitamin D3, 167
vitamin K, 120, 122

W
walnuts, 126
  Breakfast Bars, Brilliant,
    232–34
  Brownies, Black Bean,
    264–65
  Candy Bars, Crunchy
    Nut, **267**
  Dip, Pink Walnut, **262–63**
  Granola, Sprouted
    Buckwheat, **236–37**

Muffin, Real, **230–31**
Pudding, Baked Apple
    Oat, **266**
Wasa, 160, 280
water, 50–51, 60, 162
water chestnuts
  Chicken Lettuce Cups,
    254–55
weight
  healthy, 21
  inflammation and, 87–88
  obesity, 16–17
  sweeteners and, 59
Weil, Andrew, 96
West, Mae, 175
wheat berries, 180t
white beans. *see* beans,
  white
whole grains. *see* grains,
  whole
willpower, 145–46
wine. *see also* alcohol
  Sweet Potatoes, Stuffed,
    253–54
Woolf, Virginia, 194

X
xylitol, 58

Y
yams, 165
yoga, 101–2
  yogurt, 163, 166, 167,
    182t, 209
  Blueberry, Frozen, **265**,
    265
  Salad for Breakfast, **235–36**
  Slaw, Colorful Winter,
    247–48
yogurt, Greek, 163, 165

Z
zeaxanthin, 116, 122, 126
zonulin, 94
Zyflamend, 112